19·90

P9-CQB-097

METABOLISM
AND THE
RESPONSE TO INJURY

METABOLISM
AND THE
RESPONSE TO INJURY

Edited by
A W Wilkinson
and
Sir David Cuthbertson

A PITMAN MEDICAL PUBLICATION

Distributed by

YEAR BOOK MEDICAL PUBLISHERS, INC.

35 E. Wacker Drive, Chicago

First published 1976

© Pitman Medical Publishing Co Ltd, 1976

*This book is copyrighted in England and may not be
reproduced by any means in whole or in part.
Application with regard to reproduction should be
directed to the Copyright owner.*

*Distributed in Continental North, South and Central
America, Hawaii, Puerto Rico and The Philippines by*
YEAR BOOK MEDICAL PUBLISHERS, INC.

(ISBN 0–8151–9322–X)

(Library of Congress Catalog Card No: 76–48471)

by arrangement with
PITMAN MEDICAL PUBLISHING CO LTD

Reproduced and printed by photolithography and bound in
Great Britain at The Pitman Press, Bath

Foreword

The papers in this volume were contributed by friends, admirers and former pupils of Sir David Cuthbertson as a tribute in his 75th year. He has been continuously and still is active in research on the metabolic effects of injury since 1928 when he began to study the effects of fractures of the long bones of adult men on calcium metabolism and found his interests diverted into the more acute changes in protein metabolism. The concept of the 'catabolic phase' of metabolism after injury and of the 'ebb' and 'flow' components of it owe much to his imaginative approach to a biological phenomenon after injury which has been shown to occur in species as widely different as 'carcinus' the land crab, the earthworm, many kinds of animals and man. What is perhaps most strange is that until recently surgeons who have for centuries inflicted severe injury on their fellows more regularly even than war and accident have shown so little interest in the profound and lasting effects of injury on the human body. During the war of 1914–1918 the interest of surgeons was mainly centred on the control of shock and the treatment of wounds with antiseptic measures. Even in the war of 1939–1945, after relearning the forgotten lessons of the earlier Great War, surgeons tended to concentrate on the prevention and treatment of infection, and it was only when the introduction of penicillin freed them to some degree from the need to control infection that they could devote more of their time to the other effects of injury.

The studies which Sir David Cuthbertson had initiated in Glasgow in the early thirties were continued in North America in the middle forties and there and in Britain in the fifties and since, and the interest in the effects of injury has since spread more deeply into the problem and into more places in the world.

In this book there is much information which has not been published before, as well as critical reviews of particular aspects by workers of authority and especial interest who have been chosen by Sir David Cuthbertson as those most likely to have the deepest and most up-to-date knowledge of them. The effects of injury on energy requirements, various aspects of protein metabolism, the circulation, the central nervous system, endocrine function, vitamin requirements, fat and carbohydrate metabolism are reviewed and discussed. The initiation and mediation of the response and its effect on wound healing and infection are described and the requirements of amino acids and the bearing of changes in fat metabolism on intravenous feeding are discussed. There is also a chapter on the part which zinc and other essential trace elements play in the changes after injury and in wound healing.

This book will be of interest to all surgeons as well as to physiologists and others concerned with the study of all aspects of injury and wound healing.

A W Wilkinson

Contents

List of Contributors

Dr S P Allison
MD, MRCP

General Hospital, Nottingham, England

Sir David P Cuthbertson
CBE, MD, DSc, LLD, DRhc,
FRCP(Ed), HonFRCS(Ed),
HonFRCPath, HonFRCPS(Glas),
HonFIFST, FRS(Ed)

University Department of Pathological
Biochemistry, Royal Infirmary, Glasgow,
Scotland

Dr J W L Davies
PhD

MRC Industrial Injuries and Burns Unit,
Accident Hospital, Birmingham, England

Dr G S Fell
BS, PhD, MRCPath

Department of Pathological Biochemistry,
Royal Infirmary, Glasgow, Scotland

Dr A Fleck
MB, ChB, PhD, FRS(Ed)

Department of Biochemistry, Western
Infirmary, Glasgow, Scotland

Dr P Fürst
PhD

Metabolic Research Laboratory, St Eriks
Sjukhus, Stockholm, Sweden

Professor J M Kinney
MD

Department of Surgery, Columbia University,
College of Physicians and Surgeons, New
York, USA

Dr S M Levenson
MD

Department of Surgery, Albert Einstein
College of Medicine, Yeshiva University,
Bronx, New York, USA

Professor S-O Liljedahl
MD

Department of Surgery, Regionsjukhuset,
Linkoping, Sweden

Mr J R Richards
MB, ChB, FRCS

University Department of Surgery, Royal
Infirmary, Glasgow, Scotland

Dr H B Stoner
BSc, MB, ChB, MD, MRCPath

Experimental Pathology of Trauma Section, MRC Toxicology Unit, Medical Research Council Laboratories, Carshalton, Surrey, England

Mr W E Strachan
MB, ChB, FRCS(Ed)

Subregional Neurosurgical Service, Plymouth, Devon, England

Assistant Professor E Vinnars
MD

Department of Anaesthesiology and Intensive Care Unit, Stockholmas Lans Landsting, St Eriks Sjukhus, Stockholm, Sweden

Professor J C Waterlow
CMG, MB, BChir, MD, ScD, FRCP

Department of Human Nutrition, London School of Hygiene and Tropical Medicine, London, England

Professor A W Wilkinson
ChM(Ed), FRCS(Ed), FRCS, FAAP(Hon)

Department of Paediatric Surgery, Institute of Child Health, London, England

Dr D W Wilmore
MD

United States Army Institute of Surgical Research, Brooke Army Medical Center, Fort Sam Houston, Texas, USA

Professor A Wretlind
MD

Nutrition Unit, Medical Faculty, Karolinska Institutet, Stockholm, Sweden

Surgical Metabolism: Historical and Evolutionary Aspects

D P CUTHBERTSON

University Department of Pathological Biochemistry, Royal Infirmary, Glasgow, Scotland

Introduction

In animals without a circulatory system closure of a wound is by 'primary intention', the cells bordering the wound simply stretching out to span the gap. In mammals, minor wounds are closed in a similar way but with larger wounds the emergency arrest of bleeding is vital. In terrestrial vertebrates the superficial part of the clot later dries to form a protective scab. In such aquatic forms as the crustacea the clot is strengthened by a secretion with some resemblance to the normal exoskeleton. In other aquatic forms there is a 'soft clot' only.

Blood clotting is necessary to prevent excessive bleeding as well as to close and protect the wound, and has been evolved independently in different animals (Needham, 1952). It demands very necessary safeguards against clotting in the circulatory system itself. In vertebrates bleeding is also reduced by constriction of the local blood capillaries and arterioles, particularly in deep wounds. Persistend starvation of blood, however, is fatal to the tissues: the initial local pallor is but temporary. At the very edge of the wound the vessels remain dilated but the functional significance of this is not yet clear but must be regarded as part of the defence reaction.

However, it is not our intention to look into these very early phenomena but to consider the subsequent metabolic happenings. Nor is it our immediate concern to follow up interesting observations such as those of Abercrombie (1964), who described how connective tissue, if injured and the wound margins explanted into culture medium for a few days, there then results emigration of a more profuse character. There appears to be a stimulating effect on growth and cells are mobilised. There may be a specific time relationship regarding this but the precise nature of the stimulus is unknown. Although wounds of the cornea may heal

1

without mitosis there are nevertheless strong reasons for believing that there is a close physiological link between proliferation and mobilisation. In passing we also note that Dunphy (1966) found that the greatest stimulus for growth of a second wound occurs in 4 to 7 days and Linder (1966) carefully debrided, cleansed and dressed, large traumatic wounds and then somewhere about the fourth to fifth day closed the wounds in spite of a fairly heavy growth of organisms demonstrable prior to closure; only a small number broke down because of infection.

Oedema arises through the escape of fluid from blood vessels into the tissue spaces: arteriolar dilation increases the blood supply and permits leucocytes to squeeze through the endothelial cells which form around the wound. The exudate is fibrinous since it includes all the plasma proteins. It coagulates readily and isolates the area of damage.

The sensory endings of nerve-fibres carrying the sensation of pain become hypersensitive in the area of the 'flare' (dilatation of the small blood vessels). Pain discourages any exposure to further damage. The arteriolar dilatation causes a warm skin but its temperature is not higher than the rectal temperature, and is not due to a local increase in metabolic rate. There is also a systemic increase in body temperature. This is positive not accidental and may favour the host's defensive metabolism relative to that of foreign organisms and may favour healing by speeding up the regenerative processes.

Wounds are thus characterised by Galen's four cardinal signs of inflammation: calor (heat), rubor (redness), turgor (oedema) and dolor (pain).

The 'triple response' of tache, wheal and flare is established within a few minutes after injury and persists for some hours. It gives place to persisting inflammation which lasts up to five days or longer if infection is persistent.

Needham (1952) points out that in the invertebrates and protochordates defence is chiefly by phagocytosis, though some antibody formation has been shown in insects. Vascular reactions play little part except in arthropods and molluscs, and the phagocytes probably correspond chiefly to the vertebrate macrophages in their origin from a variety of tissues. In the earth worm cells of the peritoneum are phagocytic and in *Amphioxus* it is the small connective tissue cells, the blood being virtually devoid of cells. Even in the coelenterates wandering phagocytic cells play an important part in regeneration. There would seem to be a measure of agreement that in animals with a vascular system there are two types of cells, one a blood cell, the other a tissue cell which takes part in this situation.

There are two main phases in epimorphic regeneration — regressive and progressive. The former includes in sequence: 1) wound closure; 2) demolition of damaged cells and defence against foreign micro-organisms and toxic agents; 3) dedifferentiation of cells to provide new tissues for the progressive or repair phase. The latter according to Needham (1952) may be subdivided into migration, mitosis and morphogenesis (differentiation).

2

Malcolm in his classical description of the 'Physiology of Death from Traumatic Fever' published in 1893 pointed out that "shock is more part of phenomena caused by injury, whether surgical or otherwise, than a complication thereof" but it was John Hunter who a hundred years earlier in 1794 wrote in his Treatise on the 'Blood, Inflammation and Gunshot Wounds' that "There is a circumstance attending accidental injury which does not belong to disease, namely that the injury done, has in all cases a tendency to produce, both the disposition and means of cure".

Cowell (1917) in his report to the Medical Research Council described the group of symptoms which he termed 'primary wound shock' and those which developed later, particularly after prolonged transit in the cold, or after further haemorrhage, or after the onset of toxaemia, as 'secondary shock'. He noted that the latter frequently followed a moderately severe wound such as laceration of muscle or compound fracture of bone.

Much earlier Cole (1852) and Longmore (1877) had pointed out that one effect of primary shock was like fainting in that it lessened the risk of fatal haemorrhage, deadened pain "either by annihilation of function and sensation of the parts wounded, or by the state of stupor into which the shock of injury has at once thrown the patient ...... In most cases the early pain, even if severe, is evanescent, and is followed by a certain numbness ...... As a rule the graver the injury the greater and more persistent is the amount of shock".

It is interesting to search back to discover the views of these early surgeons on the treatment of battle casualties. Wisemann (1719) in his 'Chirurgical Treatise' recommended immediate amputation for mangled limbs. "It must be done suddenly upon receipt of the wound," he wrote, "while they (the soldiers) are surprised, and as it were amazed with the accident, the limb is taken off easier ...... before symptoms were upon the patient and he be spent with watchings." John Hunter (1794) described the condition of shock and Latta (1795) appears to have been the first to use the term 'shock' for the initial period of depressed vitality following injury. Bell (1798), Guthrie (1815), Hennen (1829), Cole (1852), MacLeod (1858) and many French surgeons likewise advocated early amputation. John Hunter (1794) was one of few to advise delay. He considered that on the battle field "it is almost impossible for a surgeon to make himself sufficiently master of a case, so as to perform so capital an operation with propriety; and it admits of dispute, whether at any time, and in any place, amputation should be performed before the first inflammation is over".

This question of the advisability of rapid operation on shocked cases again arose during World War 1. It was not till the later years that the improvement which followed the removal of mangled limbs in shocked cases was fully recognised. Every effort was then made to combat the condition of shock. Intravenous injections of gum and saline were claimed to be particularly useful in those cases which had lost much blood. They were not so useful in other cases of secondary wound shock.

3

Two of the earliest graphic descriptions of shock were those of Fischer (1870) and Warren (1895) who described the persistent reduced arterial pressure, the almost imperceptible thread-like pulse, the pale skin, the bluish lips, the large drops of sweat, the vomiting and occasional restlessness, the blunted sensibility, the consciousness of cold, faintness, and deadness of the extremities, the long sighing respirations alternating with superficial ones.

Almroth Wright and Colebrook (1918) pointed out that the application of restorative measures such as heat in fully developed shock must be made with caution "too rapid resuscitation by warmth ...... may be perilous to life".

Gangrene has always been a major hazard in war and wherever violence leads to bombing and to wounds of the thighs and buttocks. A recent article by two Belfast surgeons (Kennedy & Johnston, 1975) points out that it is essential that debridement should be thorough, all dead tissue being carefully excised. They firmly warn against any attempt at primary suture of a bomb wound in which muscle has been damaged as this tends to lead to gas gangrene. After debridement they advise the wounds be dressed and splinted where indicated by plaster-of-Paris. Wounds are left undisturbed until the fifth or sixth day unless pain pyrexia, odour, or soaking of the dressings dictates otherwise. If then the wound, on inspection appears clean, delayed primary suture or grafting may be carried out at the 5-day inspection. This has often to be further delayed, according to these authors, if the wound looks unhealthy or shows any signs of sepsis. All such casualties should be given tetanus toxoid and a broad spectrum antibiotic. They recommend that in the case of traumatic amputations after trimming of the skin flaps, primary closure should only be attempted when all divided muscle is seen to be absolutely healthy and uncontaminated.

The necessity for a broad conception of the pathophysiological response to injury was also stressed by Grant and Reeve (1951) who showed that there was much to be learned from a study of the reactions to injury by observers with an open mind. Both at the site of injury but in the body generally there occur phenomena, the signs of which fit in considerable measure those of inflammation. The tissue reactions exhibit Galen's classical signs, the general are early dominated by a period of depressed metabolism. Influences which come into play during the initiation and progression of this state are loss of blood plasma, or body fluid with consequent anoxia, pain and loss of body heat. Fatigue and dehydration may be additive depending on the particular situation. The oxygen supply may be sufficient for the diminished oxygen uptake but if it fails necrobiosis sets in.

THE NATURE OF THE REACTIONS TO TRAUMA

Unless the trauma be overwhelming the injury done by accident or by elective surgery almost immediately induces the beginning of a very wide range of integrated paths — first with survival and then with healing. For example, injury stimulates coagulation and fibrinolysis in direct proportion to the severity of the

4

trauma, and with effects which are both local and remote from the site of damage. William Hewson, describing the killing of a sheep in 1772, observed that "the blood which issued last coagulated first". The frequent succession of a 'positive' phase of hypercoaguability and a 'negative' phase of hypocaoguability was described as early as 1886 by Wooldridge. Depending on the damage done the homeostatic responses may or may not be adequate to bring about a full return to normality and indeed may be so far short of it that necrobiosis sets in and even death ensue. Carrel (1930) when discussing the causal relations between the loss of a fragment of tissue and its regeneration wrote: "In superficial epithelial wounds, the initiation of healing seems to be due ..... to substances set free by the traumatised cells themselves".

When reviewing these responses to injury we discern at least two compensating processes inducing both disposition and the means of cure, namely the adaptations which have evolved through natural selection in response to injury and secondly, but bound to these, the autoregulation towards normality: the preservation of the *milieu interieur* of Bernard — the homeostasis of Cannon (1923). As Moore (1972) has pointed out these two trends are to be seen in the metabolic adaptation to injury just as much as they are to be seen in the adaptation to starvation "such as the mobilisation of nitrogen compounds from protein for gluconeogenesis or wound fibroplasia". He instances the finding that after a brisk haemorrhage alone there is an increased secretion of adrenaline and noradrenaline arising in nerve synapses, and that amongst other actions, adrenaline inhibits the production of insulin, while it stimulates glycogenolysis and the hydrolysis of depot fat to free fatty acids. Insulin inhibition is considered to favour the release of amino acids from muscle, some of which pass through a 3-carbon step to glucose, other components appearing as increased nitrogen excretion in the urine. Moore also states that there is a decreased perfusion of the juxtaglomerular apparatus of the kidney, which stimulates the production of renin, angiotensin, and aldosterone, supporting the blood pressure and conserving sodium, and with it the interstitial fluid and plasma volume; a mild stimulus to the pituitary produces an increase on blood glucocorticoids that has a permissive action for the intensification of many of the foregoing changes.

Albright (1943) described many features of surgical metabolism, in particular he drew attention to the resemblance of prolonged illness and tissue injury to the results of prolonged stimulation of the adrenal cortex as seen in Cushing's syndrome.

The formation of the stress-concept by Seyle (1937) and its subsequent elaboration by him into the general adaptation syndrome has undoubtedly provided a unifying concept. But in this attempt it would seem that he outstripped the experimental evidence and by his very over-unification has tended to inhibit progress. For example, some of the confusion that surrounds the term 'shock' relates to Seyle's terminology in the 'alarm reaction', in which the first injury is referred to as 'shock' and the response thereto as 'counter-shock' even though no reduction in tissue perfusion or blood flow, in the true sense of surgical shock, is involved. Claude Bernard (1865) was only too conscious of the dangers of this when, in his 'Introduction to the Study of Experimental Medicine', he wrote: "..... the ambition to explain prematurely at one step the whole of the disease.... one loses sight of the patient, one gets the wrong idea of the disease, and by a false application of physiology, experimental medicine is hindered instead of being assisted in its progress."

The work of others such as Browne, Thorn, Hume, Ganong and Egdahl (see Moore, 1972) has elucidated the pathway by which physical injury, such as burn, fracture or surgical incision, communicates a message via the nervous system to the basal ganglia of the brain, and thence to the pituitary glands, finally stimulating the adrenal cortex to produce a variety of corticosteroid hormones.

Some of the earliest metabolic studies were those of Duval and Grigaut (1918) who noted that in the wounded there was a diminution of the N-PN of the traumatised tissues and the diminution appeared to go parallel with an increase in N-PN and residual N (i.e. N-PN minus urea N) in the blood and was related to the degree of tissue damage. The amount of these nitrogenous substances in the whole blood of those wounded, but without clinically evident shock, was at a maximum on the second day after injury, then gradually returned to normal but the rises were generally not great. In cases which terminated fatally the highest values were found just before death. Aub and Wu (1920) found somewhat similar high nitrogen values as the blood of animals shocked by muscle injury. Both urea and N-PN were increased.

In addition to the raised concentration of N-PN in the blood, the work of Wertheimer et al (1919) suggested that there was also an increased excretion of nitrogen in the urine following the initial shock phase. They found that during the first 24 hours the average excretion of the urea N might be 16g and later rise as high as 27gN. Mestrezat (1918) noted that the undetermined nitrogen in the urine was high.

There is usually some slight rise of temperature and pulse rate following moderate to severe injury, which reach their highest value during the second and third evenings following the trauma, then gradually decline. This was termed by the older writers, 'sympathetic fever'. Later it was termed 'aseptic fever'. It may remain low following a major injury yet there is evidence of increased nitrogen loss (Malcolm, 1893).

In the USA Hawk and Gies (1904) found that surgical procedures had an appreciable influence on the normal output of catabolic products in the urine. This was confirmed by Haskins (1907) who noted that the effect of a single moderate haemorrhage was to cause a temporary stimulation in urinary N excretion and that the excess of excreted nitrogen grew with each successive loss of blood and the excretion of sulphur tended to run parallel to that of nitrogen.

In 1930 and 1931 Cuthbertson reported that following fracture of one or more of the major long bones of the lower limbs excretion of nitrogen, sulphur

6

and phosphorus rose rapidly to a maximum generally within 3 to 8 days from the time of injury and that the N:S ratio suggested some relatively sulphur-rich source, such as muscle, as the main source of the material catabolised, for the level of nitrogen at the peak of this excessive catabolism might exceed 20g per day. The partition of the nitrogen and sulphur containing catabolites demonstrated that the increase in nitrogen was due to a practically proportionate increase in the urea excreted and that the increase in sulphur was due to a slightly greater proportionate increase in the excretion of inorganic sulphates and that of phosphorus of phosphate. Definite traces of creatine were observed and traces of heat-coagulable

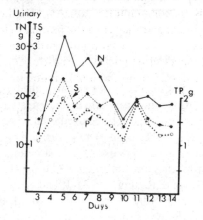

Figure 1. Youth, 16y; fracture tibia and fibula one leg

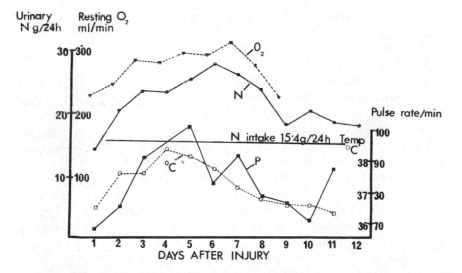

Figure 2. Man, aged 24y; fracture of tibia by kick: shock slight: no anaesthetic

7

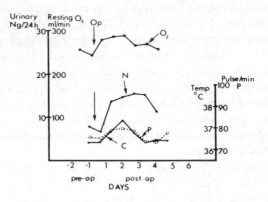

Figure 3. Man, aged 25y; meniscectomy under spinal anaesthesia

protein were occasionally found. There was an early oliguria. Later it was shown that the oxygen consumption, and heart rate increased, sometimes in parallel (Cuthbertson, 1932) and that the effect occurred even when an orthopaedic operation was done under spinal (stovaine) anaesthesia. In addition to these aforementioned catabolites there were excreted greater amounts of potassium, zinc and to a less extent magnesium and calcium (Cuthbertson, 1942; Cuthbertson et al, 1972; Cuthbertson & Rahimi, 1973). It had earlier been shown that the rat could exhibit the same order of metabolic change following a fracture (Cuthbertson et al, 1939). Some of these investigations on man are shown in Figures 1-3. The sheep likewise exhibits a catabolic response following abdominal operation (Cuthbertson, 1960) and many other observers have shown that similar changes in man follow severe burning, major sepsis, and to a less extent following operations to soft tissues (Wilkinson et al, 1949. 1950; Moore & Ball, 1952; Kinney et al, 1970 and many others).

The pathophysiological and biochemical response to moderate to severe trauma, in particular its metabolic component, thus exhibits a very complex picture. After an injury there is an immediate and well-marked disturbance of cellular vitality in the injured zone due to the actual damage done. The early reactions of tissues to local injury are dominated by vascular changes, which give rise to the classical signs of inflammation, viz swelling, redness, heat, pain and loss of function. The earliest vascular change is increased permeability. The initial permeability change in the small venules may be quite transient and is characterised by fluid exudation only. The early exudative reaction is associated with a three-fold increase of tissue resistance to infection (see review by Cuthbertson, 1964). Lymphatics also dilate and become more permeable to larger molecules during inflammation.

Two stages in the inflammatory response are identified: the initial (Burke & Miles, 1958) and delayed (Sevitt, 1958). The use of carbon labelling of vessel walls has helped to identify the sites of increased permeability (Majno, 1964) and made possible the detailed investigation of possible endogenous mediators (Spector & Willoughby, 1965; 1968 and Willms-Kretschmer & Majno, 1969). It would seem that the concensus of opinion is that the initial phase of inflammation, which may be of very short duration is brought about by increase in venular permeability through the action of an endogenous mediator such as histamine, hydroxytryptamine (serotonin), a kinin, possibly bradykinin, a prostaglandin or a combination of these. The later delayed phase of the response is more important and may appear quite slowly and persist. So far no convincing explanation has been advanced to explain the altered capillary permeability as has been done for the venular changes.

All the phenomena of inflammation can occur in denervated skin but the thresholds would seem thereby to be raised by alterations in arterial pressure and tissue perfusion (Miles & Miles, 1952; Miles & Niven, 1950).

The capillaries dilate and their permeability increases, leading to what has been termed 'reactionary oedema' and to depression of the local metabolism which I termed the 'ebb phase' (Cuthbertson, 1942). The effects of the lesion then spread more widely and there is a discharge of metabolites. Provided the injury is not immediately fatal, there is as a rule evidence of what appears to be a compensatory reaction involving the catecholamine vasoconstrictive mechanism. The local developments, on the other hand, may be such as to cause the general situation to deteriorate and lead to the development of manifest shock; the compensatory mechanism which in greater or less degree has begun to come into effect then exhibits a definite depression. The depressed stage is usually succeeded by a period when there is an increase in the local metabolism (traumatic inflammation), characterised by the increased cellular activity of the repair process, by the lysis and effluxion of the damaged tissue elements, and by what appears to be an increased and apparently generalised catabolism especially of protein with increased heat production and oxygen consumption. This I earlier described as the 'flow' phase (Cuthbertson, 1942). The injury done has thus "in all cases a tendency to produce both the disposition and the means of cure" (Hunter, 1794).

THE EBB PHASE AND FLOW PHASE

In 1942 I also took the view that 'wound shock' should be regarded as a depression in cellular vitality made more serious through loss of blood, plasma or exudate and which, if unattended and replaced, might cause the general situation to deteriorate and lead to a clinical syndrome with combinations of hypotension, hypovolaemia, tachycardia, oliguria, sweating, pallor, drowsiness etc, possibly necrobiosis and death.

The common physiological abnormality is not low blood flow with high peripheral resistance; rather it is inadequate oxygen transport due to uneven flow at tissue level or failure in tissue uptake. Nevertheless, this early reaction may help to arrest further bleeding and possibly dull pain until assistance is available,

9

but some patients do die in this condition.

That a general depression of vitality occurs early has long been recognised (Declasse, 1834; Meltzer, 1908), and this was shown by Henderson et al (1917) in burns to amount to a decrease in oxygen consumption of 45-50% in the cases studied. Davis (1936) and others also found a reduced oxygen consumption in shocked dogs. Aub (1920) found that the degree of fall in the basal metabolism of cats was roughly proportional to the severity of the shock produced, and that recovery after transfusion was usually associated with a prompt return of the metabolic rate to normal; this change in metabolic rate might precede the well-marked fall in blood pressure. This is of particular interest in view of Grant and Reeve's observations (1951) on the blood pressure of air-raid casualties.

In the classical context acute circulatory failure was recognised as the cause of death. It is now realised that the circulatory changes preceding death do not conform to a standard pattern and their clinical manifestations are very variable.

The first 'Type' of shock to be studied in detail experimentally was that due to hypovolaemia through haemorrhage with or without trauma. The tendency for the arterial pressure to fall was found to be opposed by a rise in peripheral vascular resistance due to vasoconstriction. Cournand et al (1943) confirmed in patients with various injuries that hypovolaemia is a prime cause of the clinical shock syndrome and that it causes a fall in right atrial pressure and cardiac output. Merrill et al (1946), however, showed that in patients with penetrating wounds of the chest a fall in peripheral vascular resistance sufficient to lower the arterial pressure took place even when the cardiac output was normal. Hopkins et al (1963) and Shoemaker et al (1966) have since confirmed that in haemorrhage, with or without trauma, a low cardiac output often occurs without a rise in peripheral resistance which may even fall. Variations in peripheral resistance are probably due partly to variations in sympathetic activity attributable to interacting aetiological factors, and partly to measurements made at one time not being representative of other stages of a dynamic state.

The common factor in most cases is low cardiac output but usually where there is also infection there may be many patients with normal or even high cardiac outputs. Though some may be pale, cold and sweating despite high cardiac output, many are flushed, with hot dry skin and full peripheral veins (Walters, 1972). It is essential to approach all these patients with an open mind with the object of identifying the various haemodynamic disturbances and the underlying aetiology.

Stoner (1961b) in his critical analysis of traumatic shock models has proposed that it is best to regard the body's response to injury as composed of the local response — inflammation — and a general response, which for convenience he then termed 'shock'; the initiating cause being fluid loss as the result of haemorrhage or loss from the plasma compartment, as in burns, crush injuries, and in certain infections. Blood viscosity also increases in such states and is much greater when there is haemoconcentration. While blood is obviously the ideal fluid for

10

replacing blood loss it has recently been shown that quite severe injuries can be fairly adequately treated with very large volumes of buffered saline or Ringer-lactate solutions so long as sufficient blood is given to maintain the haematocrit value at about 25 per cent (Moss, 1968). The resulting anaemia is partly compensated by increased cardiac output and appears to be well tolerated in young adults. It may not be so in old people, particularly those with pre-existing cardiovascular or pulmonary disease.

Patients with burns are commonly treated with infusions of plasma or dextran but they can also be treated by solutions of sodium salts alone. Low molecular dextran has been used to lower the viscosity of the blood.

Very large transfusions may be necessary, sometimes twice the calculated normal blood volume, but waterlogging must be avoided. A further possible reason for failure to respond to transfusion is the presence of tissue damage due to poor perfusion of the tissues in patients with severe and prolonged hypotension. Changes in lung function may lower still further the arterial Po_2: with tissue hypoxia non-volatile acid metabolites accumulate in the blood and tissues and cause acidosis. The higher the blood lactate, the worse the prognosis (Duff et al, 1969; Weil & Afifi, 1970) but the importance of the acidosis itself is not yet clear. Whether or not it acts by inhibiting the action of catecholamines is uncertain.

In shock the body temperature is in general lowered despite the diminished peripheral circulation. The reduced total metabolism and volume of circulating blood are the dominant features. Of all change produced, the tissue asphyxia is probably the most dangerous to life. It is interesting to recall here that John Hunter is reported to have advocated the use of oxygen. It may be that the hyperglycaemia which is associated with asphyxia and haemorrhage is an attempt to maintain the nourishment of the cells in the face of a failing blood supply.

Reducing the metabolic rate to create a more favourable balance between oxygen supply and demand is the principal aim of induced hypothermia. It has been found in dogs that a combination of volume expansion and mild hypothermia, effectively improved tolerance to both haemorrhage and E. coli endotoxin. In hypothermic dogs, oxygen transport was maintained at the same level as in normothermic dogs, but oxygen uptake was markedly reduced creating a more favourable 'margin of safety' between oxygen supply and demand (Halmagyi et al, 1974).

Recently attention has been directed to the finding that the preoptic centre of the anterior hypothalamic region of the brain, which is essential for thermoregulation in birds and mammals, contains large concentrations of catecholamines and that injection of catecholamines into this region affects body temperature (Bligh, 1966; Marley & Stephenson, 1972), the temperature responses being assumed to resemble those of endogenous catecholamines (Feldberg & Myers, 1964, 1965; Hori & Nakayama, 1973). In young chicks at thermoneutrality noradrenaline infused into the hypothalamus lowered body temperature and reduced oxygen consumption (Marley & Stephenson, 1970). It was noticed that this hypothermic response to noradrenaline was considerably potentiated by reducing

11

ambient temperature to 16 °C. Marley and Stephenson (1975) induced hypothermia by infusion of noradrenaline into the hypothalamus of 2-3 week old chicks
maintained within their thermoneutral range. The effect was considerably potentiated by lowering the ambient temperature.

Changes in Energy Source

Although body glycogen supplies some carbohydrate for energy in the first few
hours after injury (often associated with hyperglycaemia and traces of glycosuria)
muscle protein is mobilised to provide some energy by ultimate oxidation of the
glycogenic amino acids and it may also be that a diminution in general anabolism
provides amino acids of exogenous origin for heat production. The extent to which
fat is permitted to provide energy depends on the degree to which insulin production is restrained. Each kilogramme of fat thus mobilised yields about 1 litre of
water of oxidation. There is a rise in plasma free fatty acids and a fall in the respiratory quotient towards that occurring in fat oxidation. There may be mild keto-
anaemia with the inhibition of insulin secretion and a pseudodiabetic state sometimes referred to as 'traumatic diabetes'. The mobilisation of protein appears
related to the need for gluconeogenic amino acids such as alanine (Felig, 1973).

The patient who has been adequately resuscitated and is doing well may show
a mild alkalosis due to the inability to excrete bicarbonate with a resultant acid
urine despite plasma alkalosis. Most patients after severe injury hyperventilate
possibly due to multiple small pulmonary emboli and this adds further to the
alkalosis. Lactic acidosis occurs of the order of 3mM/l only if trauma, infection
or blood or plasma loss is severe and there is prolonged hypoperfusion of the
tissues.

Trauma Models

It has been suggested that the problems of traumatic shock can be more easily
studied by omitting the actual injury and simply studying the effects of injections
of cortisone, adrenalin, endotoxin etc. Since we know injury leads to adrenocortical stimulation such experiments do not provide valid models whose requirements
must be: 1) the site and nature of the injury must be accurately defined; 2) such
an injury must be reproducible and its intensity controllable; and, 3) it must be
measurable (Stoner, 1961a).

Limbs have been shot with bullets, explosive charges have been applied or em-
bedded and detonated, limbs have been damaged with mallets or crushed in vices,
and the gut and mesentery have been damaged either through the abdominal wall
or at open operation. While undoubtedly these reveal marked circulatory and
metabolic changes they are not readily controllable and measurable for the limits
of damage are difficult to define as for instance when infection supervenes or
more than one major tissue is affected. Where several blood vessels have been

12

damaged variable amounts of haemorrhage will occur externally or internally. Models which have been found useful are those involving:

a. Measured degrees of haemorrhage (will not be further discussed here)
b. Fractures of long bones, more particularly for the 'flow' phase
c. Burns
d. Bacterial Infections
e. Limb Ischaemia
f. Tumbling Trauma
g. Freezing
h. Cellulose Sponge-induced Granulation Tissue

These have been described at some length elsewhere by the author (Cuthbertson, 1975) and are considered also in many of the ensuing chapters. However it seems pertinent to refer briefly to two models — fracture and burn.

b. Fracture

Following observations of the disturbed metabolism in patients consequent on fractures of long bones, accidental and surgical, osteotomies, and sprains by Cuthbertson (1929, 1930, 1931, 1932, 1936) it was found that the rat replicated the phenomenon seen in man (Cuthbertson et al, 1939; Cairnie et al, 1957). These observations described the timing and extent of the nitrogen loss, its relation to different severities of trauma, to immobilisation, fever and nutrition, the associated changes in sulphur, potassium, phosphorus, and creatine metabolism, the source of them and their partition in the urine. It was recognised that the faecal nitrogen excretion was not appreciably affected by such degrees of trauma. The early period of decreased energy output was termed the 'ebb' period and the later recovery period of increased metabolic activity with increased heat production the 'flow' period (Cuthbertson, 1942). Subsequently it was shown that the increased resting heat production and protein catabolism seen after long bone fractures at ordinary environmental temperatures largely disappears if the patient or experimental animal (rat) is placed in the appropriate thermoneutral environment [30-32°C] (Caldwell, 1962,1970; Campbell & Cuthbertson, 1967; Cuthbertson et al, 1968; Tilstone & Cuthbertson, 1970; Cuthbertson et al, 1972).

That the increase in oxygen consumption following trauma in animals is a general biological manifestation is also supported by the observations of Adams and Rowan (1970) on the immediate and rapid increase in 'wound respiration' seen in ageing carrot slices. This is correlated with a characteristic sequence of activation of irreversible reactions in the glycolytic pathway. There are apparently two stages: these appear to correspond to the period of active synthesis, when ADP, produced in the cytoplasm from synthetic reactions, activates pyruvate kinase, and a period of readjustment peaking about 2 to 3 days after injury when ATP no longer reacting in synthetic reactions activates phosphofructokinase.

13

When rats are fed a protein-free diet for some time prior to fracture they do not show the characteristic pattern of increased urinary nitrogen loss, only a slight transient rise occurs (Munro & Cuthbertson, 1943). Further studies by Munro and Chalmers (1945), showed that the additional loss in urine after injury is proportional to the pre-injury levels. It was concluded that the results are due to changes in the amount of labile protein in the body at different levels of protein intake and that the urinary nitrogen largely originates in this 'depot' protein, although severe accidental injury may result in more extensive damage in protein metabolism.

Investigations in man have revealed that the urinary excretion of zinc correlated well with that of nitrogen at ordinary environmental temperatures (circa $20°C$) but not at $30°C$.

The rate of albumin synthesis in the rat was traced following fracture by my colleagues Ballantyne, Tilstone and Fleck (1973) for observations on injury in man had revealed that the concentration of albumin and transferrin falls while the concentration of α_2-macroglobulin is unchanged, and that of fibrinogen and haptoglobulin is elevated (see review by Owen, 1969). In the rat it was found that the absolute rate of albumin synthesis was significantly decreased on days 1 and 3 after fracture. On day 1 after injury the synthetic rate of albumin fell by 30%, and 60% of this decrease could be attributed to altered protein intake, the remaining 40% representing the metabolic response to trauma. Ballantyne et al suggested that impaired synthesis is a major cause of the fall in plasma albumin concentration which occurs after trauma. Likewise in man it has been shown that the fall in plasma albumin concentration after fracture of one or more long bones cannot be ascribed to increased catabolism of that protein (Ballantyne & Fleck, 1973a,b). At $30°C$ these changes were minimised.

Mourdisen (1969a,b) concluded from experiments on rabbits that losses of albumin into a wound were responsible only for 30% of the decrease in albumin concentration found and suggested that the capacity for albumin synthesis might be decreased following injury.

It seems reasonable to assume that the decrease in synthetic rate is partly due to the sensitivity of the synthesis of albumin to protein content of the diet (e.g. Kirsch et al, 1968; Morgan & Peters, 1971), but is also due to a specific response to trauma; perhaps like the acute anaemia which is invariably associated with deep extensive burns and is due partly to blood loss from the wounds and donor sites, and partly to impaired haematopoesis (James et al, 1951a,b). An important practical consequence of this anaemia is that unless the haemoglobin level is above 70% of normal by the second week, skin grafts are unlikely to take. This anaemia may require repeated blood transfusion and although sometimes this may be due to haemorrhage from gastrointestinal ulceration or infection, the cause is usually more complex. Trapping of blood within extensively burned areas of skin may be such a cause.

b. Burns

There are two types of models in general use in the study of thermal injury. One group is used to study local changes and the other to study general effects. The methods in the first group involve mostly the application of heated metal surfaces to the skin. The general response is usually studied by scalding the animal in water. It is possible, accurately, to scald known areas of skin and, by using mainly dorsal skin, limit the amount of damage to organs (Arturson, 1961; Bailey et al, 1962). A good deal of information has been acquired concerning such thermal damage but there have been fewer detailed experimental studies on the general response. In the latter the main exciting cause is loss of fluid from the circulation into the damaged tissue. Later there is an increased evaporative loss of water through the eschar despite its apparent less permeable appearance. The absence of blistering and the type of eschar formed in the fur-bearing skin of animals is important and this makes it difficult to compare such skin with human skin, particularly in relation to infection.

An intact eschar decreases the total nutritional cost of a full-thickness burn by decreasing evaporative heat loss while it is still intact. Excision of burn wound eschars and closure of the resultant wounds result in a metabolic and nutritional response to full-thickness burns quite similar to that seen after major trauma. Excising the burn wound eschar and leaving the resultant wound open results in far greater body weight loss and urinary nitrogen excretion than is seen if the eschar remains intact.

Recently Caldwell (1962) reported on the effect of raising the environmental temperature from around 20°C to 30°C, on the outcome of full-thickness skin burns in rats. On a food intake fixed at the level of the pre-injury period, the rats with burns and housed at 20°C ambient lost weight by up to 40%, but those at 30°C ambient gained weight. The latter showed reduced negative nitrogen balance, markedly improved wound healing, and reduced mortality. Later studies showed that rats with full-thickness skin burns and subsequently housed at 30°C ambient did not show a negative energy balance, unlike injured rats housed at 20°C (Caldwell et al, 1966). Moyer (1962) has shown that the excessive oxygen consumption in burned rats can be prevented by covering the burned areas with an impermeable material.

Many of the above observations have been shown to apply to man.

Parallel Studies in Cold Blooded Species (Crustacea and Oligochaetes)

So far I have dealt with the reaction to injury in homeotherms but in a most interesting series of experiments on the aquatic poikilothermic crustacean *Carcinoides maenus* Needham (1955) found that amputation of appendages in fasting specimens caused an immediate increase in nitrogen output which then declined along an exponential type of curve, during the next 12 days or so. Superimposed on this

curve were cyclic fluctuations in output, with a period of six days. The excess
output over the first ten days was proportional to the normal output before
operation, the relative excess being independent of diet. Later, however, carbohydrate reduced output and protein increased the short-term oscillation in output. Excess nitrogen output was related to the amount of damaged tissue
remaining but not to the amount of tissue removed and it did not come entirely

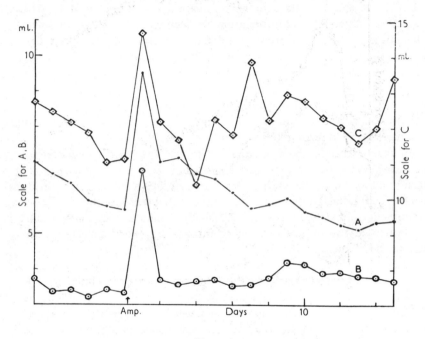

Figure 4

from the demolished tissues. Removal of the sinus gland region of the eye-stalks
caused an increase in output by one order of magnitude over that due to limb
amputation. After excision of portions of the body-wall this pattern of output
differed from that following amputation of the appendages and was more similar
than the latter to that following skin and bone trauma in man. These fluctuations
or cycles of nitrogen output are of interest for I found two in man and in the
rat (Figure 4).

In the earthworm Needham (1958) has also found evidence of increased nitrogen excretion following amputation of the tail, the increase being proportional
to the degree of injury and the amount of tissue amputated. Feeding reduced
both the normal output and the excess nitrogen due to injury. (See Figure 5 for
data on *Esenia foetida* (Savigny.)

16

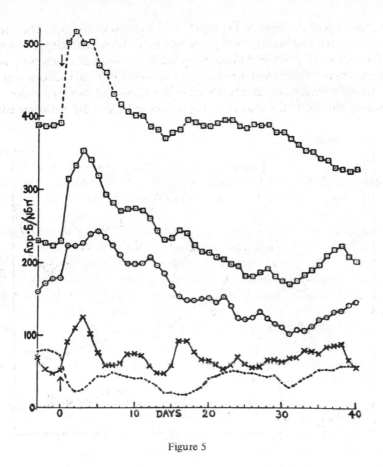

Figure 5

THE METABOLIC RESPONSE TO INJURY

This response can be divided into two phases in terms of heat production or by oxygen consumption, as measured by heat loss in a direct calorimeter and by metabolic activity in general. The terms 'ebb' and 'flow' describe simply the dwindling and rising tides of such activity (Cuthbertson, 1942; Cairnie et al, 1957; Stoner & Pullar, 1963). The former may last up to 24 to 72 hours: the latter is generally mostly over with in two weeks but in more severe injuries may last up to eight weeks or longer. The ebb phase corresponds to the period of traumatic shock. Through its circulatory depression, shock may have the adaptive functions of reducing haemorrhage, and pain, and of conserving energy and material for the following phase. But people may die if, for example, the haemorrhage is massive and not compensated by transfusion, and if sepsis spreads and a condition of septic shock supervenes: the organism may then pass into a state of necrobiosis and may die. Generally in the ebb phase there is adequate oxygen to

17

meet the diminished demands of the tissues — at least to begin with. This period is not to be confused with the lag, or latent, period preceding visible growth. The latter is longer in duration since it includes the 'flow' period.

The time-relationships of the changes in activity of the various metabolites and in terms of heat production can be viewed in terms of a definite sequence [Figure 6] (see Cuthbertson, 1970).

Protein Metabolism

This would appear to be the most important aspect of metabolism during any morphogenetic process for the tissues are mainly protein in nature. Extensive proteolysis characterises the regressive phase and protein synthesis the repair phase of regeneration.

There appears to be, in addition to reflex wasting and autolysis, a generalised increase in catabolism to meet the exigencies of the enhanced metabolism of the recuperative process. If it is assumed that excess nitrogen following fracture comes from muscle, then the loss of muscle substances in the rat can account for four-fifths of the total loss of body-weight (Cuthbertson et al, 1939). The presumption is that in addition the reserves of carbohydrates and fat are also called on to meet the demand for readily oxidisable material.

Early Studies on the Effect of Diet and Pituitary Extract on Nitrogen Balance and Healing

A few experiments were made to determine how far this loss of tissue substance, as indicated by increased excretion of certain catabolites, could be spared by the ingestion of additional food, in particular carbohydrate. It was hardly to be expected that the natural reparative processes could be materially influenced by dietary means but this could not be assumed with certainty until proof was forthcoming. Morgan's early experiments (1906) on salamanders demonstrated that the influence of diet on the regeneration of tissues can be of only secondary importance, for salamanders receiving no food regenerate their amputated limbs just as rapidly as do well-fed animals. Howes et al (1933) found, too, that the rate of healing of stomach wounds of adult rats was not noticeably affected by complete starvation or by a half-adequate diet. The healing rate in young rats was, however, affected. Cuthbertson et al extended their observations to rats with fractures but difficulties were encountered for the animals were readily put off their basic diet, which had to be kept slightly below the optimal level in order to allow the animal to continue on a constant intake throughout the whole preoperative and postoperative period. It was found impossible to make the animals eat more food during the first few days after the operation. Later, evidence was obtained that additional carbohydrate exercised a definite sparing effect on the general loss of tissue substance, although it did

18

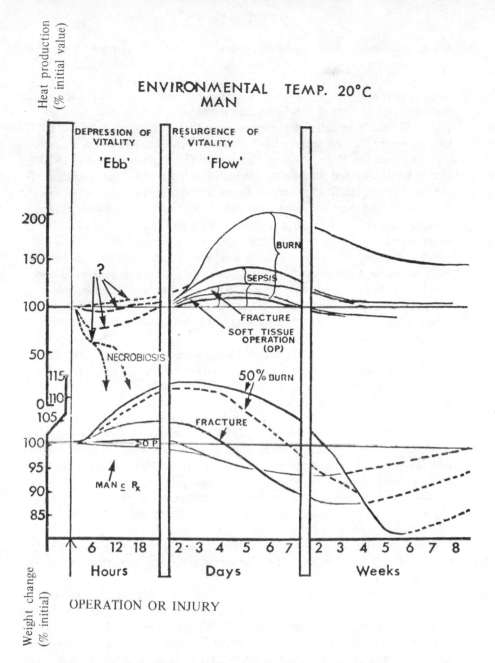

Figure 6. Diagram depicting effects of different types of injury on 'man' nursed at normal ward temperatures (around 20°C) in respect of his total heat production and weight changes under orthodox treatment, both during the first 48 hours after injury or operation and the weeks that then follow (Cuthbertson, 1970, reproduced by permission of The Ciba Foundation, London)

not appreciably affect the local tissue wastage. Further experiments were necessary and obviously they were this time made applicable to the human being.

Patients with fractures of the femur or of the bones of the legs due to direct violence were selected (Cuthbertson, 1936) and within a day or two after trauma they were given diets rich in protein, calories or both. It was found that these diets considerably modified the urinary losses. Diets rich in first-class protein and containing the maximum number of calories which the patient could consume (as much as 230 g protein were consumed daily by one patient and 4100 kcal by another) failed to eliminate a negative nitrogen balance at the height of the catabolic process. There occurred first a period of retention of nitrogen while the nitrogen excretion was rising, then a period of loss, to be followed later by another period of retention. The failure to attain nitrogen equilibrium at the height of catabolism in our cases is the more extraordinary since there was relatively little, if any, disturbance of body temperature, and since we found that when excess food was given to a normal uninjured person a well-marked retention of nitrogen and sulphur takes place, temporarily at least (Cuthbertson et al, 1937; Cuthbertson & Munro, 1937). In some of our injuries caused by indirect violence, where there was not the same extent of soft tissue damage, nitrogen retention was observed on surplus diets.

In passing it should be noted that in wound healing experiments Clark (1919) found that a high protein diet eliminated the quiescent period which precedes construction and epithelialisation, whereas a high fat diet lengthened this period to six days and carbohydrate and mixed diets gave intermediate values. Thomson et al (1938) have shown that the hypoproteinaemic dog is frequently incapable of normal fibroplasia, and Rhoads et al (1942) demonstrated that fibroplasia can occur if the dog is given ample amounts of acacia intravenously to maintain the colloid osmotic pressure of the plasma. Acacia solution was not recommended for hypoproteinaemia in patients.

Although some workers consider that the temporary loss of appetite which often follows injury is mainly the causative factor for negative nitrogen balance of the post-injury period and in severe injuries, especially burns, may be an important factor, the observations of Wilkinson (1966) and Clark (1967) have shown that injury, super-imposed on starvation following operation, induces an additive catabolic effect.

Conditions which undermine the general nutrition, such as prolonged vitamin deficiency and particularly lack of vitamin C, also retard wound healing. There is a considerable, though not unanimous body of experimental evidence in support of this thesis. Crandon's experiment (Lund & Crandon, 1941) on himself suggested that a very prolonged deprivation of vitamin C (six months) is necessary in the healthy subjects before effects on intercellular substance and collagen formation affect wound healing. It was obvious that patients with peptic ulcer on an ill-balanced diet might exhibit such a deficiency in wound healing.

In the course of an investigation into the action of a crude extract of anterior

20

pituitary tissue of the ox we noticed that the extract had definite nitrogen-retaining properties when injected into the rat (Cuthbertson et al, 1941a). Experiments showed that this particular extract, when injected daily into rats suffering from a fractured femur, produced by open operation, prevented the loss in body-weight and excessive loss of nitrogen and creatine which were the usual concomitants of such an injury. The effect of the extract on the metabolism of the injured animals was general rather than local, and possibly represented the normal growth response to this extract, superimposed on and thereby masking the increased catabolism following injury. Observations of the rate at which the atrophied muscles were restored under the influence of the pituitary extract showed that, although the animal as a whole grew more rapidly under the pituitary stimulus and the total protein catabolism was in general covered by a protein anabolism, a greater rate of restitution of the atrophied muscles of the injured limb was not thus induced. In other words, the promotion of a general protein anabolism provided no special stimulus for the restoration of the muscles of the injured limb. Further, the extract had no significant effect on the total time required to heal superficial wounds (Cuthbertson et al, 1941a,b).

This experiment demonstrated that the rate of wound healing was not significantly accelerated by a substance which induced an acceleration of general growth – that is, local anabolism was not affected by general anabolism. Could it be that a general catabolism might influence local anabolism? We later showed that the feeding of dried thyroid accelerates the rate of wound healing (Barclay et al, 1944).

Earlier we suggested that the increased catabolism which we had noted may intimately be concerned in the healing process. Carrel (1921) considered that 'slight infection' of an experimental wound by staphylococci in bouillon or 'irritation by such substances as turpentine and chick embryo extracts' shortens the latent period of healing of experimental wounds in the dog (to less than two days) as compared with a 'non-irritating antiseptic dressing'.

The wound itself, as we have already noted, affects the organism in many ways including local loss of blood and fluid, partial or total destruction of tissues with release of cellular products into the circulation direct, pain with instantaneous efferent neural stimuli to the brain and endocrine organs. Moore (1972) holds that the wound initiates catabolism and a continuously open wound inhibits anabolism. It is widely recognised that most wounds heal during the period of negative nitrogen balance and that there is sufficient restoration of tensile strength in the tissue(s) affected to permit artificial supports to be withdrawn. This enables stitches to be withdrawn from the skin, the functioning of gastrointestinal anastomoses, and the healing of blood vessels and visceral suture lines.

The restoration of tensile strength in fractured bones requires many months, especially in major lower third to midshaft long bone fractures. Because of the need for stricter immobilisation fractures are associated with larger alterations in calcium and phosphorus metabolism than are most other forms of trauma. The

21

early healing of a fracture does not involve calcification of collagen (Moore, 1972) and calcium changes in the fracture itself, after a period of acute bone resorption are not observable for many weeks. In fractures, the final restoration of tensile and weight bearing strength occurs during the anabolic phase of convalescence. This is likewise the period of calcification of osteoid matrix, a process which involves only a fraction of the body's total calcium and small compared to the effects of immobilisation. In all wounds there is continuous metabolic activity for weeks, months and years. The wound has a high demand for substrate even in late cancer.

Moore (1972) distinguishes between the acute effects of injury "without a low flow or state" such as he attributes results from injuries associated with civilian or military casualties (burns, fractures) or from major operations involving widespread dissection or visceral removal, in distinction to those changes that are due to prolonged hypoperfusion of tissue or prolonged low flow states. As in the latter he is really describing tissue anoxia through failure of oxygen transport, it should be our purpose to avoid this situation of the low flow state as this leads to necrobiosis. Obviously there can occur many intermediate states.

As to the compositional changes Moore had considered these under four headings: 1) body cell mass; 2) conservation of extracellular fluid; 3) change in energy source, and 4) alterations in neutrality regulation.

The tissues most prominently involved are skin and muscle depending on the degree or the nature of the trauma. The changes occurring in muscle are reflected in the rapid decrease in the bulk of palpable muscles. Transient immobilisation and starvation add to this reduction. The release of cellular products to the extracellular fluid and the subsequent excretion of their metabolic end products are characteristic of this 'flow' stage, e.g. increased urinary N, S, P, K, Mg, Ca, Zn, Cu, creatine. Urea is still the major end product of nitrogen metabolism and sulphate that of sulphur metabolism (Cuthbertson, 1931).

It seems that the body is early geared to an antianabolic state in the ebb phase with the consequence of excessive catabolism of absorbed amino acids of dietary origin. Moore (1972) also considers that the body exhibits an inability to synthesise new muscle protein after injury and there is a loss of intracellular electrolytes (particularly potassium, phosphate and sulphate) in the urine. Though muscle cells may suffer such changes there is no apparent residual effect suggesting impaired function even when very severe injury and infection cause very considerable losses amounting to 50 to 60 per cent of the muscle mass. Even after moderate grade injury in the adult this may amount to about 30 g nitrogen corresponding to 220g protein and approximately 1 kg wet lean tissue. Despite this evidence of catabolism most wounds heal during it to reach eventually their former tensile integrity in the area affected. The abolition of nitrogen and fat loss, if it can be affected on a balance sheet scale, has no demonstrable effect upon convalescence according to Moore (1972). By contrast prolonged post-trauma starvation has an adverse effect upon all aspects of convalescence.

22

The extent of this metabolic response depends both on the nature and severity of the injury being slight for uncomplicated surgery, greater for major skeletal trauma, and considerable in sepsis and major burns (Kinney et al, 1970). Accidental bone injuries appear to give a greater response than osteotomies and arthroplasties. Pain at injury, and subsequently, may be a factor. Of those injuries associated with sepsis there is a greater increase in body temperature, and burns cases also present a unique situation because of extrarenal losses. In an early series of 19 cases of fracture (Cuthbertson, 1936), 15 male patients lost an average 60g nitrogen, equivalent to some 375g body protein (3.4% of the total protein content of the body during the first 2 to 12 days), but in 4 cases there were more extensive losses, and one patient excreted an excess of nitrogen over the first 10 days after injury equivalent to 9 per cent of his total body protein. These observations were generally conducted over the first 10-14 days post-injury. In a more recent series (Cuthbertson et al, 1972) the losses of nitrogen over a similar period were of the order of 53 g at ordinary ward temperature. The protein catabolic responses can be practically eliminated if there is depletion of the labile protein reserves before injury so that there is apparently no further labile protein to lose (Munro & Cuthbertson, 1943; Munro & Chalmers, 1945). This observation negatives the suggestion that the extra nitrogen is largely from damaged tissue elements and effused blood. After adrenalectomy, the protein catabolic effect of injury disappears. Supporting doses of corticoids will permit the return of the effect of injury (Ingle et al, 1947; Campbell et al, 1954).

As already noted, the effect of thyroidectomy on the catabolic response to injury is conflicting and thereby confusing, but Richards believes that the degree of excessive catabolism is related to the amount of free thyroxine in the blood (Richards et al, 1973).

In the chapters which follow there will be adequate discussion of recent advances in our knowledge of the energy stores and whole-blood energetics but some reference will be made to weight loss and the effects of environmental temperature.

WEIGHT LOSS FOLLOWING THERMAL INJURY

The severe weight loss frequently associated with thermal injury has been attributed to a combination of hypermetabolism and inadequate caloric intake. Energy expenditures as much as twice normal have been recorded during the first three weeks after such injury (Gump & Kinney, 1971; Zawacki et al, 1970), and negative nitrogen balance may persist for 5-6 weeks (Soroff et al, 1961). At the same time, oral administration may be restricted by paralytic ileus, disorientation, facial burns, associated injuries or the need for respiratory support via an endotracheal or tracheostomy tube. Prior to the recent developments of techniques for complete intravenous nutrition feeding, administration of nutrients by the venous route was also limited. Even with the administration of 4000-8000 kcal/

23

day by a combination of intravenous and oral routes, actual weight gain was seldom achieved in the first few weeks, although weight stabilisation may be attained (Wilmore et al, 1971).

THE EFFECT OF ENVIRONMENTAL TEMPERATURE ON METABOLISM AFTER INJURY IN MAN

Reference has been made earlier in this paper to the effect of an environmental temperature of 30°C on the protein metabolism following injury in experimental animals: such a temperature falls within the zone of thermo-neutrality 28-32°C. Studies have also been made on man following fracture of long bones, arthroplasties, and burns. The observations of Barr et al (1968), Davies and Liljedahl (1970) on burns, and Cuthbertson et al (1968, 1972) on fractures, have shown that the increased protein catabolism and resting heat production, normally seen at around 20°C, largely disappears at an environmental temperature around 30°C, as it does in the rat. In the case of the patients with burns, a dry sterile air flow is blown on the wounds; this keeps them dry and avoids the need for dressings. In the case of bone injuries, a relative humidity of 35-45 per cent has been employed in the patient's cubicle. With this treatment the more severely injured showed a greater reduction in catabolism, and the ameliorating influence of the higher temperature was more noticeable in them.

In the rat, and to a considerable extent in man, the increased utilisation of protein for gluconeogenesis and subsequent oxidation following fracture as calculated during the first 99 days after injury from the extent of the nitrogen loss, parallels the increased heat loss (production) at ordinary environmental temperature (circa 20°C — Cairnie et al, 1957), and at the higher environmental temperature of 30°C this increase in protein utilisation with heat loss (production) largely disappears in the rat and is reduced in man. Erici (1954) and Cuthbertson and Tilstone (1967) have shown, respectively, that at such a temperature superficial wounds in the rabbit and rat heal more quickly.

In general, the patients tolerate the warm, dryish conditions fairly well, and the nutritive state of severely burned patients is easier to sustain. By the application of such heat the skin temperature of the extremities can be raised several degrees: that of the toes by as much as 12°C. By the use of extra bed coverings heat losses can undoubtedly be diminished, particularly at normal ward temperatures. The advantage of the higher environmental temperature over extra bed coverings is presumed to be mainly related to the reduction of total resting heat production to basal values provided by the thermo-neutral conditions.

Reference has already been made to the ameliorating influence of this environment of 30°C on the disturbances of the plasma proteins, tending to reduce the changes. However, the response of the adrenal cortex of the rat as evinced by levels of corticosterone in the blood is not inhibited at this higher temperature (Tilstone & Roach, 1969).

In the case of burns, at least part of the effect of temperature within the zone of thermal neutrality (ZTN) is due to the sparing of heat, normally used by the body to maintain the temperature gradient between the body and its surroundings to meet the energy demand due to the great evaporative loss of water from the burned surface; but such an explanation does not hold for simple fractures with no exudate or exposed underlying tissues.

CONTROL OF THE METABOLIC RESPONSE TO INJURY

Injury, by physical or chemical agents, is a threat to homeostasis. It will produce a temporary upset in the otherwise well-controlled functioning of many major physiological and biochemical systems, and unless adequate regeneration of the damaged tissue is effected, it may result in some degree of permanent malfunction in the injured area.

Hormonal Influences

All endocrine systems so far studied are stimulated at some stage in the body's response to trauma as are local tissue hormones. Of the hormonal factors which play a part in affecting the issue in this delayed phase, cortisol and/or its analogues appear to play a permissive role in the metabolic response in terms of the protein catabolic effect, but the catabolic response is not proportional to the level of hormone in the plasma (Selye & Collip, 1936; Ingle, 1951; Ingle et al, 1947; Campbell et al, 1954). The electrolyte response is controlled by the secretion of aldosterone.

Of the hormonal components of the anterior pituitary the anabolic properties of an alkaline extract of the anterior pituitary can overwhelm the protein catabolic effect induced by fracture of a femur in the rat (Cuthbertson et al, 1941a) without necessarily accelerating wound healing (Cuthbertson et al, 1941b). The rather contradictory evidence about the action of pure STH on man has been reviewed (Cuthbertson & Tilstone, 1969).

The changes in energy metabolism after trauma such as thermal burns and long bone fracture immediately suggest a possible connection between the observed effects and thyroid activity but the response of this gland seems light according to some investigations. The reports are also somewhat conflicting. Some have found only a very brief increase in thyroid activity immediately after operation in previously well patients. In 1968 Miksche and Caldwell showed that the catabolic response to bilateral femur fracture and to burning is absent in thyroidectomised rats. But any alteration in thyroid activity seems insufficient to account for the timing of the observed increase in metabolic rate and protein loss after injury. Richards et al (1973) found evidence that the degree of negative nitrogen balance in the rat following injury is directly related to the steepness of the slope of disappearance of administered radio-thyroxine.

The administration of large doses of insulin and the administration of concentrated solutions of glucose intravenously have been shown to effect a marked reduction in urinary nitrogen and potassium loss in severely burned patients (Hinton et al, 1973).

The recent observations of Wilmore et al (1974) on burned patients bring together an integrated set of findings. To quote "Glucagon secretion is stimulated by sympathetic activity and by catecholamines. Increased adrenergic activity may well mediate the hypergluconemia which occurs after burns. Catecholamines suppress insulin release, and low insulin levels have been reported after burn injury and in severe trauma. The return of insulin and glucagon to normal levels after burn trauma occurs with closure of the burn wound, a period during which urinary catecholamines decrease to normal levels. Catecholamines may therefore direct the islet-cell response, which, in turn, controls the disposition of the key substrates under their control."

The hormonal changes measured could represent independent rate-change effect related to time after injury, without meaningful relations to each other and to the concurrent metabolic events. However, the fact that manoeuvres, which increase insulin and suppress glucagon release tend to reverse the catabolic state is compatible with the role of these hormones in influencing nitrogen balance in markedly catabolic burn patients. The therapeutic maintenance of an anabolic insulin/glucagon ratio by providing exogenous insulin plus glucose when necessary is a theoretically rational measure in catabolic states.

Robinson et al (1973) consider that there appears to be a failure in the enhanced compensatory production of the hormone erythropoetin in severe burns and this accounts for the refractory anaemia that persists until wound closure.

Other useful reviews have been prepared by Moore, 1972; Johnston, 1972; Allison, 1975 and Cuthbertson, 1975.

The work of Ryan et al (1974) suggests that the net protein catabolism associated with haemorrhagic shock may be promoted by removal of leucine from the cellular synthetic amino acid pool through irreversible combustion. Catecholamines have been shown by Wool (1960) to suppress protein synthesis and Ryan et al have shown that this also holds for corticosterone. These changes persist for at least three days following haemorrhage. Such an effect would shift the dynamic balance of breakdown and resynthesis towards net protein catabolism. Amino acids not combusted by muscle, as well as the alanine produced by transfer of the leucine to pyruvate are probably released to the liver as gluconeogenic and ureagenic precursors (Felig, 1973). This effect is greater than that due to fasting.

It may be that the unexpected anticatabolic effects of infused amino acids without carbohydrate (Blackburn et al, 1973) or amino acid keto analogues in ameliorating the usual nitrogen excretion of injury or fasting to a degree that cannot be accounted for by their caloric value, may possibly be due to replacement of the combusted leucine.

It is suggested by Ryan et al (1974) that the similarities of the effects of haemorrhagic shock and of glucocorticoid hormones on leucine metabolism

26

raises the possibility that shock stimulated adrenal cortical and adrenal medullary secretions may contribute to the observed effects of haemorrhage shock on leucine metabolism.

O'Keefe, Sender and James (1974) have studied the fate of an infusion of ^{14}C leucine as a means of measuring the synthetic and breakdown rates of body protein before and at three days after abdominal surgery. They found at post injury stage a consistent fall in protein synthesis. They concluded that the 'catabolic' response to operative stress involves a fall in protein synthesis without an acute rise in breakdown rates of body protein. The method used was developed from Waterlow's (1967) original method. This involves an infusion of ^{14}C leucine to measure the synthetic and breakdown rates of body protein. The post operative loss of nitrogen was associated with a consistent fall in protein synthesis. The breakdown rates also fell but to a smaller extent in 3 of 4 patients. They concluded that the 'catabolic' response to operative stress involves a fall in protein synthesis without an acute rise in breakdown rates of body protein. These findings do not agree with the early work of Madden (1950) who investigated the effect of ^{35}S labelled methionine on the metabolic response to turpentine abscesses in dogs in respect of the urinary excretion of sulphur and corporation of sulphur into plasma protein and various other tissue proteins in the dog. The organic nitrogen and sulphur intakes were constant (oral, pre-injury, parenteral, post-injury). The tagged methionine was given one day after injection of the turpentine. The dogs were sacrificed 24 hours later. There was an increased output of both sulphur and nitrogen as compared with control dogs, but no increase in urinary excretion of ^{35}S. The appearance of ^{35}S (in terms of specific activity) in various tissue proteins was generally comparable in the abscessed and normal animals, though there was distinctly higher activity in the plasma protein of the abscessed dogs.

Levenson et al (1966) reported on somewhat similar experiments carried out on normal and burned rats, using ^{15}N labelled glycine. When rats are deeply burned over about one-third of their body surfaces, there is an increase in urinary excretion that reaches a peak 3 to 4 days after injury and then gradually returns to normal in about 14 to 16 days. This response is similar to that seen in injured patients, but of shorter duration, an observation which the writer had also noted.

The last authors found like the writer that in the rat the faecal N is not appreciably affected by injury and the same holds for man (Cuthbertson, 1936; Cuthbertson et al, 1939).

AMINO ACID TRANSPORT

In contrast to gut and kidney the amino acid flow is not unidirectional in the main bulk of the other tissues: there is both efflux and influx.

After a meal containing protein the amino acid concentrations in portal blood increase, but in peripheral blood the changes are quite small — the liver exercising a homeostatic effect although in the case of the branched-chain amino acids their metabolism mainly occurs in muscle. Only small changes in amino acid concentration occur in peripheral blood, and diurnal rhythms have been described for some amino acids, for example tryptophan and tyrosine.

In protein deficiency the pattern of free amino acids is altered; the concentrations of the essentials, notably the branched-chain amino acids, are reduced while those of the non-essentials are maintained or even increased. The plasma amino acid pattern is also influenced by the energy supply. It would be of interest to know if moderate to severe trauma covers the alanine concentration required through increased demand for gluconeogenesis as in fasting. The investigations of Bergström et al (1975) of needle biopsies of the *muscularis quadriceps femoris,* following an overnight fast in patients undergoing routine uncomplicated operation, revealed that though the total amounts of free amino acids in the plasma and muscle were not changed, the amino acid profiles differed from those in normal subjects. In plasma, as compared to controls, the most significant changes were an increase in phenylalanine and tyrosine and a decrease in serine, proline, histidine and isoleucine. In muscle the greatest decrease occurred in the concentrations of glutamine, arginine and lysine followed by proline and glutamic acid. The increases in taurine, valine and phenylalanine were all highly significant and in serine, glycine, alanine and leucine significant, whereas tyrosine showed only a moderate rise. The shift in methionine was somewhat less. It is of interest that the alterations in the muscle free amino acid pool are not reflected in the values found in plasma.

Using the term 'apparent' flux to give a general indication of the overall rate of amino acid or protein turnover by determining with labelled amino acids measurements on urine (in the case of ^{15}N-amino acids) or on plasma or respiratory carbon dioxide (in the case of ^{14}-labelled amino acids) a steady state has been achieved by continuous infusion, it was found that the amino acid flux in the adult is some three times greater than the normal amino acid supply from the food.

INTRAVENOUS NUTRITION

Whereas there are undoubtedly indications of diminished metabolism during the 'ebb' phase and increased catabolism during the 'flow' phase the respective contributions of antianabolism of ingested protein and excessive catabolism of endogenous sources of protein are still imperfectly understood throughout both periods, nevertheless wounds in general heal. There is thus doubt in the minds of some on how effective can be the use made of absorbed nutrients at this stage. Obviously the patient's nutritional state should not be allowed to deteriorate to his detriment if it is known that counter measures can be effective. With the emergence of safe means of intravenous nutrition it is obvious that when the patient is unable to ingest, digest or absorb a sufficiency of all the nutrients and energy by the normal oral gastrointestinal route over such a period as will begin to jeopardise adequate recovery then recourse must be made to intravenous or direct enteral feeding depending on the cause of the disorder. When all are given intravenously this is termed complete intravenous nutrition. In a subsequent chapter by Professor Wretlind a fully documented account of the present highly proficient stage of such a nutritional regime is given and it is shown that young children can make good growth and older patients maintained on it for periods up to several years.

The mixture consists of an adequate supply of water, amino acids (in the L-form), carbohydrates (glucose is preferred), a suitable fat emulsion, twelve electrolytes or minerals and thirteen vitamins. In some cases where oral intake is only partially sufficient supplementary intravenous nutrition with all, or some special nutrients may be indicated.

Dudrich et al (1968, 1972) have, for shorter periods, used an intravenous system of 'hyperalimentation' with hypertonic glucose and amino acids. This can only be given satisfactorily through a central vein catheter.

Blackburn et al (1973) in order to depress insulin secretion and enhance fat mobilisation limits the intravenous supply to amino acids for short periods. The 'pros' and 'cons' of these systems are dealt with in succeeding chapters.

Protein Turnover in Relation to Trauma

The urinary excretions of total N, S, P, K, Zn and Cu and to a lesser extent those also of Ca and Mg are increased following moderate to severe injury: that of Na shows early reduction due to Na retention. The increased excretion of these constituents and creatine is mainly related to:

a) the severity and nature of the injury: the more severe the injury the greater the negative balances

b) the nutritive state of the body at the time of injury and during the immediate pre-injury period, particularly in respect of the protein and total energy content of the diet.

c) the environmental temperature of the individual following the injury.

d) the presence of a certain but not necessarily increased level of circulating corticosteroid, e.g. cortisone.

e) age and sex. The healthy young male responds significantly more than does the child and the elderly: women up to the menopause appear to present a reduced catabolic response.

There is no question that as wounds heal there we have the obvious evidence of a local protein anabolism. But the observations of Fleck and his collaborators (Ballantyne & Fleck, 1073a,b; Ballantyne et al, 1973) have shown that there is reduced synthesis of plasma albumin following injury, but a rise in fibrinogens, α-globulins and acute phase reactant proteins. The question which is still being debated is how far the above increases in urinary catabolites — and to these should

29

be added creatine — are due primarily to an increased general catabolism of:

a) endogenous substances mainly of muscle and liver origin, possibly also from skin, *or*

b) of absorbed nutrients of the food which are largely rejected by the body which is in an anti-anabolic phase, that is there as a reduced synthesis of protein in general, which normally compensates for 'wear and tear'.

During the 'ebb' phase the response generally is geared towards antianabolism; later — in the 'flow' phase — it is apparently mainly a mixture of both a) and b) with b) predominating in the more severely injured.

If the rate of protein turnover be reduced to conserve energy costs to the injured then the now surfeit amino acids will largely be oxidised by the usual catabolic channels yielding heat and mainly urea and inorganic sulphate as end products of the oxidation. The energy yielded from the oxidation of the amino acids is presumably not different from that arising during normal turnover nor will the end products be different. Such oxidation of amino acids is thermodynamically a less efficient process for the generation of ATP than the oxidation of carbohydrate or fat and so more energy is wasted (SDA). The other explanation of SDA, namely that the entry of amino acids into the body stimulates protein synthesis and, since this requires energy oxygen consumption increases. This alternative does not seem tenable in the light of the preceding argument.

References

Abercrombie, M (1966) In *Wound Healing.* (Ed) C Illingworth. Page 61
Adams, PB and Rowan, KS (1970) *Plant Physiol., 45,* 490
Albright, F (1943) *Harvey Lect., 28,* 123
Allison, SB (1975) *Brit. Med. J., 1,* 860
Arturson, G (1961) *Acta chir. scand. Suppl.274*
Aub, JC (1920) *Amer. J. Physiol., 54,* 358
Aub, JC and Wu, H (1920) *Amer. J. Physiol., 54,* 416
Bailey, BN, Lewis, SR and Blocker, TG (1962) *Tex Rep. Biol. Med., 20,* 30
Ballantyne, FC and Fleck, A (1973a) *Clinica chim. Acta, 44,* 341
Ballantyne, FC and Fleck, A (1973b) *Clinica chim. Acta, 46,* 139
Ballantyne, FC, Tilstone, WJ and Fleck, A (1973) *Brit. J. exp. Path., 54,* 409
Barclay, THC, Cuthbertson, DP and Isaacs, A (1944) *Quart. J. exp. Physiol., 32,* 309
Barr, PO, Birke, G, Liljedahl, SO and Plantin, LO (1968) *Lancet, i,* 164
Bell, C (1798) *Wounds loc cit,* Guthrie, GJ (1815) *Gunshot Wounds.* London
Bergström, J, Furst, P, Noreé, L-O and Vinaars, E (1974) *J. appl. Physiol., 36,* 693
Bernard, C (1865) *An Introduction to the Study of Experimental Medicine.* Translated by HC Greene (1927). Macmillan, New York
Blackburn, GL, Flatt, JP, Clowes, GMA, O'Donnell, TF and Hensle, TE (1973) *Ann. Surg., 177,* 588
Bligh, J (1966) *Biol. Rev., 41,* 317
Burke, JF and Miles, AA (1958) *J. Path. Bact., 76,* 1
Cairnie, AB, Campbell, RM, Pullar, JD and Cuthbertson, DP (1957) *Brit. J. exp. Path., 38,* 504

Caldwell, FT (1962) *Ann. Surg., 155,* 119

Caldwell, FT (1970) In *Energy Metabolism in Trauma. Ciba Foundation Symposium.* (Ed) R Porter and J Knight. Churchill, London. Page 23

Caldwell, FT, Hammel, HJ and Dolan, F (1966) *J. appl. Physiol., 21,* 1665

Campbell, RM and Cuthbertson, DP (1967) *Quart. J. exp. Physiol., 52,* 114

Campbell, RM and Cuthbertson, DP (1970) *Quart. J. exp. Physiol., 55,* 338

Campbell, RH, Sharp, G, Boyne, AW and Cuthbertson, DP (1954) *Brit. J. exp. Path., 35,* 566

Cannon, WB (1923) *Traumatic Shock.* Appleton, New York

Carrel, A (1921) *J. exp. Med., 34,* 425

Carrel, A (1930) quoted by Arey, LB (1936) *Physiol. Rev., 16,* 327

Clark, AH (1919) *Bull. Johns Hopk. Hosp., 30,* 117

Clark, R (1967) *Brit. J. Surg., 54,* 445

Cole, JJ (1852) *Military Surgery.* London

Cournand, A, Riely, RL, Bradley, SE, Breed, ES, Noble, RP, Lausen, HD, Gregersen, MI and Richards, DW (1943) *Surg., 13,* 964

Cowell, EM (1917) *Report Spec. Ctee. Surg. Shock, MRC, No 25, Nos I-VII,* 99

Cuthbertson, DP (1929) *Biochem. J., 23,* 1328

Cuthbertson, DP (1930) *Biochem. J., 24,* 1244

Cuthbertson, DP (1931) *Biochem. J., 25,* 236

Cuthbertson, DP (1932) *Quart. J. Med., 25,* 233

Cuthbertson, DP (1936) *Brit. J. Surg., 23,* 505

Cuthbertson, DP (1942) *Lancet, i,* 433

Cuthbertson, DP (1960) In *The Biochemical Response to Injury.* (Ed) HB Stoner and CJ Threlfull. Blackwell, Oxford. Page 193: (1975) *Progr. Food Nutr., 1,* 263

Cuthbertson, DP (1964) In *Mammalian Protein Metabolism, Vol.2, Chapter 19.* (Ed) HN Munro and JB Allison. Academic Press, New York. Page 373

Cuthbertson, DP (1970) In *Energy Metabolism in Trauma. Ciba Foundation Symposium.* (Ed) R Porter and J Knight. Churchill, London. Page 155

Cuthbertson, DP (1975) *International Encyclopaedia of Food and Nutrition, Vol. 16, Chapter 25, 1.* Pergamon, Oxford: (1975) *Progr. Food Nutr., 1,* 263

Cuthbertson, DP and Munro, HN (1937) *Biochem. J., 31,* 694

Cuthbertson, DP and Rahimi, AG (1973) *Brit. J. Surg., 60,* 421

Cuthbertson, DP and Tilstone, WJ (1967) *Quart. J. exp. Physiol., 52,* 249

Cuthbertson, DP and Tilstone, WJ (1969) *Adv. clin. Chem., 12,* 1

Cuthbertson, DP, McGirr, JL and Robertson, JSM (1939) *Quart. J. exp. Physiol., 29,* 13

Cuthbertson, DP, Webster, TA and Young, FG (1941a) *J. Endocrin., 2,* 459

Cuthbertson, DP, Shaw, GB and Young, FG (1941b) *J. Endocrin., 2,* 468

Cuthbertson, DP, Smith, CM and Tilstone, WJ (1968) *Brit. J. Surg., 55,* 513

Cuthbertson, DP, Fell, GS, Smith, CM and Tilstone, WJ (1972) *Brit. J. Surg., 59,* 925

Davies, JWL and Liljedahl, S-O (1970) In *Energy Metabolism in Trauma. Ciba Foundation Symposium.* (Ed) R Porter and J Knight. Churchill, London. Page 59

Davis, HA (1936) *Proc. Soc. exp. Biol., NY, 34,* 21

Declasse, JA (1834) *loc. cit. Mann FC (1914) Bull. Johns Hopk. Hosp., 25,* 205

Dudrick, SJ, Wilmore, DW, Vars, HM and Rhoads, JE (1968) *Surg., 64,* 134, (1969) *Ann. Surg., 169,* 974

Dudrick, SJ, MacFadyen, BV, Buren, CT van, Rubert, RL and Maynard, AT (1972) *Ann. Surg., 176,* 259

Duff, JH, Groves, AO, McLean, APH, Lapointf, R and MacLean, LD (1969) *Surg., Gynec., Obstet., 128,* 1051
Dunphy, JE (1966) In *Wound Healing.* (Ed) C Illingworth. Churchill, London. Page 283
Duval, P and Grigaut, A (1918) *CR Soc. Biol., Paris, 87,* 873
Erici, I (1954) *Svensk Kir. Foren. Fch.* Page 34
Feldberg, W and Myers, RD (1964) *J. Physiol., 173,* 226
Feldberg, W and Myers, RD (1965) *J. Physiol., 177,* 239
Felig, P (1973) *Metabolism, 22,* 179
Fischer (1870) *loc. cit.* WB Cannon *Traumatic Shock.* New York. Page 2
Grant, RT and Reeve, EB (1951) Spec. Ref. Blackwell, London. *Ser. Med. Res. Comm. London, No 277*
Gump, FE and Kinney, JM (1971) *Arch. Surg., 103,* 442
Guthrie, GJ (1815) *Gunshot Wounds of the Extremities.* London
Halmagyi, DFJ, Broell, J, Gump, FR and Kinney, JM (1974) *Proceedings of the 1st International Congress on Intensive Care, London, June 1974.* Page 24
Haskins, HD (1907) *J. biol. Chem., 3,* 321
Harkins, HN (1941) *Surgery, 9,* 1
Hawk, PB and Gies, WJ (1904) *Amer. J. Physiol., 2,* 171
Henderson, Y, Prince, AL and Haggard, HW (1917) *J. Amer. Med. Assoc., 69,* 965
Hennen, J (1829) *Principles of Military Surgery.* London
Hewson, W (1772, repr. 1846) In *The Works of William Hewson.* (Ed) G Gulliver. Sydenham Society, London. Page 46
Hinton, P, Allison, SP, Littlehohn, S and Lloyd, J (1971) *Lancet, i,* 767 *Lancet, ii,* 218
Hori, T and Nakayama, T (1973) *J. Physiol., 232,* 71
Howes, EL, Briggs, H, Shea, R and Harvey, SC (1933) *Arch. Surg., 27,* 846
Hunter, J (1794) *A Treatise on the Blood, Inflammation and Gunshot Wounds.* Nicol, London
Ingle, DT (1951) *Recent Progr. Hormone Res., 6,* 159
Ingle, DT, Ward, EO and Kuinzenga, MH (1947) *Amer. J. Physiol., 149,* 570
James, GW, Purnell, OJ and Evans, EI (1951a) *J. Clin. Invest., 30,* 181
James, GW, Purnell, OJ and Evans, EI (1951b) *J. Clin. Invest., 30,* 191
Johnston, IDA (1972) *Adv. clin. Chem., 15,* 255
Kennedy, TL and Johnston, GW (1975) *Brit. med. J., 1,* 382
Kinney, JM, Long, CL and Duke, JH (1970) In *Energy Metabolism in Trauma. Ciba Foundation Symposium.* (Ed) R Porter and J Knight. Churchill, London
Kirsch, R, Frith, L, Black, E and Hoffenberg, R (1968) *Nature (Lond), 217,* 378
Latta, J (1795) *A Practical System of Surgery. Vol.2.* Edinburgh
Levenson, SM, Pulaski, EJ and Del Guerico, LRM (1966) In *Physiologic Principles of Surgery, Chapter 1.* Samden, Philadelphia. Page 1
Linder, F (1966) In *Wound Healing.* (Ed) C Illingworth. Churchill, London. Page 135
Longmore, T (1877) *Gunshot Wounds.* London
Lund, CC and Crandon, JH (1941) *J. Amer. Med. Assoc., 116,* 663
Macleod, GHB (1858) *Notes on the Surgery of War in the Crimea.* London
Madden, SC (1950) In *Plasma Proteins. Vol.2.* (Ed) J Youmans. Charles C Thomas, Springfield, Illinois. Page 62
Majno, G (1964) In *Injury, Inflammation and Immunity.* (Ed) L Thomas, JW War and L Grant. Williams and Wilkins, Baltimore. Page 58

Malcolm, JD (1893) *The Physiology of Death from Traumatic Fever.* Churchill, London
Marley, E and Stephenson, JD (1970) *Brit. J. Pharmac., 40,* 639
Marley, E and Stephenson, JD (1972) In *Handbuch der Experimentellan Pharma-kologie. Vol.33. Catecholaminer.* (Ed) H Blaschko and E Muscholl. Springer-Verlag, Berlin. Page 463
Marley, E and Stephenson, JD (1975) *J. Physiol., 245,* 289
Meltzer, SJ (1908) *Arch. intern. Med., 1,* 571
Merrill, AJ, Warren, JV, Stead, EA and Brannon, ES (1946) *Our Heart J, 31,* 413
Mestrezat, W (1918) *CR Soc. Biol. Parts, 81,* 888
Miksche, LE and Caldmell, ED (1968) *Amer. Surg., 54,* 455
Miles, AA and Miles, EM (1952) *J. Physiol. Lond., 118*
Miles, AA and Niven, JSF (1950) *Brit. J. exp. Path., 31,* 73
Moore, FD (1972) In *Homeostasis: Bodily Changes in Trauma and Surgery. Chapter 2. David-Christopher Text Book of Surgery.* (Ed) Sabiston. Saunders, Philadelphia. Page 26
Moore, FD and Ball, MR (1952) *The Metabolic Response to Injury.* Charles C Thomas, Springfield, Illinois
Morgan, EG and Peters, T (1971) *J. biol. Chem., 246,* 3500
Morgan, TH (1906) *J. exp. Zool., 3,* 457
Moss, GS (1968) In *Combined Injuries and Shock.* (Ed) B Schildt and L Thoren. Intermedes Proceedings of the Swedish Research Institute of National Defence, Stockholm, *80,* 291
Mourdisen, HT (1969a) *Clin. Sci., 37,* 431
Mourdisen, HT (1969b) *Scand. J. clin. lab. Invest., 23,* 235
Moyer, CA (1962) In *Research in Burns.* (Ed) CP Artz. American Institute of Biological Sciences, Publ.9, Washington
Munro, HN and Chalmers, M (1945) *Brit. J. exp. Path., 26,* 396
Munro, HN and Cuthbertson, DP (1943) *Biochem. J., 37,* xii
Needham, AE (1952) *Regeneration and Wound Healing.* Methuen, London
Needham, AE (1955) *J. Embryol. exp. Morphol., 3,* 189
Needham, AE (1958) *J. exp. Zool., 138,* 369
O'Keefe, SJD, Sender, PM and James, WPT (1974) *Lancet, ii,* 1035
Owen, JA (1969) *Adv. clin. Chem., 9,* 1
Rhoads, JE, Fliegelman, JT and Panzer, LM (1942) *J. Amer. Med. Assoc., 118,* 21
Richards, JR, Harland, WA and Orr, JS (1973) In *Hormones, Metabolism and Stress: Recent Progress.* Slovak Academy of Science, Bratislava. Page 151
Robinson, H, Monafo, WW, Saver, SM and Gallacher, NI (1973) *Ann. Surg., 178,* 565
Royal College of Pathologists (1972) *Pathology of Injury. Report of Working Party.* (Ed) AC Hunt. Miller and Metcalf, London
Ryan, NT, George, BC, Odessey, R and Egdahl, RH (1974) *Metabolism, 23,* 901
Sevitt, S (1958) *J. path. Bact., 75,* 27
Seyle, H (1937) *Endocrinology, 21,* 169
Seyle, H and Collip, IP (1936) *Endocrinology, 20,* 672
Shoemaker, WC (1966) *Shock; Chemistry, Physiology and Therapy.* Charles C Thomas, Springfield, Illinois
Soroff, HS, Pearson, B and Aritz, CP (1961) *Surg., Gynec., Obstet., 112,* 159
Spector, WG and Willoughby, DA (1965) In *The Inflammatory Process.* (Ed) BW Ziveifach, L Grant and RT McClusky. Academic Press, New York. Page 427

Spector, WG and Willoughby, DA (1968) In *The Pharmacology of Inflammation*. English Universities Press, London

Thomson, WD, Raudin, IS and Frank, IL (1938) *Arch. Surg., 36,* 500

Tilstone, WJ and Cuthbertson, DP (1970) In *Energy Metabolism in Trauma. Ciba Foundation Symposium.* (Ed) R Porter and J Knight. Churchill, London

Tilstone, WJ and Roach, PJ (1969) *Quart. J. exp. Physiol., 54,* 341

Walters, G (1972) Haemodynamics — general. In conference on *Shock*. (Ed) I McA Ledingham and TA McAllister. Kimpton, London

Warren, IC (1895) *Surgical Pathology and Therapeutics*. Philadelphia. Page 278

Waterlow, JC (1967) *Clin. Sci., 33,* 507

Weil, MH and Afifi, AA (1970) *Circulation, 41,* 989

Wertheimer, Fabre and Clogne (1919) *Bull. et Mem. de la Soc. Chirur., 45,* 9

Wilkinson, AW (1966) In *Wound Healing*. (Ed) C Illingworth. Churchill, London. Page 153

Wilkinson, AW, Billing, BH, Nagy, G and Stewart, CP (1949) *Lancet, i,* 640

Wilkinson, AW, Billing, BH, Nagy, G and Stewart, CP (1960) *Body Fluids in Surgery, 2nd Edition*

Willms-Kretschmer, K and Majno, G (1969) *Amer. J. Path., 54,* 327

Wilmore, DW, Curreri, PW, Spitzer, KW, Spitzer, ME and Pruitt, BA (1971) *Surg., Gynec., Obstet., 132,* 881

Wilmore, DW, Lindsey, CA, Moyland, JA, Falcoona, GR, Pruitt, BA and Unger, RH (1974) *Lancet, i,* 73

Wiseman, R (1719) *Chirurgical Treatise, loc. cit,* Guthrie, GJ (1815) *Gunshot Wounds of the Extremities.* London

Wool, IG (1960) *Ann. J. Physiol., 198,* 54

Wooldridge, LC (1866) *Arch. Anat. Physiol. (Physiol. Abth.),* 397

Wretlind, A (1972) *Nutr. Met., 14, Suppl.1*

Wright, A and Colebrook, L (1918) *Lancet, i,* 763

Zawacki, BE, Spitzer, KW, Mason, AD and Johns, LA (1970) *Ann. Surg., 171,* 236

Zweifach, BW and Thomas, L (1957) *J. exp. Med., 106,* 385

The Response to Injury as Affected by Age, Particularly in the Neonate and the Young Child

A W WILKINSON

Institute of Child Health, University of London, England

Introduction

It is often said that in babies and young children wounds heal better or faster or more easily than in older children or adults, but there is very little evidence to support this kind of statement. Indeed there seems to be no biological reason why this should be the case, or why there should be any difference in the response to injury or in the healing of injury because of age, except for the very important fact that the foetus and young baby are growing rapidly and the requirements for growth as well as for healing must be satisfied. It seems unlikely that there should be any harmful competition between growth and healing because survival of the organism depends on a good inflammatory response to injury and normal healing of the damaged tissues, and growth appears to continue unaffected by the infliction of injury. It is well known that healing of gangrenous bowel can occur in the foetus long before birth. There are many clinical observations, which have been confirmed by animal experiment, that the small intestine may undergo a volvulus or be the site of an intussusception during intra-uterine life and that this is made more likely by associated abnormalities such as meconium obstruction. Gangrene of the twisted or intussuscepted bowel is followed in the sterile environment of the foetal abdomen by absorption of the infarcted tissue, and healing and sealing off of the ends of the intact bowel with the production of an intestinal atresia. The presence of meconium in the distal bowel is good evidence of the prior continuity of the bowel. When the two ends of the bowel have been sealed off the contents of the distal bowel are expelled normally and this part of the intestine then becomes contracted and empty. The proximal segment of intestine is completely obstructed and its contents accumulate and cause dilatation of the bowel, while the continued attempt to force these contents out of the obstruction at the blind end lead to hypertrophy of the muscle wall.

Up to 45 per cent of babies born with atresia of the oesophagus, duodenum or rectum are small at birth or are born prematurely or both. Babies who weigh 1.5 kg or less at birth survive laparotomy or thoracotomy 8 weeks or more before the end of normal gestation. While the mortality rate of such babies is very high death is seldom due to the failure to produce an inflammatory reaction or normal healing of the surgical injury.

NEONATAL PHYSIOLOGY

The newly born baby is completely at the mercy of the environment and the doctors and nurses who look after him or her. The baby cannot complain as the older child and adult do of pain and discomfort, of feeling too hot or too cold, of hunger or of thirst. Those looking after the newly born baby must, therefore, understand and anticipate all that the baby needs in order to survive in the best possible condition. Like the adult and older child, the baby loses heat to the environment by radiation, conduction and convection. Rather less than 25 per cent of the total heat loss from the body is due to the insensible loss of water by evaporation from the body surface and in the expired air. The older child and adult can pull on more clothes and bedding when they feel too cold because of an unfavourable environment; the baby cannot and is thus liable to an increased heat loss which in turn imposes an increased energy and oxygen consumption. The surface area of a newborn infant has never been accurately measured but is said to be only 15 per cent of that of an adult weighing 70 kg but its weight is only 5 per cent of that of the adult, so surface area may be three times as great per kilogram body weight in the neonate as in the adult. At full term the fat content of a newly born baby is between 12 to 16 per cent body weight, but a baby born weighing only 1.5 kg contains only 12 per cent as much fat as it would at term. Even so, the human neonate is remarkable amongst mammals for its high fat content at birth since most other mammals contain only 1 or 2 per cent of fat. The newborn baby can maintain a stable body temperature when the difference between rectal or deep body temperature and the environmental temperature does not exceed 2 or 3°C. When the environmental temperature of a naked premature baby falls by 2°C heat production and oxygen consumption must be increased by 25 per cent to prevent a fall in body temperature (Hill & Rahintulla, 1965; Scopes, 1966). This loss of heat can be reduced also by clothing the infant or simply by covering the body with a single layer of material.

The 'neutral thermal environment' is defined as one in which the deep body temperature of the baby is within the range of 36.5 to 37.5°C but the heat production and oxygen consumption are minimal. The range of neutral temperature

36

is about 32 to 34°C at 50 per cent humidity for infants and is higher for small babies weighing less than 2.5 kg (Brück, 1961; Oliver & Karlberg, 1963); in adults it is 26 to 31°C. The nearer the ambient temperature is to the upper range of neutral temperature the more difficult it is to control the ambient temperature and prevent overheating, which is perhaps more deleterious to the baby than cooling. Most babies and certainly almost all premature babies are nursed in incubators after major surgical operations and the control of temperature within the modern incubator leaves a good deal to be desired. The fitted thermometers are often inaccurate and methods of indicating the relative humidity are usually so crude and unreliable as to be useless. The lower limit of the neutral thermal zone for any particular baby is called the 'critical temperature' and below this heat production must be increased to maintain body temperature. When the temperature within an incubator is above the neutral range heat loss must be increased by greater evaporation of water and the capacity of the neonate to sweat is limited. Hey and O'Connell (1970) showed that in the first month of life a draught-free temperature of 24°C would provide a neutral thermal environment for a clothed baby in a cot.

It is uncertain how much influence the maintenance of a neutral thermal environment has on the energy requirements of a baby after a major operation, and exact control of the temperature within the neutral thermal zone is extremely difficult with the incubators which are available for clinical use. Nevertheless it seems likely that the attempt should always be made to maintain the baby within the neutral thermal zone for an operation, in the hope that it will reduce oxygen consumption and the associated catabolism of muscle during starvation after injury to the minimum. There is some support for this belief. Losses of up to 10 per cent of birth weight during the first few days of life are not uncommon in normal infants and can be related partly to the restriction of water and milk intake; these losses can be reduced by offering either water or milk soon after birth providing the baby will consume these liquids. An energy expenditure of 60 kcal per kg per 24 hours by an infant weighing 3.5 kg would result in the consumption of 210 kcal per 24 hours; the dissipation of 25 per cent of the resulting heat production would impose an insensible water loss of 90 g per 24 hours. Zweymuller (1970) found that under basal conditions the insensible water loss was 32.6 to 38.9 g per 24 hours for a 3 kg baby, and was increased by crying and other activity and was lowest in those who slept during most of the time of observation.

There are considerable differences in the body composition of the neonate and the adult and it is not possible to extrapolate by simple calculation the constituents of either to the other (Table I). The neonate contains 14 per cent more water but a third less nitrogen, a quarter less potassium and half as much calcium as the adult when the theoretical composition of the neonate is scaled up to that of a 70 kg adult. In the same way when the composition of a 70 kg adult is scaled down to a weight of 3.5 kg the water content is 12 per cent less,

37

TABLE I. The Effect of Dividing the Weight and Constituents of the Adult Body by 20 to Reduce a Total of 70 kg to 3.5 kg and, Secondly, of Multiplying the Constituents of the 3.5 kg Neonate by 20 to give a 70 kg Body

	Water kg	Total nitrogen g	Na mM	K mM	Cl mM	Ca g
Baby wt. 3.5 kg	2.4	66	243	150	160	28.2
Same baby x 20 (Wt. = 70kg)	48	1320	4860	3000	3200	564
Adult wt. 70 kg	42	2000	5150	4050	2940	1320
% Difference	+14	−34	−4	−26	+9	−57
Adult wt. 70 kg	42	2000	5150	4050	2940	1320
Same adult ÷ 20 (Wt. = 3.5 kg−	2.1	100	257.5	202.5	147	66
Baby wt. 3.5 kg	2.4	66	243	150	160	28.2
% Difference	−12.5	+51	+6	+48	−8	+140

the total nitrogen and potassium are half as great again, whereas the calcium content is one and a half times and the sodium and chloride are much the same. Perhaps the most important difference between the neonate and the older adult is that the neonate is growing rapidly; the more prematurely the baby is born the greater is the rate of growth just after birth and the requirements for it. The energy value or requirement of this growth is far more than the energy value of the fat and protein laid down in the normal baby. Energy is also needed for swallowing, digestion, absorption and conversion of the constituents of milk into various kinds of body tissue. After operation or other injury all these requirements are additional to those for the production of an inflammatory reaction and for healing. Moreover, because of the wide species differences in the metabolism of young mammals, the only way in which they can be studied is in the human infant after surgical operations.

Widdowson (1973) has calculated that in the first month of life in the rat 80 per cent of the energy intake as fat, protein and carbohydrate in the food can be accounted for by the increments of fat and protein in the body tissues, but in the pig these increments amount to only 50 per cent of the total calorie intake; yet in the first four weeks of life the body weight of the pig increases nearly seven times and its fat content by 20 times. Another important difference perhaps is that both pigs and rats are born together in large numbers, and their homeostatic capacities and limitations are very different to those of the human baby who is usually born single and into a different kind of environment. The human baby may start feeding after a longer interval after birth and has a very much slower rate of growth as judged by increments of weight.

The natural food of the newborn human baby is human milk and even when this is offered *ad libitum* from a few hours after birth not all babies behave in the same way. Some begin to feed without delay but others may take little or no milk for up to four days after birth (Wilkinson et al, 1962). There is no good explanation for this variation in behaviour but it is clear that there is in the baby some type of appetite mechanism which determines when consumption of milk will begin and how much will be taken, and that the volume of milk produced by the mother is not the only factor to be considered. This variation in the consumption of milk is independent of any obstetric injury which may have been inflicted during delivery of the child, and of such other early disturbances as the respiratory distress syndrome. This variation in milk consumption during the early days after birth has a considerable influence on the metabolism of the newly born child. It should also be remembered that when a major operation is necessary during the first few days of life it may be the second severe injury which the child has received, the first being during the process of delivery.

The renal function of the newly born baby has been regarded by many as both immature and ineffective and by simple direct comparison with adult standards this is certainly the case. It must be remembered however that the kidneys of the newly born baby have to deal with quite different excretory requirements to those of the adult. Normal food for the human baby is human breast milk. At the end of the first week of life the human neonate may be consuming about 400 ml of human milk of which about 85 per cent is absorbed from the bowel and 65 per cent of the absorbed substances are retained within the body; the total intake is about 1 g of nitrogen, 8 mM of potassium, 5 mM of sodium and 3 mM of magnesium of which about two-thirds are retained (Wilkinson et al, 1962). Even when breast milk is fed from the first day only small quantities of urine are passed on the second and third days and the osmolality of this urine is about 400 to 500 milliosmoles per litre of urine water, about the maximum possible for the newly born baby's kidneys.

As the water intake rises towards the end of the first week the urine volume rises and the urine osmolality and the concentrations of sodium, potassium and nitrogen in the urine all fall. Human milk imposes a much smaller osmotic load on the kidneys, about 12 milliosmoles per 100 calories compared with the 30 milliosmoles per 100 calories of cow's milk.

One of the most remarkable features of renal function during the first week of life is the capacity of the kidneys of the neonate to restrict the excretion of sodium, potassium and magnesium in the urine to very small quantities at very low concentrations, and in this respect the kidneys of the neonate are more than equal if not vastly superior to those of the adult. What the kidneys are unable to do during the first week of life is to excrete excessive volumes of water or quantities of sodium administered by intravenous infusion. Lasch(1923) showed that in the first month of life infants could excrete only 55 per cent of a water load. McCance et al (1954) found that although infants aged 6 to 18 days who were given a water load equivalent to 6 per cent of their body weight at first increased their urine volume rapidly, they could not excrete within four hours as adults could, a volume of urine equal to the dose of water. These quantities are equivalent to water loads of 210 ml in a 3.5 kg neonate and 4.2 litres in a typical 70 kg male adult. This inability to produce diuresis in the first few days after birth occurs whether the water is given by mouth or by intravenous infusion. Four weeks after birth most babies who were born at term could excrete the whole of a water load equal to 3-5 per cent of the body weight within three hours.

The calorific value of new tissue laid down in the body in each 24 hour period is highest soon after birth and in smaller babies. It is much reduced after the age of four months from 33 kcal per kg per 24 hours for protein and fat at birth to 7 kcal per kg per 24 hours after four months. Widdowson (1973) calculated that a small premature baby born weighing 1.1 kg after 28 weeks of gestation would lay down fat and protein with a calorific value of 35 kcal per kg per 24 hours if it grew to 3.5 kg body weight in twelve weeks. This is equivalent to just over 25 per cent of the total calorie intake. She has also calculated that on an energy intake of 126 kcal per kg per 24 hours at the age of two months 48 kcal per kg of the total intake are used for basal metabolism, 33 to provide for the calorific value of the increments of tissue in the body and 45 for the further heat production needed for normal activity and for the energy cost of growth.

Metabolic balance studies can provide a good deal of useful information in the study of growth and the effect of injury in the newly born baby and young infant. The observations made in such studies must be interpreted with considerable care and their limitations must be recognised because of the considerable cumulative errors inherent in the method no matter how carefully the measurements are made. For example, how should the large outputs of various constituents in the meconium in the first two or three days of life be interpreted since these materials are probably all in the intestine at the time of birth. The delay before the consumption of adequate quantities of milk is established also has an important bearing on the total metabolic balance, and particularly on the incorporation of materials into the body tissues. We assumed that the onset of a positive balance of potassium was a suitable indication of net growth. The apparently irregular onset of potassium retention is related to the time at which milk feeds are well established. If the zero day for plotting the potassium retention is made the day on which potassium balance first became positive then a remarkable similarity is found in the retentions by individual babies, and an apparently haphazard behaviour is wiped out. What is more difficult to explain is the variation in the potassium—nitrogen ratio of the retentions of different babies. There is some appearance of regularity but the differences are considerable and interpretation of metabolic balances in patients after operation must be modified by this knowledge of the differences in the behaviour of normal babies. Indeed, it is difficult to find an entirely normal baby since there is so much individual and obstetric variation and the number of balances which can be carried out is limited and it is difficult to obtain a satisfactory mean.

There is a very consistent pattern of concentrations in the urine of sodium, potassium and nitrogen in neonates when these are plotted according to the day in which potassium balance first becomes positive. When the urinary concentrations of sodium, potassium and nitrogen of adults subjected to partial gastrectomy are compared with those of a normal baby and one operated on for duodenal atresia there is some similarity in the pattern but the urinary concentrations in the neonate are very much smaller than in the adult, a reflection both of the remarkable powers of conservation in the neonate in the case of sodium and potassium, and of the much smaller scale of turnover and excretion in the normal baby and a baby with duodenal atresia.

POST-OPERATIVE CHANGES

The total daily output of potassium and nitrogen per kg body weight have been compared in 10 normal neonates and 10 neonates born with congenital abnormalities which required relief by thoracotomy or laparotomy within the first few days of life; one other neonate was included who suffered from a myelomeningocoele which was treated by operation. The normal babies were offered *ad libitum* feeds of expressed breast milk from 4 hours after birth. The neonates who were operated on were fed either by a transanastomotic tube (3 with oesophageal atresia; 2 with duodenal atresia) often from 24 hours after operation, or by mouth usually within 48 hours of operation (2 jejunal atresia; 2 volvulus of midgut, 1 gastroschisis, 1 myelomeningocoele); there was a variable length of delay and starvation from birth to operation. The mean daily output by the 10 normal neonates in the urine for the first 5 days after birth was 0.15 mM/kg/24 hours potassium and 43.4 mg/kg/24 hours nitrogen. After 13 operations on 11 patients the mean daily output for 5 days after operation was 0.54 mM/kg/24 hours potassium and 179 mg/kg/24 hours nitrogen. The potassium to nitrogen ratio was 2.9 : 1 for the normals and 3.01 : 1 after operation but the mean daily outputs per kg body weight were more than 3 times as large for potassium and 4 times for nitrogen after operation as in the normal babies.

There are much larger losses of nitrogen and potassium in the urine after major operations in the neonate than in the normal baby during the first 5 days after birth. The potassium to nitrogen ratios suggest that much of this loss could be attributed to the potassium and nitrogen in the urine being derived from skeletal muscle, whether the catabolism of that muscle is due simply to starvation or to catabolism as part of a response to injury, such as is seen in well nourished adult males. Most of our balance studies have been made in neonates who were being nursed in incubators at a mean temperature of about 28°C and

41

not in a neutral thermal environment. It is impossible to say how much difference such an environment would make.

Summary

Although the quantities of materials excreted in the urine after operation by the neonate are very small these balance studies suggest that the metabolic response to injury in the neonate is similar to that of the adult, an increased output of nitrogen and potassium, accompanied by conservation of sodium. The response is modified by the earlier consumption of milk after operation by the babies compared with adults and by growth. There has been much discussion on what is a valid basis to compare metabolism in the neonate and the older child or adult. Probably the best would be lean tissue mass since this would imply the metabolically active tissue of the body regardless of age, nutritional state or total body weight. It might not avoid complications due to the effects of rapid growth in the premature baby but it would avoid the errors inherent in body weight due to variations in body water content and distribution and fat content. Unfortunately there is no way of measuring lean body mass in patients except indirectly by estimating total body water content and this was not possible when most of these studies were made and its use is limited by ethical restrictions. However, if comparison is made on the basis of body weight an increased daily urinary output of 180 mg nitrogen per kg per 24 hours by a neonate would be equivalent to 12.6 g nitrogen per 24 hours in a 70 kg adult male which is not much above the normal average of 11.0 g. Similarly an increased output of 0.54 mM of potassium per kg per 24 hours by a neonate would be equivalent to one of only 37 mM in a 70 kg adult. Comparisons of this kind are perhaps not valid and it is more realistic to remember that the outputs of nitrogen and potassium in the urine are three times as great in the 5 days after operation as they are in the normal neonate for 5 days after birth. These reactions are, of course, modified in premature babies by the different stage of development at birth, by the different total body composition and by the differences in rate of growth of organs and tissues and thus of the availability of materials for growth,maintenance of metabolism and repair. In spite of this the production of an inflammatory response to injury and of the means of repair of damage and healing clearly are provided in spite of the demands of continuing metabolism and growth.

Acknowledgments

I am indebted to the members of my department, in particular Miss Iris Harris for the analytical work on which the balances are based; to the Nursing Staff of The Hospital for Sick Children for the collections of materials; and to the children and parents whose metabolism was studied.

References

Brück, K (1961) *Biologia Neonat., 3,* 65
Hey, EN and O'Connell, B (1970) *Arch. Dis. Childh., 45,* 335
Hill, JR and Rahimtulla, KA (1965) *J. Physiol., 180,* 239
Lasch, W (1923) *Z. Kinderheik., 36,* 42
McCance, RA, Naylor, NJB and Widdowson, EM (1954) *Arch. Dis. Childh., 29,*104
Oliver, TK and Karlberg, P (1963) *Amer. J. Dis. Childh., 105,* 427
Scopes, JW (1966) *Brit. Med. Bull., 22,* 88
Widdowson, EM (1973) In *Therapeutic Aspects of Nutrition.* (Ed) JHP Jonxis,
    HKA Visser and JA Troelstra. Stenfert Kroese BV, Leiden. Page 3
Wilkinson, AW, Stevens, LH and Hughes, EA (1962) *Lancet, i,* 983
Zweymuller, E (1970) *Arch. Dis. Childh., 45,* 815

The Influence of the Nature, Severity and Environmental Temperature on the Response to Injury

A FLECK

Department of Biochemistry, Western Infirmary, Glasgow

Introduction

The clearest evidence that the metabolic response to injury is proportional to the degree of injury has been obtained in studies on burned patients, in whom the area of the body surface affected gives a measure of the extent of the injury (Davies & Liljedahl, 1970). The nature of the injury may modify the response. Burning injury leads to considerable increases in catecholamine excretion and the greatest increase in resting metabolic expenditure (RME) of all injuries (Kinney et al,1970a). Sepsis is also associated with considerable increases in RME and fractures usually give a lesser response (Kinney et al, 1970b). In contrast, after abdominal surgery, there may be no detectable increase in RME although it is usual to find weight loss of 7-10% in males after abdominal surgery.

NATURE AND SEVERITY OF INJURY AND THE RESPONSE

Direct Comparison of Two Injuries

Because of the influence of the nature and severity of the injury and environmental temperature on the response, especially the acute phase reactants of the plasma proteins, and the components of the urine losses and variations in the severity of the injury in accidental fractures of long bones, we chose rather to study patients undergoing hip arthoplasty by the Charnley procedure which is a fairly standard severe injury. The influence of environmental temperature in such patients undergoing this operation was compared with other patients who had suffered acute myocardial infarction (AMI).

We compared food intake, urinary outputs of nitrogen, potassium, magnesium

44

and creatine and the serum protein changes in the two groups. The net nitrogen loss (i.e. food nitrogen-urine nitrogen) of the two groups is summarised in Table I. Food intake was decreased in all groups in the early days after injury. The net nitrogen loss, however, is considerably greater after THR than after AMI and prolonged for 14 days. Similarly there was a significant increase in creatine

TABLE I. Comparison of N Metabolism of Two Injuries: Total Hip Replacement (THR) and Acute Myocardial Infarction (AMI) at 20° Environmental Temperature

| | Nitrogen g/d | | | | | |
| | Day 1-4 | | Day 5-7 | | Day 8-10 | |
	AMI	THR	AMI	THR	AMI	THR
Intake N	7.5	7	9	9.5	9.7	9.5
Urine N	13.1	15	9.2	14.5	9.5	13.5
Net N (Food N minus Urine N)	-5.6	-8	-0.2	-5	+0.2	-4

excretion after THR but only a transient response in the patients who had suffered AMI. The excretion of potassium and magnesium followed similar patterns.

The changes in the plasma proteins: albumin, C-reactive protein (CRP), α_1-acid glycoprotein were consistent with those described previously (Fleck, this volume). However, again the changes after AMI were less than after THR and, in the case of α_1-acid glycoprotein, the level remained within the normal range after AMI (Table II).

TABLE II. Comparison of Changes in Plasma Proteins after AMI and Fracture of a Long Bone

| | Albumin | | C-reactive protein | | α_1-acid glycoprotein | |
	AMI	Fractures	AMI	Fractures	AMI	Fractures
Day 1	35	34	0.04	0.12	0.9	1.4
3	32	31	0.09	0.10	1.3	1.6
5	31	27	0.05	0.08	1.2	1.8
10	34	30	0.02	0.06	1.2	1.9

Limit of accepted (lower) 35g/l   not detectable   (upper) 1.4g/l
'normal' range   in 'normal'

Note: Values are quoted in g/l

It was concluded that the magnitude of the response is greater in the injury leading to the greater amount of tissue damage (THR).

Comparison with Severe Injury

In terms of net nitrogen loss, AMI is a relatively minor injury causing a response of the same order as the surgical treatment of duodenal ulcer (Table III). The response to THR although much greater than AMI, is similar to that of accidental long bone injury and significantly less than after sepsis, major skeletal trauma or burns (Table III).

TABLE III. Nitrogen Loss and Increase in Relative Metabolic Energy Expenditure (RME) after Injury

Injury	Approximate Net N loss (g/d) (mean of first 4 days)	Increase in RME (%) [1]
Acute myocardial infarction	3	—
Elective abdominal surgery	2-4 [2,3]	not significant
Total hip resection	6-81	—
Long Bone Injury [4]	3-7	
Sepsis	2-8	+25-45
Major skeletal trauma	4-10	+10-30
Burns[5]	8-20	+40-100

[1] from Kinney et al (1970)
[2] Moore and Ball (1955)
[3] Kinney, Long and Duke (1970)
[4] Tilstone and Cuthbertson (1970)
[5] Davies and Liljedahl (1970)

ENVIRONMENTAL TEMPERATURES AND THE RESPONSE

Direct Comparison of Three Temperatures

The food intake and the urine nitrogen excretion were determined in patients nursed at 20°C environment, i.e. the normal ward temperature; at 28°C and at 30°C temperature. At both the higher environmental temperatures of 30° and 28°

46

TABLE IV. The Influence of Environmental Temperature after Injury on Nitrogen Metabolism

| | Day 1–4 | | | Day 5–7 | | | Day 8–10 | | |
	20°	28°	30°	20°	28°	30°	20°	28°	30°
Intake	7	9	8.5	9.5	12.2	9.8	9.5	13	10
Urine N	15	13.5	13	14.5	14	12	13.5	12	11
Net N (Food N minus Urine N)	-8	-4.5	-4.5	-5	-1.8	-2.2	-4	+1	-1

there is considerable reduction in the loss of urinary nitrogen and net nitrogen loss (Table IV). It is also apparent, however, that there is an influence on food intake which was maximal in the small group of patients nursed at the 28° environmental temperature after injury. From these preliminary observations we could conclude that the influence of the 28°C environmental temperature is equally beneficial to the 30° temperature but has the additional advantage that the patients and nurses tolerate 28° much better than the 30° environment.

Direct Comparison of Three Temperatures

Low Environmental Temperature

Tilstone (1968) using a standard dorsal wound in mice to examine the rate of wound healing found that the healing of the wound was delayed in mice maintained at -3°C in comparison with those caged at the more usual 20° environmental temperature. Unfortunately, no additional metabolic studies were possible at that time.

Increased Environmental Temperature

There is little direct comparative evidence on the metabolic response in individuals acclimatised to a tropical environment close to the thermoneutral zone (28-30°C). Elebute (1974), however, reports some studies from Lagos in Nigeria where the environmental temperature was in the region of 27-32°C and relative humidity from 80-90%. Patients who had undergone elective abdominal surgery (vagotomy and drainage) showed a response of increased urine nitrogen of the same order as would be anticipated in temperate (i.e. about 20°C) zones. He did suggest, however, that increased environmental temperatures (28-30°C) and high humidity led to an increase in the 'catabolic' response.

47

Discussion

There is good evidence that the degree of the metabolic response is in accord with the extent or severity of the injury. However, the response is modified by age, sex and previous nutritional status (Cuthbertson, 1964). It is also modified by environmental temperature. Extremes increase the response or delay wound healing whereas when the temperature is close to the thermoneutral zone, the response as demonstrated in several ways, is minimised.

Whether the minimising of the metabolic response is of significant benefit to the patient has not been demonstrated except in severe burns. When the burned area is greater than 70% of the body surface, the probability of survival when patients are nursed at 20°C is very small, but when the environmental temperature is raised to the thermoneutral zone, the body weight loss is markedly reduced and the metabolic changes in plasma proteins, nitrogen loss etc are minimised (Davies et al, 1969).

References

Cuthbertson, DP (1964) In *Mammalian Protein Metabolism, Vol.II, Chap.19.* (Ed) HN Munro and JB Allison. Academic Press, New York and London

Davies, JWL and Liljedahl, S-O (1970) In *Energy Metabolism in Trauma. Ciba Foundation Symposium.* (Ed) R Porter and J Knight. Churchill, London

Davies, JWL, Liljedahl, S-O and Birke, G (1969) *Injury, 1,* 43

Elebute, EA (1974) *Brit. J. Surg., 61,* 60

Kinney, JM, Duke, JH Jr, Long, CL and Gump, FE (1970a) *J. clin. Path., 20,* Suppl. (Roy. Coll. Path.), 4, 65

Kinney, JM, Long, CL and Duke, JH (1970b) In *Energy Metabolism in Trauma. Ciba Foundation Symposium.* (Ed) R Porter and J Knight. Churchill, London

Moore, FD and Ball, MR (1955) *The Metabolic Response to Surgery.* Charles C Thomas, Springfield, Illinois

Tilstone, WJ (1968) *Studies on Wound Healing and the Metabolic Response to Injury.* PhD Thesis, University of Glasgow (1968)

Tilstone, WJ and Cuthbertson, DP (1970) In *Energy Metabolism in Trauma. Ciba Foundation Symposium.* (Ed) R Porter and J Knight. Churchill, London

The Spinal Cord in Relation to the Effects of Injury

W E STRACHAN

Subregional Neurosurgical Service, Plymouth, Devon, UK

Introduction

The management of spinal injury in the past 25 years has been conditioned by
the proven ineffectiveness of one operative technique — decompressive laminec-
tomy and by the persuasiveness of the conservative school of thought. There is
fairly general agreement regarding the necessity for debridement in penetrating
cord wounds and most surgeons accept the need for the removal of compressive
bone fragments in lesions below L1, where the neurological deficit is due to root
involvement rather than cord. However, the treatment of the majority of cord
injuries is less obvious, particularly when the neurological lesion is subtotal. Many
surgeons take the progression of neurological deficit as an indication for surgical
interference. Nonetheless, it remains a fact, that the majority of patients with
immediate sensori-motor loss below the level of the injury seldom gain significant
functional recovery in spite of all therapeutic measures available.

PATHOLOGICAL CHANGES IN ACUTE SPINAL INJURY

It would seem reasonable to assume that in all such cases the spinal cord had been
anatomically transected by the violence of the injury. This, in fact is not so, as
the cord in its tough dural sheath displays a surprising resilience, even in the face
of massive fracture dislocations. The midcervical region, being one of the more
mobile areas of the spinal column, is particularly prone to injury. Patients so
injured frequently present with a paraplegia plus distal upper limb involvement
and a sensory level, say at C5/6 dermatome. It is not uncommon for such patients
to develop in the ensuing 24 hours, what has been termed loosely, ascending

myelitis, with progression to tetraplegia and diaphragmatic paralysis. Not surprisingly, death may occur even with artificial respiration. Usually examination of the cord shows enlargement due to swelling — this has a spindle-shaped appearance tapering upwards and downwards over several segments. Sections show central haemorrhagic necrosis, with, in the region of the tracts, axonal debris and fat droplets from fragmented myelin, along with large fluid filled spaces.

Similar features are present in severe injuries in experimental animals. Lesser injuries and study of the spinal cord at varying intervals after injury help to explain the mechanism (Ducker et al, 1971; Osterholm & Mathews, 1972a,b). Examination of sections taken 30 minutes after a 500 g/cm injury reveals small petechial haemorrhages in the central grey matter. After 2 hours these have enlarged considerably and there is evidence of neuronal disintegration. By 4 hours this process has extended to coagulative necrosis of up to 40% of the grey and the surrounding white matter. After 24 hours, apart from a rim of white matter, the whole section appears amorphous and necrotic. Electron microscopy studies show that the earliest changes are in the microvasculature with damage to the endothelium, particularly in the post-capillary venules. From these studies it has been suggested that neuronal degenerative change may be secondary to vascular change and hypoxia. The appearances are similar to those found in ischaemia due to multiple radicular artery ligation.

Lock et al (1971) studied CSF lactate accumulation following experimental cord injury and circulatory arrest and the correlation they found supports the view of ischaemia and hypoxia. Injections of minute quantities of various substances (noradrenaline, histamine and serotonin) by a traumatic method produced histopathological changes of haemorrhagic necrosis in the spinal cord.

There are two theories as to the nature of the mechanisms involved — on the one hand some observers (Dohrmann et al, 1972) believe that the vascular smooth muscle contracts, thereby narrowing the lumen, increasing resistance and obstructing the blood flow. On the other hand Osterholm and Mathews (1972a) hold that catecholamines are responsible for the vascular change.

IMPLICATION OF CATECHOLAMINES

Although there appears to be good evidence for accumulation of amines at the site of spinal cord trauma (Naftchi et al, 1974), the precise nature of the product has not been clarified completely. Noradrenaline and dopamine seem to be the most likely, but the source of the catecholamine also awaits final proof. Osterholm and Mathews (1972a,b) have carried out a great deal of experimental work and propose that noradrenaline is the active substance responsible for the vascular change and that it is released in excessive quantities in the cord neurovascular system.

Noradrenergic fibres have been associated with the peripheral sympathetic nervous system for many years, but in the past decades the presence of a noradrenergic fibre system in the cord has been demonstrated by various groups of workers (Dahlstrom & Fuxe, 1965). The fibres descend from the cell bodies in the reticular medulla and end in synaptic relationship with neurones and vessels of the spinal grey matter where accumulations of catecholamines have been demonstrated by histofluorescent techniques (Osterholm, 1974).

In supporting their neurotransmitter theory against that of the effect of direct vascular disruption, Osterholm and Mathews (1972a,b) sectioned cats' spinal cords at T1 and a week later subjected the T8 level to a standard 500 g/cm injury. Sections examined two hours after injury showed that oedema was present. Haemorrhages occupied under 1% of the cord area instead of the 23% found in previous experiments where prior section at the higher level had not been carried out. Preliminary sectioning of the dorsal roots 6–9 bilaterally also had some protective action.

Protective Effects Against Noradrenaline

Further proof of the implication of noradrenaline was obtained by examining the protective effects of a series of drugs with known anti-noradrenaline properties (Osterholm & Mathews, 1972b). Alphamethyltyrosine was found to be the most effective — but an optimal dosage of 200 mg/kg caused toxic renal damage with anuria in 50% of the cats. Also effective were reserpine, which interferes with the formation of noradrenaline from dopamine, and phenoxybenzamine which is a specific receptor blocker.

However, other workers (Hedeman et al, 1974) using basically similar techniques in dogs and cats have failed to find this increase in noradrenaline but have reported that dopamine was increased. They found also that alpha-methyltyrosine had no protective effect. On the other hand, Vise et al (1974), using dogs, studied the vascularity and blood brain barrier function with fluorescent microscopy following injury to the spinal cord and demonstrated a perivascular fluorescence which appeared to be the same as that seen in the catecholamine stores of the adrenal medulla. They feel that the mechanism for intrinsic CNS production of noradrenaline proposed by Osterholm and Mathews (1972a) lacks credibility — particularly on the grounds of the time scale — as it was reported that there was a two-fold increase in noradrenaline after thirty minutes and a seven-fold increase in two hours. Vise et al (1974) suggest that the spinal injury disrupts the normal blood brain barrier and permits the circulating catecholamines to pass across. It has been shown (Muelheims et al, 1969) that following C2 section in dogs, the circulatory noradrenaline levels are increased ten-fold in 3 minutes.

Although there is still much clarification to be done, the implications for the clinician treating spinal injury are clear. For the first time there is hope. There may be technical problems ahead if the theorists are correct — time may be vital — so we may have to produce methods whereby delay in instituting anti-catecholamine therapy is reduced to a minimum. It may come that the geographical situation of the accident may govern the prognosis.

THERAPY IN THE ACUTE PHASE

Hypothermia

A slightly earlier attempt to overcome the prevailing attitude of clinical helplessness in spinal cord injury followed the observation by Albin et al (1968) of the beneficial effects of hypothermia in experimental injury to monkeys. However, the results from a number of laboratories have been mixed and the application to the clinical situation has been difficult. White (1973) has been able to produce a system using a heat exchanger which appears to be capable of maintaining a cord surface temperature of around $20°C$. There have not been a sufficient number of reports under controlled conditions to assess the true efficacy of this technique. Osterholm (1974) in applying hypothermia to his standard experimental technique, found a 50% reduction in noradrenaline and a corresponding protective action against haemorrhagic necrosis. Recently, Tator and Deecke (1973) found perfusion under normothermic conditions to be more effective than hypothermia in experimental lesions in monkeys.

Steroids

High dosages of steroids — usually Dexamethasone® — have been given empirically by most neurosurgeons for some years on the basis of their effectiveness on cerebral oedema. In the laboratory the mode of action has not been demonstrated and the effects have been questioned — particularly where the damage to the cord has been most severe. An interesting recent study by Lewin et al (1974) has shown that Dexamethasone had little measurable effect on oedema, but prevented the loss of potassium from the injured cord substance and all the treated animals were reported to show significantly better functional recovery.

Hyperbaric Oxygen

Kelly et al (1972) showed that while the PO_2 of the spinal cord responded to ventilation with 100% oxygen and carbogen (95% O_2 5% CO_2) the traumatised spinal cord responded only to hyperbaric oxygen at 2—3 atmospheres. Dogs so treated made a significantly greater functional recovery than the control group.

CLINICAL DEVELOPMENTS FOLLOWING INJURY

Following severe damage to the spinal cord, there develops a complete flaccid motor paralysis below the site of the lesion — a condition known as 'spinal shock'. This bears no relation to surgical shock. It may be produced temporarily in experimental animals by cord cooling or by procaine injection.

Clinically there is paralysis, loss of reflexes, both superficial and deep, sensory loss and abolition of autonomic activity below the site of damage. Bladder and bowel function are lost with resultant urinary retention, meteorism and ileus. Sweat secretion is likewise lost below the lesion. The duration of spinal shock varies from a few days to weeks, although in lower animals the length may be much less (e.g. in the frog, minutes; cat and dogs, hours).

With recovery from spinal shock, reflex activity returns. This usually commences with response to plantar stimulation and genital reflexes. Later, withdrawal responses become more vigorous and mass reflexes may result from minor stimulus — giving violent withdrawal and visceral autonomic effects with evacuation of bladder and bowel and profuse sweating. The loss of autonomic reflexes leads to disturbance of vasomotor control. Postural hypotension is a problem. There is neither vasoconstriction in response to cold, nor sweating in response to heat.

PROBLEMS IN MANAGEMENT OF THE SPINALLY INJURED

Obviously the level of involvement has an important part in determining the management and the development of complications. The higher the lesion, the more complex the problem.

Respiratory

One of the most serious traumatic injuries is involvement at mid-cervical level. Quite apart from the devastating sensori-motor paralysis, complex respiratory changes occur, frequently leading to death. Kadoya et al (1974) showed that following direct C4 trauma, spontaneous respiration ceased. This apnoea was transitory in mild trauma, and, providing the respiratory support was used at this stage, spontaneous respiration was regained. With more severe injury, most animals developed delayed respiratory paralysis, due to oedema and haemorrhagic necrosis.

In the management of the acute tetraplegic there are many problems and the earliest of these are usually respiratory. Some of these may be attributed directly to cord damage and associated injuries, others to secondary respiratory and metabolic effects. The end product from whichever cause, is hypoventilation, which in itself, may precipitate secondary effects and thereby a vicious cycle. With the aid of clinical, radiological and respiratory test evidence, a decision can be made as to the magnitude of the primary factors and the policy arrived at as to whether a tracheostomy is necessary to reduce the dead space. However, it must be realised that the ventilatory capacity of an established tetraplegic is considerably lower than in the active individual. In an average individual in the supine position, about 40% of tidal volume comes from diaphragmatic action and 60% from the rib cage. In the tetraplegic, the diaphragm is the only major functioning muscle of respiration and also it is required to carry out nine times more work in displacing the abdominal viscera.

53

Cheshire and Coats (1966) have shown that a tidal volume of 200 ml or a vital capacity of 800 ml may be adequate to maintain a tetraplegic under basal conditions and that an isolated, seemingly high pCO_2 does not in itself constitute an indication for tracheostomy, as blood gases in tetraplegia require to be interpreted in the light of the reduced activity of the patient.

Certain factors predispose to hypoventilation, in particular pulmonary collapse from aspirated gastric contents, pulmonary oedema from overhydration and sputum retention due to ineffectual coughing as a result of paralysis of the intercostals and diaphragm. In the presence of an unstable fracture, vigorous physiotherapy is impracticable. In such circumstance, the early stabilisation of a mid-cervical fracture by the anterior route may be indicated.

Postural Hypotension

The effects on the systolic and diastolic blood pressure of change of position from the erect to supine in some individuals may be considerable. In spinal man the C5 level appears to be critical. Guttmann (1973) showed that tilting on an inclined table patients with lesions below this level did not give any different results from other non-spinal convalescent patients, whereas above this level there was profound vascular maladaptation as a result of interruption of splanchnic control.

Metabolic and Acid-Base Disturbance

There is on the whole, a tendency to overtransfuse patients with spinal injury, with resultant fluid overloading. This is possibly the result of confusion of the hypotension of spinal shock with surgical shock.

Potassium requirements after spinal injury may be high: up to 300 mEq in 24 hours may be necessary. Failure to restore the potassium deficiency following injury, leads to impairment of cardiac and smooth muscle function. Calcium tends to be mobilised from the bones due to inactivity, so the administration of calcium is unnecessary. The same is probably true of magnesium.

Nutrition

The body's continuing caloric requirements must be met; 1500 to 1800 kcal per day is probably the base line for the average adult, but it is advisable to aim at a total daily caloric intake of 2000 or more kcal. Nutrients are needed also to provide high energy substrate for tissue repair and the conversion of a negative to a positive nitrogen balance. As a general principle, it is always preferable to give fluid and nutrients by the oral route where possible. However, in the tetraplegic patient, the consequences of spinal shock are such that smooth muscle function almost invariably ceases for some time and oral feeding is impracticable. In such circumstances it is necessary to resort to intravenous nutrition. If there is excessive nasogastric aspirate, the volumes and electrolyte concentrations should be determined for balance purposes. However, in most cases, by the fourth or fifth day after injury, bowel sounds return and the gradual introduction of oral feeding may be commenced.

Thermal Regulation

The inability of the tetraplegic to control his body temperature is well known, particularly in the immediate post-accident period. In hot climates, environmental hyperthermia may have serious metabolic effects and therefore an air-conditioned environment becomes essential. It has been shown that with a complete tetraplegic, nursed without blankets in a constant temperature of 21°C, the body temperature will stabilise between 34 and 35°C (rectal). There are theoretical benefits in the slight reduction of body temperature, as experiment has shown that the oxygen requirements at 34°C are approximately 20% less than at 37°C.

FUTURE PROSPECTS

A relatively small part of the rehabilitation progress of a tetraplegic is essentially medical. It is only by the use of a multidisciplinary team that the excellent results obtained by Guttmann (1973) and others may be achieved.

It seems likely, however, in the next decade answers may come in the early management of spinal injury. Unfortunately although regeneration and even restitution of function appears to occur after spinal cord severence in experimental animals, there is no convincing evidence of recovery following anatomical transection in mammals.

References

Albin, MS, White, RJ, Acosta-Rua, GJ and Yashon, D (1968) *J. Neurosurg.,* 29, 113
Cheshire, DJE and Coats, DA (1966) *Paraplegia, 4,* 1
Dahlstrom, A and Fuxe, K (1965) *Acta Physiol. Scand., 64, Suppl.274,* 1
Dohrmann, GJ, Wagner, FC and Bucy, PC (1972) *J. Neurosurg., 36,* 407
Ducker, TB, Kindt, GW and Kempe, LG (1971) *J. Neurosurg., 35,* 700
Guttmann, LG (1973) *Spinal Cord Injuries.* Blackwell Scientific, Oxford
Hedeman, LS, Shellenberger, MK and Gordon, JH (1974) *J. Neurosurg., 40,* 37
Kadoya, S, Massopust, LC Jr, Wolin, LR, Taslitz, N and White, RS (1974) *J. Neurosurg., 41,* 455
Kelly, DL Jr, Lassiter, KRL, Vongsvivut, A and Smith, JM (1972) *J. Neurosurg., 36,* 425
Lewin, MG, Hansebout, RR and Pappius, HM (1974) *J. Neurosurg., 40,* 65
Locke, GE, Yashon, D and Feldman, RA (1971) *J. Neurosurg., 34,* 614
Muelheims, GH, Walter, KE and Billy, L (1969) *Proc. Soc. exp. Biol. Med., 130,* 574

Naftchi, NE, Demeny, M, De Crescito, V, Tomasula, JJ, Flamm, ES and
    Campbell, JB (1974) *J. Neurosurg., 40,* 52
Osterholm, JL (1974) *J. Neurosurg., 40,* 5
Osterholm, JL and Mathews, GJ (1972a) *J. Neurosurg., 36,* 386
Osterholm, JL and Mathews, GJ (1972b) *J. Neurosurg., 36,* 395
Tator, CH and Deecke, L (1973) *J. Neurosurg., 39,* 52
Vise, WM, Yashon, D and Hunt, WE (1974) *J. Neurosurg., 40,* 76
White, RJ (1973) *Clin. Neurosurg., 20,* 400

The Circulatory Response to Energy Metabolism in Shock, Injury and Infection

J M KINNEY and F E GUMP

Department of Surgery, Columbia University College of Physicians and Surgeons, New York, USA

Introduction

Any examination of energy metabolism is intimately related to the circulation since oxygen is the most flow-limited of all substances carried by the blood. The fact that approximately one-fourth of the arterial oxygen is removed during the course of a single transit through the resting body results in a unique dependence on an adequate circulation for continuing energy exchange. When metabolic requirements are altered, circulatory adjustments play a major role in the body's efforts to restore equilibrium conditions. Additional oxygen can be supplied to the tissues in only two ways: by increased extraction of oxygen from arterial blood or by augmented blood flow. The relationship between oxygen consumption and blood flow is, therefore, of critical importance in many clinical situations. Furthermore, measurements of blood flow and oxygen consumption become even more significant when it is possible to examine specific organs. Fragmentary clinical studies have suggested that changes in cardiac output and oxygen consumption are not uniformly distributed throughout the body and the relationship between blood flow and oxygen consumption may vary widely in different vascular beds. In surgical patients the relationship between circulation and energy metabolism is of particular importance in shock, sepsis, and injury.

Ever since the regulation of cardiac output has been studied, it has been recognised that output increases approximately in proportion to the increase in metabolic rate. Normal values for cardiac output and oxygen consumption are traditionally presented in terms of body surface area (BSA) while blood oxygen content is usually recorded as volume per cent (ml O_2/100 ml of blood). Three litres/min/m² is a generally accepted normal value for cardiac output (Brandfonbrener et al, 1955), and when this is multiplied by the normal oxygen content of

57

arterial blood it is possible to calculate the oxygen transported to the tissues (3000 ml/min/m^2 x 19 ml O_2/100 ml blood = 570 ml O_2/min/m$_2$, or approximately one-fifth of the oxygen delivered. Under these resting conditions average mixed venous blood contains 14.8 vol % oxygen, is 73% saturated and the A-V difference is 4.1 vol %.

A variety of conditions will change both resting metabolic expenditure and cardiac output, as well as the relationship between them. Increases are more common and partial listing of these conditions, often referred to as hyperdynamic states, would include: exercise (Chapman & Fraser, 1954; Roncoroni et al, 1959), pregnancy (Bader et al, 1955), sepsis (Clowes et al, 1966), hyperthyroidism (Graettinger et al, 1959), anaemia (Branon et al, 1945), A-V fistula (Epstein et al, 1953), Paget's disease (Rapaport et al, 1957), cirrhosis (Del Guercio et al, 1964; Kowalski & Abelmann, 1953), beriberi (Blacket & Palmer, 1960), glomerulonephritis (DeFazio et al, 1959), and hypertension (Finkielman et al, 1965). Decreased cardiac output has been described in congestive heart failure (Sarnoff, 1955), valvular heart disease (Braun et al, 1959), anaesthesia (Snyder, 1938) and shock (Cournand et al, 1953).

Hyperdynamic circulatory states have received increasing attention. Clowes (1963) suggested that patients with large areas of tissue necrosis or inflammation demand a far higher level of cardiac output than is the case in uneventful convalescence and subsequently presented evidence that the ability of the septic patient to increase cardiac output is an important factor in survival (Clowes et al, 1966). Wilson et al (1965) directed attention to the elevated cardiac output seen in some patients with septic shock and since then haemodynamic studies in trauma, shock, and sepsis have been vigorously pursued. The list of hyperdynamic conditions referred to previously will serve to illustrate features that are unique to the surgical patient.

DECREASED CARDIAC OUTPUT

The pioneering haemodynamic studies in shocked patients of Cournand et al (1953) stressed a decrease in cardiac output associated with peripheral vasoconstriction. Oxygen consumption was maintained in the face of decreased blood flow by greater normal O_2 extraction, as judged by an increase in the A-V oxygen difference. The increased oxygen extraction seen in these patients represented a familiar compensatory mechanism since Donald et al (1955) had found that the oxygen saturation of mixed venous blood fell as soon as exercise started, and that increased oxygen extraction enabled the body to double oxygen supply to the tissues without any increase in cardiac output. The extraction percentage for oxygen has been shown to increase approximately threefold in exercising subjects in contrast to the increase of slightly more than twofold in patients with haemorrhagic shock (Wade & Bishop, 1962).

A similar increase in oxygen extraction has been repeatedly described in

58

experimental shock but it is important to appreciate that despite increased oxygen extraction, experimental shock studies consistently report less than normal values for oxygen consumption. Therefore lactate levels, or possibly excess lactate, might serve better to predict survival in clinical shock. While this is true of lactate levels that remain elevated after appropriate therapy (Broder & Weil, 1964), it has become apparent that blood lactate levels are the sum of complex metabolic events (Duff et al, 1969). Measurable lactate production has been demonstrated in well-perfused resting striated muscle (Andres et al, 1956), producing potential uncertainty in the evaluation of elevated lactate levels. Despite continuing efforts, the ideal indicator of overall tissue oxygenation has yet to be discovered. This is not surprising considering the varied tolerance to hypoxia among different organs.

To summarise, when cardiac output is reduced, the normal relationship between blood flow and oxygen consumption is altered so that up to two to three times as much oxygen is extracted during each circulation through the tissues. As a rule, this compensatory mechanism will keep oxygen consumption within normal levels. It is not clear how long patients can survive with subnormal levels of oxygen consumption but this ability must be very limited. The 'oxygen debt' concept as described in exercise or experimental shock has not been well documented in clinical shock associated with a decreased cardiac output (Wilson et al, 1972; Shoemaker et al, 1973).

INCREASED CARDIAC OUTPUT

The normal relationship between blood flow and oxygen consumption is also modified when cardiac output is increased. The hyperdynamic conditions listed previously fall into this category as do patients with sepsis. Initial studies in this area focused on haemodynamic data and the work of Clowes (1966) and Wilson (1965) has already been mentioned. Udhoji and Weil (1965), MacLean et al (1967) and Kho and Shoemaker (1968) confirmed that in septic shock cardiac output could be normal or even elevated. Border et al (1966) studied a group of critically ill patients with high cardiac outputs and commented on the decreased A–V oxygen difference and increased right atrial oxygen tension. These authors postulated systemic arteriovenous shunting as an explanation for their findings. Similar reports by Hopkins et al (1965) and Del Guercio et al (1968) discussed the possible significance of A–V shunts in septic shock while the work of Siegel et al (1967) suggests that A–V shunting might explain the low oxygen consumption in some septic shock patients. These authors examined the relationship between oxygen consumption and total blood flow. They noted increased venous oxygen saturation in hyderdynamic shock patients resulting in an abnormally narrow A–V oxygen difference and a decreased level of oxygen consumption. Large increases in cardiac output may occur with much smaller changes in oxygen consumption. The discrepancy between a large increase in blood flow and a relatively small increment in oxygen consumption has also been observed in septic

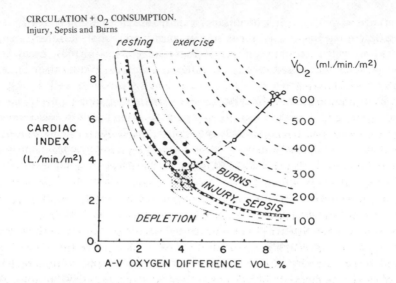

CIRCULATION + O_2 CONSUMPTION.
Injury, Sepsis and Burns

Figure 1. The circulatory response to the hypermetabolism of exercise is compared with the response to the resting hypermetabolism of major injury and infection. The heavy dashed line represents average normal values for adult man. The data for exercise is taken from Wade and Bishop (1963)

shock and must result from blood flow through tissues that do not take up oxygen. However, the recent interest in arteriovenous shunts should not obscure the fact that other mechanisms may be responsible for these findings.

Data are presented in Figure 1 to emphasise the contrast between the circulatory response to exercise from that in major injury or infection without shock. The surgical patients exhibit various degrees of resting hypermetabolism and increases in oxygen delivery with no increase in oxygen extraction. Unlike the exercising subject, the resting hypermetabolic patient is showing evidence of circulatory or ventilatory failure when the central venous oxygen concentration begins to drop.

Blood flow can vary independently of oxygen consumption in both physiological and pathological states. The ability to increase cutaneous blood flow is important in heat transport and has no relationship to the metabolic needs of the skin. Similarly, renal blood flow is large because of decreased renal vascular resistance rather than renal tissue O_2 requirements. Changes in blood viscosity due to anaemia will affect flow far more than oxygen consumption. In fact, anaemia probably represents the original hyperdynamic state since it was recognised to increase heart action long before cardiac output could be measured (Bamberger, 1857). The increased cardiac output of hyperthyroidism has also been obvious for more than 100 years but there has been controversy as to whether cardiac output is increased in proportion to oxygen uptake. However, in

60

studies where A—V oxygen difference measurements are available they are usually narrowed (Kontos et al, 1965) indicating that blood flow increases to a greater extent than does oxygen consumption. This finding has been ascribed to peripheral vasodilation and the need to dissipate excess heat rather than to arteriovenous shunting.

The situation in anaemia is more complex because the severity of the anaemia plays a major role in determining the circulatory response. Although many investigators have stressed the importance of peripheral compensatory mechanisms in anaemia whereby the percentage of oxygen extraction is increased, examination of their data reveals that this does not take place until haemoglobin levels fall below 7 g/100 ml (Leight et al, 1954; Sharpey-Schafer, 1944). Increased cardiac output is the primary response to moderate anaemia and the decreased oxygen content of both arterial and venous blood results in a narrowed A—V oxygen difference. Sharpey-Schafer (1944) showed that increased extraction (increased A—V oxygen difference) is not a factor when haemoglobin levels are above 7 g/100 ml. Since moderate anaemia has no effect on oxygen consumption, such patients will have increased blood flow without an increase in oxygen consumption. There is no need to invoke arteriovenous shunting to explain these findings.

In surgical practice sepsis with or without shock, remains the prime example of a hyperdynamic circulation. In such patients cardiac output is increased to a greater extent than oxygen consumption and A—V oxygen difference is less than normal (Gump et al, 1970). Although these changes suggested arteriovenous shunting once decreased haemoglobin levels were taken into account, increased blood flow was seen to be related to additional metabolic demands for oxygen. Clearly haemoglobin concentration is an important variable in any evaluation of the circulatory alterations associated with sepsis since anaemia is commonplace and can be additive with infection to increase cardiac output and narrow A—V oxygen difference.

The contribution of increased cutaneous blood flow to the increased cardiac output seen in sepsis is difficult to measure. Febrile septic patients have increased skin blood flow and since little oxygen is extracted from this blood, some narrowing of the whole body A—V oxygen difference will result. If thyrotoxic patients can be taken as a guide, increased circulatory requirements for heat dissipation exist in the presence of hypermetabolism even without an increase in body temperature. While the relationship between sepsis and oxygen consumption is complex, significant infections are usually associated with an increased metabolic rate so that the need for heat transport undoubtedly plays a role in the circulatory response.

Increased blood flow and a decreased peripheral resistance are consistent features of the hyperdynamic circulatory state associated with sepsis. These haemodynamic responses are well established but associated changes in oxygen consumption are more variable. There is general agreement that cardiac output increases to a greater extent in sepsis, with and without shock, than does oxygen consumption. In septic patients who are not in shock, oxygen consumption falls below predicted normal values only when oxygen consumption is calculated from the product of cardiac output and A–V oxygen difference. When oxygen consumption is measured by analysis of expired air resting values have been normal or moderately increased. Our studies show that major sepsis (excluding burns) usually results in less than a 50% increase in oxygen consumption while cardiac output is often increased to a far greater extent. The disproportionate increase in blood flow implies flow through tissues that do not extract oxygen but, as noted previously, this may be due to fever or anaemia rather than A–V shunting. However, since typical hyperdynamic circulatory changes can exist in afebrile patients with normal haemoglobin levels, other mechanisms have to be considered. In a recent study of hind limb sepsis in the dog, the extra cardiac output was found to be due to the release of a powerful vasodilator from the septic region (Hermreck & Thal, 1969). A–V shunting, in the sense of non-nutritional flow, was not thought to be a factor since lactate measurements failed to provide evidence of cellular hypoxia.

We have recently reported (Gump et al, 1970a) similar findings in a group of patients with major burns studied 6–26 days after injury and prior to skin grafting. The burned patients were contrasted to other febrile surgical patients and haemoglobin values and temperature elevations in both groups were comparable.

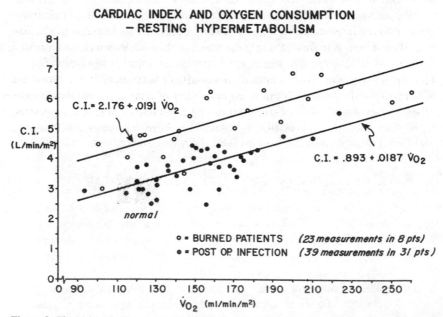

Figure 2. The rising cardiac output in relation to the rising oxygen consumption of patients with major infection is represented by the lower line. The upper line represents the corresponding data for patients with third degree burns (Gump et al, 1970)

Despite this fact, blood flow tended to be higher at any level of oxygen consumption in the burned patients (Figure 2), indicating the presence of flow through non-metabolising tissues in these patients. Whether this was due to blood flow through newly opened arteriovenous channels or simply vasodilation is not clear. However, the disproportionate increase in cardiac output is again illustrated and in these burned patients more than fever and anaemia was involved. Similar findings have, of course, been reported in other kinds of infection, although the contributions of decreased haemoglobin levels or fever cannot easily be distinguished.

Recently shifts in the oxyhaemoglobin dissociation curve have been suggested as an explanation for decreased oxygen extraction in sepsis (Watkins et al, 1974). Red blood cell levels of 2,3 diphosphoglycerate (2,3 DPG) are a major determinant of the affinity of haemoglobin for oxygen; in hypoxaemic states 2,3 DPG levels increase with a proportional shift of the oxyhaemoglobin dissociation curve to the right (Valeri & Fortier, 1969). This implies that more oxygen can be released to the tissues at a given oxygen tension. In sepsis, despite the increased tissue requirements for oxygen 2,3 DPG levels are low making it more difficult for haemoglobin to release its oxygen. Under these circumstances the oxygen content of venous blood would be increased and oxygen consumption would not reflect increased blood flow. The haemodynamic sum of these events, increased cardiac output and decreased A—V oxygen difference, has frequently been described in septic patients.

Cardiac failure is a recognised complication of sepsis and septic shock and underlines the importance of high circulatory requirements in these conditions. Since blood flow is increased to a greater extent than is oxygen consumption, it is clear that elevated energy requirements due to infection and fever cannot account for the extra cardiac output. If vasodilator substances or red blood cell abnormalities are involved it raises the possibility of pharmacologic modification of the hyperdynamic state. Before this can be considered a practical suggestion, blood flow, oxygen consumption, and evidence of cellular hypoxia will have to be examined in individual organs and vascular beds.

REGIONAL BLOOD FLOW AND OXYGEN CONSUMPTION

The ability to measure cardiac output in critically ill patients has led to a better understanding of circulatory requirements in sepsis and shock, especially of blood flow but oxygen transport and consumption have also been receiving increasing attention. Unfortunately, whole body measurements neglect internal distribution of flow and oxygen consumption as well as the fact that not all vascular beds are equally important in survival. There are also significant variations in oxygen extraction in different organs under normal resting conditions. The normal 40% oxygen extraction in the myocardium limits the ability of this organ to extract additional oxygen when demands are increased and under these circumstances additional oxygen can be supplied only be increased blood flow.

Clinical studies dealing with regional circulatory responses to whole body changes are extremely limited because of the technical problems involved. However, a number of studies have been carried out in congestive heart failure and thyrotoxicosis (Kontos et al, 1965; Schweitzer et al, 1967; Theilen & Wilson, 1967). Unequal distribution of the increased cardiac output seen in anaemia has been suggested on the basis of animal studies, but no efforts have been made to confirm this in anaemic subjects (Murray, 1964).

When cardiac output is decreased by heart disease, tissue oxygenation is maintained by increased oxygen extraction. This is evident both on examination of mixed venous blood as well as blood draining either upper (Mason & Braunwald, 1964) or lower (Hlavavoa et al, 1966) extremity. It has been suggested that most of the decrease in extremity blood flow seen in CHF is due to cutaneous vasoconstriction and that muscle blood flow is reasonably well preserved. When arm blood flow was related to cardiac output it was found that cardiac output decreased more than did flow to the arm so that the ratio of arm to total flow was higher than normal despite the decreased absolute value (Schweitzer et al, 1967). The splanchnic bed may be the first to feel the effect of decreased cardiac output in heart failure as judged by Myers' reports of marked decreases in splanchnic blood flow determined by hepatic vein catheterisation (Myers, 1955).

When cardiac output and oxygen consumption are increased in thyrotoxicosis the splanchnic bed also appears to play an important role (Myers et al, 1950). In the myocardium, on the other hand, oxygen consumption and blood flow are increased proportionately (Regan & Hellems, 1956; Rowe et al, 1956). Peripherally, muscle blood flow and oxygen consumption increase together; the increased cutaneous blood flow, ascribed to heat transport, has been mentioned previously.

SPLANCHNIC METABOLISM AND SURGICAL FEVER

The increase in resting heat production associated with fever has never been clearly identified as to the tissues involved and the chemical reactions that are responsible. Studies on non-shivering thermogenesis in small animals emphasise the increased peripheral utilisation of fatty acids. Yet the hypermetabolism of clinical fever may not be equivalent to non-shivering thermogenesis induced by environmental changes.

The old observation of increased heat production following protein ingestion (specific dynamic action) has been linked to the deamination of certain amino acids. Cuthbertson and co-workers (Cairnie et al, 1957) have suggested that the increased heat production after skeletal injury in the rat might be due to an 'endogenous specific dynamic action' that was underlying the increased nitrogen excretion. Since urea synthesis is increased in protein feeding, injury, and a variety of febrile conditions, and the liver is the sole organ to synthesise urea, is the hypermetabolism of clinical fever limited to the liver?

The gastrointestinal blood supply under normal resting conditions could conceivably determine hepatic function through its domination of the substrate supply. However the hepatic blood supply appears to be adjusted to the metabolic requirements of the body as a whole. The hepatic blood flow has been shown to increase after a protein meal in proportion to the rise in cardiac output and blood flow to the entire body that occurs at the same time. Similar changes in systemic and hepatic circulation have been detected in man during febrile reactions to pyrogenic agents that increase total oxygen consumption. Liver temperature rises after protein feeding and during fever, presumably as a result of augmented hepatocellular metabolism. Myers (1955) has confirmed that the relationship between cardiac output and arteriovenous oxygen difference for the whole body has a similar pattern to that which exists for the liver. This investigator found that the rapid intravenous injection of amino acids caused a prompt rise in the splanchnic oxygen consumption as a result of widening the arteriovenous oxygen difference without increasing hepatic blood flow. This pattern differs from that following the administration of an intravenous pyrogen to normal man, in which the arteriovenous oxygen difference remains

TABLE I. The circulatory response of the liver in man is divided into conditions depending upon both the change in blood flow and oxygen consumption of the liver (Myers, 1955)

| Hepatic | Per Cent Oxygen Removed from Blood | | |
	Low	Normal	High 'hypoxaemia'
High	Increased plasma volume — variable	Pyrogen Epinephrine	(Anaemia)
Normal	(Erythremia) Glucose infusion	Normal Portal cirrhosis Diabetes mellitus Hypertension Pregnancy	Hyperthyroidism Leukaemia Amino acids
Low		Myxoedema Portal cirrhosis	Cardiac failure Portal cirrhosis ? Hepatitis ? Obstructive jaundice Orthostasis Exercise Anaesthesia

65

essentially normal while the hepatic blood flow is promptly increased (Table I). Myers (1955) has summarised the circulatory response of the liver to various conditions, depending upon whether the oxygen extraction is altered for a given hepatic blood flow.

The extent of increase in splanchnic blood flow and oxygen consumption was studied by Gump et al (1970b) in 15 patients who were febrile as a result of intraperitoneal infection. Whole body and splanchnic blood flow were measured together with whole body and splanchnic oxygen consumption, and showed that about one-third of the patients had no increase in oxygen consumption despite fever, and small increases in cardiac output with no significant change in the proportion of blood flow or oxygen consumption across the splanchnic bed. The patients with an increase in resting oxygen consumption always had an increased cardiac output and increased splanchnic blood flow. The increase in blood flow and oxygen consumption across the splanchnic viscera accounted for only 40 to 50 per cent of the total increase, establishing that the hypermetabolism of this form of surgical fever involved tissues other than the liver, and chemical reactions other than deamination and urea synthesis. It is of interest that three burn patients studied in a similar fashion revealed much larger increases in resting oxygen consumption; however, the resting blood flow to the liver was of the same order of magnitude as that seen with intra-abdominal infection (Gump et al, 1970a). This is consistent with the fact that the fever and increase in nitrogen excretion of burn patients are of the same order of magnitude as those seen in cases of major peritoneal infection.

Summary

The relationship between energy expenditure and the circulation has been reviewed for conditions involving a decrease or an increase in resting cardiac output. The normal resting cardiac output may be considered to be divided approximately in three parts: tissues with a high, steady metabolism (60%), the muscle mass at rest (20%) with large capacity for increases during exercise, and the remaining tissues with low, steady metabolism (20%). The normal resting body has an $A-V\ O_2$ difference of approximately 4 vol%, but this varies from 1.0 vol% (skin) to over 11.0 vol% (heart). Data is summarised to emphasise that increasing the normal $A-V\ O_2$ difference in disease or injury is an abnormal and serious development, in contrast to the prompt widening of $A-V\ O_2$ difference in normal exercise.

The hyperdynamic circulation in surgical infection is discussed and the need is emphasised for better understanding of the correlation between the circulation and O_2 consumption of individual tissues and organs. Rapid infusion of amino acids has been shown to widen acutely the $A-V$ difference of the splanchnic blood flow. The association of an increased energy expenditure and an increased urea excretion in the catabolic phase of injury or infection, has suggested that the liver might be the site of the increased energy expenditure. Studies in febrile patients with abdominal sepsis demonstrated that only 40 to 50% of the elevated blood flow and O_2 consumption in the hyperdynamic state could be accounted for in the splanchnic area. Thus the clinical conditions with increased blood flow require further study to determine which tissues, in addition to the splanchnic area, have increased blood flow to meet increased O_2 demands, and how much additional blood flow is required for heat transport to the body surface.

References

Andres, R, Cader, G and Zierler, KL (1956) *J. clin. Invest., 35,* 671

Bader, RA, Bader, ME, Rose, DJ and Braunwald, E (1955) *J. clin. Invest., 34,* 1524

Bamberger, H (1857) *Lehrbuch der Krankheiten des Herzens.* Baunmuller, Vienna

Bendixen, HH, Egbert, LD, Hedley-Whyte, J, Laver, MB and Pontoppidan, H (1965) *Respiratory Care.* CV Mosby Co, St Louis

Blacket, RB and Palmer, AJ (1960) *Brit. Heart J., 22,* 483

Border, JR, Gallo, E and Schenk, WG Jr (1966) *Surgery, 60,* 225

Brandfonbrener, M, Landowne, M and Shock, NW (1955) *Circulation, 12,* 557

Branon, ES, Merrill, AJ, Warren, JV and Stead, EA Jr (1945) *J. clin. Invest., 24,* 332

Braun, K, Rosenberg, SA and Schwartz, A (1959) *Amer. J. Cardiol., 3,* 40

Broder, G and Weil, MH (1964) *Sciences, 143,* 1457

Cairnie, AB, Campbell, RM, Pullar, JD and Cuthbertson, DP (1957) *Brit. J. exp. Path., 38,* 504

Chapman, CB and Fraser, RS (1954) *Circulation, 9,* 57

Clowes, GHA Jr (1963) *J. Trauma, 3,* 161

Clowes, GHA Jr, Vucinic, M and Weidner, MG (1966) *Ann. Surg., 163,* 966

Cournand, A, Riley, MD, Bradley, SE, Breen, ES, Noble, RP, Lauson, HD, Gregerson, MI and Richards, DW (1953) *Surgery, 13,* 964

DeFazio, V et al (1959) *Circulation, 20,* 190

Del Guercio, LR, Commaraswamy, RP, Feins, NR, Wollman, SB and State, D (1964) *Surgery, 56,* 57

Del Guercio, LR, Cohn, JD, Greenspan, M, Feins, NR and Kornitzer, G (1968) In *Third International Conference on Hyperbaric Medicine.* National Academy of Sciences, Washington, DC

Donald, KW, Bishop, JM, Cumming, G and Wade, OL (1955) *Clin. Sci., 14,* 37

Duff, JH, Groves, AC, McLean, APH, LaPointe, R and MacLean, LD (1969) *Surg., Gynec., Obstet., 128,* 1051

Epstein, FP, Shadle, OW, Ferguson, TB and McDowell, ME (1953) *J. clin. Invest., 32,* 543

Finkielman, S, Worcel, M and Agrest, A (1965) *Circulation, 31,* 356

Graetting, JS, Muenster, JJ, Selverstone, LA and Campbell, JA (1959) *J. clin. Invest., 38,* 1316

Grande, F (1961) In *Techniques for Measuring Body Composition.* (Ed) J Brozek and A Henschel. National Academy of Sciences — National Research Council, Washington, DC. Page 168

Gump, FE, Price, JB Jr and Kinney, JM (1970) *Curr. Topics surg. Res., 2,* 385

Gump, FE, Price, JB Jr and Kinney, JM (1970a) *Surg., Gynec., Obstet., 130,* 23

Gump, FE, Price, JB Jr and Kinney, JM (1970b) *Ann. Surg., 171,* 321

Hermreck, AS and Thal, AP (1969) *Ann. Surg., 170,* 677

Hlavavoa, A, Linkart, J, Prerovsky, I, Ganz, V and Fronek, A (1966) *Clin. Sci., 30,* 377

Hopkins, RW, Sabaga, G, Penn, I and Simeon, FA (1965) *JAMA, 191,* 731

Kho, LK and Shoemaker, WC (1968) *Surg., Gynec., Obstet., 127,* 81

Kontos, HA, Shapiro, W, Mauck, HP Jr., Richardson, DW, Patterson, JL Jr and Sharpe, AR (1965) *J. clin. Invest., 44,* 947

Kowalski, HJ and Abelmann, WH (1953) *J. clin. Invest., 32,* 1025

Leight, L, Snider, TH, Clifford, GO and Hellems, HK (1954) *Circulation, 10,* 653

Maclean, JD, Mulligan, WG, McLean, APH and Duff, JH (1967) *Ann. Surg., 166,* 543

Mason, DT and Braunwald, E (1964) *J. clin. Invest., 43,* 532

Murray, JF (1964) *Amer. J. Physiol., 207,* 228

Myers, JD, Brannon, ES and Holland, BC (1950) *J. clin. Invest., 29,* 1069

Myers, JD (1955) *Circulation in the Splanchnic Area in Shock and Circulatory Homeostatis.* Josiah Macy Jr Foundation, New York

Rapaport, E, Kuida, H, Dexter, L, Henneman, PH and Albright, F (1957) *Amer. J. Med., 22,* 252

Regan, TJ and Hellems, HK (1956) *Circulation, 14,* 90

Roncoroni, AJ, Aramendia, P, Gonzales, R and Tagnini, AC (1959) *Acta physiol. Lat. Amer., 9,* 55

Rowe, GG, Huston, JH, Weinstein, AB, Tuchman, H, Brown, JL and Crumpton, CW (1956) *J. clin. Invest., 35,* 272

Sarnoff, SJ (1955) *Physiol. Rev., 35,* 107

Sharpey-Schafer, EP (1944) *Clin. Sci., 5,* 125

Schweitzer, P, Pironka, M and Klvanova, H (1967) *Z. ges. exp. Med., 143,* 126

Schweitzer, P, Pironka, M and Klvanova, H (1967a) *Z. ges. exp. Med., 143,* 131

Shoemaker, WC, Montgomery, ES, Kaplan, EK and Elwyn, DH (1973) *Arch. Surg., 106,* 630

Siegei, JH, Greenspan, M and Del Guercio, LRM (1967) *Ann. Surg., 165,* 504

Snyder, JC (1938) *J. clin. Invest., 17,* 571

Theilen, EO and Wilson, WR (1967) *J. appl. Physiol., 22,* 207

Udhoji, VN and Weil, MH (1965) *Ann. intern. Med., 62,* 966

Valeri, CR and Fortier, NL (1969) *New Engl. J. Med., 281,* 1452

Wade, OL and Bishop, JM (1962) *Cardiac Output and Regional Blood Flow.* Blackwell Scientific Publications, Oxford

Watkins, GM, Rabelo, A, Pizak, LF and Shelden, GF (1974) *Ann. Surg., 180, 2,* 213

Wilson, FW, Christensen, C and LeBlanc, LP (1972) *Ann. Surg., 176,* 801

Wilson, RF, Thal, AP, Kindling, PH, Grifka, T and Ackerman, E (1965) *Arch. Surg. Chicago, 91,* 121

Metabolism of Fat Emulsion for Intravenous Nutrition

ARVID WRETLIND

Nutrition Unit, Medical Faculty, Karolinska Institutet, Stockholm, Sweden

Introduction

A supply of food energy is necessary to cover the body requirements for resting metabolism, synthesis of body tissues, excretory processes, maintenance of thermal balance, physical activity and specific dynamic action. The most important *sources of energy* are carbohydrates and fat. In many patients on intravenous nutrition it is — for different reasons — difficult to infuse the required amount of energy in the form of carbohydrates and other water soluble energy yielding substances such as alcohol and sorbitol. However, with intravenous fat emulsions — in combination with not less than 20 cal per cent of carbohydrate — the required amount of energy can readily be supplied. The advantage of fat emulsions is that a large amount of energy can be given in a small volume of isotonic fluid. The combustion of fat produces 9 kcal per g which is more than twice the energy obtained from either carbohydrate or protein. Because of their isotonicity, the fat emulsions may be given into peripheral veins, in contrast with the concentrated glucose solutions, which have to be given through a catheter in a central vein. Thrombophlebitis occurs very infrequently with an isotonic fat emulsion. The infusions do not cause diuresis and are not lost either in the urine or faeces. Fat emulsions also supply the body with essential fatty acids and triglycerides, which are a part of ordinary food. In this way the normal lipid composition of the body may be maintained.

BIOCHEMICAL BACKGROUND

Both fats and oils are glyceryl esters of fatty acids or neutral fats. Quantitatively, they comprise the most important group of the larger class of food components

69

known as lipids. The lipids include a heterogeneous group of substances which are insoluble in water, but dissolve in the so-called fat solvents. Besides the common neutral fats, there are a large number of other lipids. Phospholipids have an orthophosphate group as an integral part of the structure, and they form essential constituents of all cells. The different kinds of cerebrosides and gangliosides occur in the nervous system, as is evident from their names. Other lipids are found in small amounts in several other tissues.

Transport of Fat in the Body

The digestion and absorption of dietary fat occur in the small intestine. The fatty acids with chain lengths shorter than 12 carbon atoms are transported directly to the liver via the portal vein without re-esterification. The longer-chain fatty acids are re-esterified after absorption. In order to be transported further, the triglycerides, synthesised in the mucosa cells, are covered by a phospholipid and protein layer to form chylomicrons (Fraser, 1958). The chylomicrons, which are one micron or less in diameter, are carried in the lymphatic vessels to the thoracic duct and so to the subclavian vein and into the general circulation. The chylomicrons are disintegrated mainly by the enzyme lipoprotein lipase. The lipoprotein lipase hydrolyses the triglycerides of the chylomicrons. This reaction makes the free fatty acids of the chylomicrons available. Serum albumin will serve as an acceptor for the free fatty acids formed. When the triglycerides are hydrolysed, the chylomicrons disrupt, and the milky, lipaemic plasma rapidly clears up, and therefore the lipoprotein lipase is also called 'the clearing factor'. This enzyme may be activated by heparin and released into the blood stream (Engelberg, 1956).

The free fatty acids form a labile fraction bound to the serum albumin. The amount of free fatty acids in plasma is very small, 20 mg per cent, but is very rapidly metabolised. The turnover rate is about 30 per cent per minute. As plasma contains about 0.5 mmol/litre, and the molecular weight of a fatty acid, such as oleic acid, is 283, the energy released from 3 litres of plasma may be about 1.1 kcal/minute or 1.7 Mcal/day ($283 \times \frac{0.5}{1000} \times 3 \times \frac{30}{100} \times 9 = 1.14$ kcal). That energy will cover the basal metabolism. The body can easily increase the total turnover of free fatty acids. In fact, 80-90 per cent of the total energy consumption of the body may be derived from free fatty acids.

An excess of the free fatty acids forms triglycerides in the adipose tissues or other tissues, including the liver. In the liver some of the triglycerides are more firmly combined with protein, phospholipid and cholesterol to form the various groups of lipoproteins circulating in the blood. The chylomicrons may be considered a borderline group of lipoproteins of particularly low density. The chylomicrons, lipoproteins and free fatty acids are used as energy sources, or stored in the tissues.

70

Storage of Fat in the Body

Lipids are present in all the cells, where they perform special functions, such as those concerned with structure and cell permeability. These functional, lipid components of the cell represent a relatively stable fraction. Other fats represent the large quantities of depot fats.

When the lipases in the adipose tissue are activated, the triglycerides provide free fatty acids for the blood. There is considerable evidence that triglyceride breakdown and resynthesis are continuous, although the products of lipolysis, free fatty acids and glycerol, are not the immediate substrates for the re-esterification reaction. The free fatty acids must first be activated to form acyl-coenzyme A derivatives, which then react with α-glycerophosphate derived from glucose — not glycerol — to initiate glyceride synthesis. Glycerol cannot be utilised by adipose tissue to form triglycerides. The release of triglyceride glycerol can be used as one indication of the fat turnover in the adipose tissue.

A major function of adipose tissue is to store fats. The predominant fatty acids in the body have a chain length of 16 and 18 carbon atoms. This remains true even when large amounts of fatty acids of shorter chain length are ingested.

The body may contain from 4 to 18 kg of fat in men, and from 7 to 30 kg of fat in women. The fat of the body forms the largest energy store. Only one kilogram, or less than 10 per cent of the body fat, seems to be essential for life.

Oxidation of Fat in the Body

The stored neutral fat in different parts of the body is mobilised by lipolytic enzymes into glycerol and free fatty acids. Glycerol is metabolised along the same pathways as carbohydrate. It is converted into triosephosphate, pyruvate and, finally, oxidised through the three carboxylic acid cycle.

Fatty acids are oxidised by a process of successive β-oxidations via the acyl-coenzyme (acyl-CoA). Pairs of carbon atoms are removed, and acetyl-coenzyme-A (acetyl-CoA) is formed and finally acetic acid. The carnitine derivatives are essential for the transport of acyl-CoA to the fatty acid oxidising system. The acetyl-coenzyme A (acetyl-CoA) either joins the Krebs' cycle to be completely oxidised, or unites, in pairs to form the ketoacid, acetoacetic acid (CH_3COCH_2COOH). Acetoacetic acid and other ketone bodies, β-hydroxybutyric acid and acetone, formed by the liver, circulate in the blood and are oxidised by various tissues, forming carbon dioxide, water, and energy (heat or physical activity).

On a high fat, and low carbohydrate diet, an insufficient amount of oxaloacetic acid from pyruvic acid by the *Wood-Werkman reaction* may be available to initiate the Krebs' cycle for the oxidation of the acetyl-CoA. The accumulating acetyl-CoA forms a surplus of ketone bodies, and ketosis develops. This

71

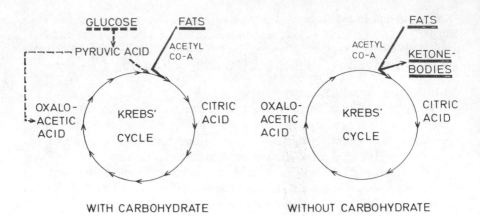

Figure 1. Diagram showing that 'fat can only be burnt in the fire of carbohydrate'

This is the modern biochemical explanation of the phrase, that 'fat can only be burnt in the fire of carbohydrate' (Figure 1).

A number of factors control the hydrolysis of the triglycerides (lipolysis) in the adipose tissue. Powerful lipolytic agents are epinephrine, norepinephrine and human growth hormone. Hypoglycaemia produces a substantial secretion of human growth hormone, bringing about an increase in lipolysis, and thus a rise in the production of free fatty acids and glycerol.

Importance of Essential Fatty Acids

In 1930 it was reported by Burr and Burr that, certain polyunsaturated fatty acids were essential for growth and survival of rats. The fatty acids which can not be produced in the body have been found to be linoleic acid and linolenic acid with 2 and 3 double bonds respectively. Some of the various symptoms produced by deficiency of essential fatty acids are summarised in Table I.

TABLE I. Symptoms of Essential Fatty Acid Deficiency
1. Decreased growth
2. Sterility and abortion
3. Dermatitis
4. Increased permeability
5. Increased water evaporation
6. Increased mitochondrial oxidation
7. Increased energy requirement
8. Formation of abnormal fatty acids
9. Fatty liver
10. Increased tendency to thrombosis

72

A diet deficient in linoleic acid increases the energy requirement. Adam et al (1958) found that 155 kcal/kg were necessary for infants when the diet contained less than 0.1 energy% of linoleic acid (Figure 2). The energy requirement decreased to 85 kcal/kg at a linoleic acid content of more than 4 energy%.

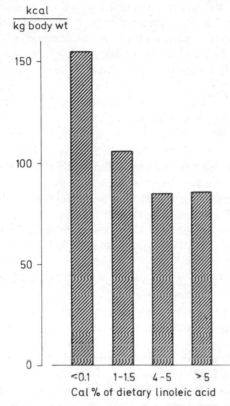

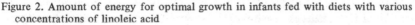

Figure 2. Amount of energy for optimal growth in infants fed with diets with various concentrations of linoleic acid

Hansen et al (1963) showed that 6.3kcal were required per g gain in body weight with a linoleic acid content in the diet of less than 0.1 energy%. The energy requirement decreased to 3.9 kcal/g of gain when the linoleic acid content increased to 4-5 energy%. One explanation for this effect may be an increased metabolic rate caused by greater activity of the oxidative enzymes from the mitochondria, resulting from a changed permeability of the mitochondrial membranes caused by essential fatty acid deficiency. This condition also results in an increased water loss by evaporation through the skin.

Both linoleic (ω6) and linolenic acid (ω3) exhibit essential fatty acid activity. However, the two acids are not physiologically interconvertible. This means that it is hard to accept that the essential fatty acid need could be satisfied only with

73

linoleic acid. Rivers and Davidson (1974) found that second-generation mice fed a diet containing not only linoleic but also linolenic acid had a lower, fasting, metabolic rate than mice given a diet including linoleic acid but no linolenic acid. Sinclair et al (1974) showed that the addition of linseed oil containing linolenic acid could cure skin lesions occurring in monkeys on a diet rich in linoleic acid. The fatty infiltration of the liver, observed histologically in the monkeys, also disappeared when linolenic acid was added to a linoleic acid rich diet. The total lipid in the liver was reduced from 300 to 600 g to 190 and 240 g/kg dry matter respectively. Both these investigations seem to indicate that linolenic acid is essential.

The importance of essential fatty acids in nutrition has recently been demonstrated by the fact that linoleic acid, via arachidonic acid, forms the hormone-like substances called prostaglandins. One of their effects is the antilipolytic property, which results from the inhibition of the adenyl cyclase. The prostaglandin also prevents aggregation of platelets, and possibly, thrombosis. The thrombotic tendency in vivo can be reduced by increasing the polyunsaturated fatty acid intake at the expense of saturated fatty acids (Hornstra, 1974). Linoleic acid, and possibly, linolenic acid, appear to be much more active than oleic acid.

The requirement of essential fatty acids (linoleic acid) has been estimated to 0.4 g/kg/day in infants and 0.1 g/kg/day in adults.

Metabolism of Fat in Starvation, after Trauma and after Operation

During starvation after operations, trauma, etc, the main source of energy is the body fat (Figure 3). Lipolysis is a major pathway for the metabolism of the fat and for the supply of fatty acids to the blood stream. The metabolic pathways of fat oxidation seem not to be impaired in the postoperative period and in other conditions with increased energy requirements. The largest site of lipolytic activity is in adipose tissue with its large stores of triglycerides. Its importance is due to fatty acids being the direct metabolic fuel for tissues during starvation. The oxidation of fatty acids can account almost entirely for the total caloric expenditure.

The metabolic controls of lipolysis include a rapid-acting hormonal component which activates lipolysis in a few minutes. There is also a slower-acting hormonal component which induces new lipolytic enzymes during a period of some days. The first step in the activation of lipolysis is the combination of the catecholamines with a receptor on the plasma membrane of the adipocyte. This interaction activates a membrane-bound enzyme, adenyl cyclase. The latter produces the unique nucleotide, cyclic adenosine monophosphate, which has been termed the second messenger (Robison et al, 1971). The cyclic adenosine monophosphate combines with a receptor in the adipocyte which is closely linked to an enzyme, protein kinase, which in this way is activated. The activated kinase enzyme phosphorylates another enzyme, triglyceride lipase, converting it from

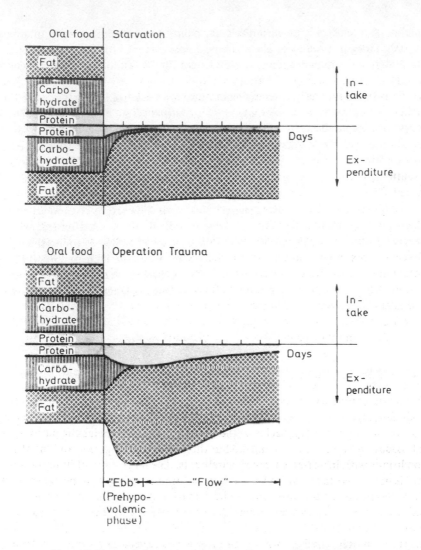

Figure 3. Energy balances in starvation, after operation and trauma

an inactive to an active form. The latter is responsible for the initial breakdown of triglycerides to fatty acids for delivery to the blood stream. This sequence of three enzymes (cyclase, kinase and lipase) acting on each other creates interesting cascade properties (Galton, 1971). Since an enzyme can convert many times its own weight of substrate, linkage of enzymes together functions as a chemical amplifier. A small amount of the initial effector is required to trigger off the first enzyme in the cascade, which activates many times its own weight of the next enzyme, and so on along the series. It allows a small input signal of hormone in blood, to result in a large output of fatty acids. An amplication factor of about 100,000 may be produced. There is now ample evidence for the occurrence of each step in the human adipocyte (Burns et al, 1971; Tulloch et al, 1972; Gilbert & Galton, 1974).

Several local tissue mechanisms are available to control lipolysis and prevent excessive release of fatty acids into the bloodstream from adipose tissue. The enzyme phosphodiesterase actively destroys cyclic adenosine monophosphate by its conversion to 5-adenosine monophosphate. Prostaglandins are released by the adipocyte during lipolysis and powerfully inhibit adenyl cyclase (Shaw & Ramwell, 1968) and prevent further formation of cyclic adenosine monophosphate.

Lipolysis is increased postoperatively (Schultis & Geser, 1970) and after burns. The plasma content of free fatty acids is accordingly increased after trauma and burns (Allison et al, 1968; Wadström, 1959). Birke et al (1965) found the increase to be in direct proportion to the severity of the burn. The increased lipolysis serves a metabolic purpose. Rodewald (1962) showed that the respiratory quotient was decreased postoperatively, indicating that the great need of energy was mainly covered by fat combustion.

COMPOSITION OF FAT EMULSIONS

Two of the commercial fat emulsions now available — Intralipid and Lipofundin S — contain soybean oil as fat (Table II). Egg yolk-phospholipids are used as emulsifiers in Intralipid, and soybean phospholipids in the other emulsion. The fatty acid contents in the soybean oil and the egg yolk-phospholipids are shown

TABLE II. Composition of Fat Emulsions

	Intralipid *	Lipofundin S †
Soybean oil	100 or 200 g	100 or 200 g
Egg yolk phospholipids	12 g	
Soybean phospholipids		7.5 or 15 g
Glycerol	25 g	
Xylitol		50 g
Distilled water to a volume of	1000 ml	1000 ml

* Vitrum, Stockholm, Sweden

† Braun, Melsungen, Germany

TABLE III. Fatty Acids in Soybean Oil and Egg yolk phospholipids in Intralipid

		Soybean oil %	Egg yolk phospholipids %
Myristic acid	C_{14}	0.04	0.09
Palmitic acid	C_{16}	9.2	32.5
Palmitoleic acid	$C_{16:1}$	0.03	0.4
Stearic acid	C_{18}	2.9	15.7
Oleic acid	$C_{18:1}$	26.4	32.0
Linoleic acid	$C_{18:2}$	54.3	11.3
Linolenic acid	$C_{18:3}$	7.8	0.3
Arachic acid	C_{20}	0.1	0.1
Arachidonic acid	$C_{20:4}$	–	0.2
Behenic acid	C_{22}	0.06	3.4
Unidentified acids		–	0.2

in Table III. Isotonicity results from the addition of glycerol or xylitol. The greatest experimental and clinical experience has been obtained with Intralipid. There are also some preparations containing fat as an emulsion mixed with amino acids and sorbitol.

Schoefl (1968) and Fraser and Håkansson (1974) have made electron-microscopic studies on Intralipid and chylomicrons. These investigations showed that the size of the fat particles in Intralipid 10% (mean diameter 0.13 μm) was about the same as found in chylomicrons (the mean diameter varied between 0.096 and 0.21 μm). The particles in Intralipid 20% were somewhat larger (mean diameter 0.16 μm). These and a number of other investigations have shown many physical and biochemical similarities between chylomicrons and the fat emulsion Intralipid.

However, great biological differences have been found to exist between different fat emulsions. For a fat emulsion to be used clinically it must be non-toxic, without side effects when given for a long time, and must not affect the respiration, circulation, the blood picture etc.

TOLERANCE OF FAT EMULSION

Tolerance during long-term infusions is of the greatest interest and significance, as fat emulsions, when used clinically have often to be given for long periods. In a number of investigations on dogs it has been shown that only when using the fat emulsion Intralipid could 9 g of fat per kg and day be administered for a planned period of 4 weeks without side effects (Håkansson, 1968). The amount of fat infused corresponded to the total energy requirement of the dogs. The other emulsions (Lipofundin S and emulsions containing cottonseed oil) which were investigated caused severe toxic effects and all the dogs died before the end of the investigation period. The causes of death were bleeding from the gastro-intestinal tract, liver damage, and fat embolism.

ELIMINATION OF FAT EMULSION FROM THE BLOODSTREAM

It is desirable that the particles in an artificial fat emulsion should have the same biological properties as those of the natural chylomicrons as regards transport in the blood, and distribution and utilisation in the body. The chylomicrons and

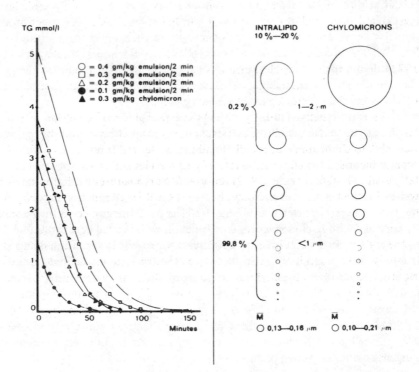

Figure 4. The elimination of the fat from the bloodstream after injection of Intralipid and natural chylomicrons (Hallberg, 1965b). The injection was made in dog with various amounts of Intralipid. The ordinate shows the concentration of triglycerides in the blood. The abscissa indicates the time. The sizes of the fat particles in the Intralipid and of the chylomicrons are shown to the right of the elimination curves.

the fat particles in the fat emulsion Intralipid seem to be metabolised in the same way.

Temporary hyperlipaemia occurs after every fat infusion. According to investigations by Hallberg (1965a,b) the kinetic principle for the elimination of fat particles in Intralipid in the dog and man is practically identical with that for the elimination of natural chylomicrons (Figure 4). The kinetic principle is characterised by the fact that above a certain 'critical particle concentration', the elimination is maximal. Below the critical concentration elimination is exponential. The maximal elimination in a person who has fasted overnight, corresponds to 3.8 g of fat per kg and 24 hours (35 kcal/kg/24 hours). After starving for 38 hours the elimination capacity is increased to 52 kcal/kg/24 hours. During the postoperative period while starving for 48 hours the elimination capacity rises to 100 kcal/kg/24 hours. Wilmore et al (1973) have also confirmed this increased fat elimination capacity in the excessively catabolic state of patients suffering from burns.

On infusion of 10% Intralipid for 4 hours, maximum serum triglyceride levels were found at the end of the infusion, returning to preinfusion levels within 2 hours, whereas serum free fatty acids gradually reached a maximum within 4 hours post-infusion and fell to pre-infusion levels by 6-8 hours (MacFayden et al, 1972). Serum triglyceride clearance was independent of the amount of energy in the simultaneous parenteral nutrition. However, the disappearance rate of serum free fatty acid was increased by larger energy supply.

Coran and Nesbakken (1969) studied the effect of the fat emulsion Intralipid on plasma triglycerides and free fatty acid in neonates. They found that neonates were able to eliminate fat as rapidly as adults. Moreover, it was observed that heparin increased the elimination rate of triglycerides and raised the level of free fatty acids. Gustafsson et al (1972) reported that prematures, with normal birth weight for the length of pregnancy, had a maximal fat elimination capacity from the bloodstream of approximately 6 g of fat/kg per 24 hours, i.e. as high a value as that for healthy, adult subjects. For neonates with a birth-weight that was light-for-date the maximum fat elimination capacity was lower. These infants showed a distinct tendency, with each dose of fat to accumulate lipids in the plasma, and mostly in the chylomicron fraction. In some cases Gustafsson et al (1972) found that an intravenous heparin dose of 50 IU/kg appreciably improved the infant's capacity to eliminate fat. This finding supports the assumption that in neonates who have been undernourished during their intrauterine life, the functions of the lipoprotein lipases are in some way defective. However, it should be possible to improve the elimination capacity by combining the supply of Intralipid with heparin, and in this way enable a large intravenous supply of energy to be administered.

On the basis of observations regarding the elimination of Intralipid from the bloodstream an Intra-Venous Fat Tolerance Test (IVFTT) has been developed by Carlson and Hallberg (1963), Boberg et al (1969) and Carlson and Rössner (1972).

In this connection it was found that the exponential elimination was especially slow in persons with a tendency to hypertriglyceridaemia.

The effect of intravenous supply of fat on the triglyceride concentration in blood has been studied. One group of patients with burns was given intravenously 100 g of fat daily, as 500 ml of Intralipid 20% (Carlson & Liljedahl, 1971). There were no significant differences in the mean concentration of plasma triglycerides between the group given fat, and the group without fat infusions, but the free fatty acid level in blood decreased when fat was given. These investigations show that burn patients tolerated and cleared the fat emulsion from the bloodstream and used artificial fat emulsion in about the same way as dietary fat. Further evidence of this statement is the great success in treatment of burns with fat emulsions as part of a complete intravenous nutrition (Birke et al, 1972; Lamke et al, 1974).

INFLUENCE OF FAT EMULSION ON THE RETICULOENDOTHELIAL SYSTEM AND IMMUNOLOGICAL FACTORS

Gigon et al (1966) have shown by studies on man that, after infusion of Intralipid some of the fat particles are absorbed by the endothelial cells in the pulmonary vessels. They did not observe any sign of aggregation of the fat particles.

Fat particles from certain fat emulsions are taken up by the reticuloendothelial (RES) cells. Thus Scholler (1968) and Lemperle et al (1970) have shown by means of experiments on both animals and human beings that fat particles in Lipofundin S are phagocytosed by Kupffer's cells and other RES cells. By direct experiments on animals and man, however, Scholler (1968) and Lemperle et al (1970) found that fat particles in *Intralipid,* when occasional injections are given, are not phagocytosed by Kupffer's cells, nor is the production of antibodies affected.

These and other tolerance studies show that there are great biological differences between the various fat emulsions. *On account of these pronounced differences it is not correct to speak of fat emulsions in general. The name of the fat emulsion should always be given and its exact composition stated.*

Carpentier et al (1974) has shown that fat emulsion (Intralipid) causes no reduced formation of immunoglobulins.

FAT EMULSION AND THE COAGULATION SYSTEM

The influence on the coagulation mechanism has been thoroughly studied by several researchers. According to Amris et al (1964) and Brøckner et al (1965) on subjecting fat emulsions to a thrombin generation test, changes occurred in the clotting time, which were interpreted as hypercoagulability. On this account the authors recommended 5 IU of heparin per ml of infused fat emulsion in order to hasten the elimination of the fat from the bloodstream by the release of the 'clearing factor' or lipoprotein lipase. Duckert and Hartmann (1966), Hartmann (1967), Cronberg and Nilsson (1967) and Kapp et al (1971) found as a result of very extensive experimental and clinical investigations that Intralipid did not have any effect on coagulation or on the fibrinolytic system. There is no reason to anticipate a greater disposition to thrombosis after fat infusions. Consequently it did not seem necessary to administer heparin together with the fat infusions. This concept was supported by the investigations made by Huth et al (1967). Thrombophlebitis occurs extremely rarely when fat emulsions are given in a peripheral vein.

EMULSION AND PULMONARY FUNCTION

Measurement of steady state pulmonary diffusion capacity and membrane diffusing capacity in normal human volunteers before and after administration of 500 ml of 10% Intralipid intravenously have shown a significant decrease in those functions for at least 4 hours following the infusion in 6 of 10 subjects. These changes returned to control levels within 24 hours in all six subjects. Simultaneous infusion of heparin with Intralipid prevented the decrease in both the steady state pulmonary diffusion capacity and membrane diffusing capacity (Greene et al, 1972). This finding might support the concept of adding heparin to Intralipid postoperatively, when the pulmonary function is often impaired. Jacobson (1974) recommends a supply of 2,500 IU of heparin per 500 ml of 20% Intralipid.

The pulmonary diffusion capacity, determined by [133] Xenon perfusion-diffusion and carbon monoxide rebreathing technique, was found to be normal following the infusion of Intralipid (Wilmore et al, 1973). Blood gas levels did not change after infusion of single or multiple units of the fat emulsion.

TABLE IV. Osmolality of Solutions for Intravenous Nutrition and of Plasma

Solution	mOsm per kg water
Plasma	290
0.9% NaCl	308
10% Intralipid	280
20% Intralipid	330
5% Glucose	278
10% Glucose	523
20% Glucose	1,250
30% Glucose	2,100
50% Glucose	3,800
3.3% Aminosol	555
10% Aminosol	925
Vamin	1,275

81

In intravenous nutrition it is important that the osmotic pressure of the blood is not altered. Consequently isotonic solutions should be used. If hypertonic solutions are used they must be given slowly during the whole 24 hours according to the technique described by Dudrick et al (1969). Table IV gives a survey of the osmolality of different infusion solutions. For comparison the plasma osmolality has been given. It is evident that large amounts of energy can be given by means of fat emulsions without changing the osmotic pressure of the blood. An example of the significance of this has been given by Bernhoff (1970). He showed that the contraction strength of the myocardium is reduced when hypertonic infusion solutions are used. On the other hand iso-osmotic solutions such as 5.5% glucose and 10% and 20% Intralipid had no negative effect on the myocardium.

NUTRITIONAL ASPECTS OF FAT EMULSIONS

Energy Source

Investigations have shown that intravenously supplied fat emulsions are utilised, in principle, in the same way as alimentary fat. It is evident from studies that have demonstrated that fat emulsions can be used as a source of energy to improve the nitrogen balance (Schärli, 1965; Abbott et al, 1955; Wadström & Wiklund, 1964; Larsen & Brøckner, 1965; Hallberg et al, 1966; Reid, 1967). Moreover, it has been found that intravenously administered fat emulsions are oxidised in the body as calculated (Geyer et al, 1948; Lerner et al, 1949; Eckart et al, 1973,1974). Reid (1967) found a decrease in the respiratory quotient when fat emulsions were administered, which showed a combustion of the fat supplied. When a positive energy balance was attained in intravenous nutrition with Intralipid, the expected weight increase was obtained, which also shows that the fat is utilised in the same way as the fat in our usual diet (Jacobson & Wretlind, 1970).

The amount of fat that has to be supplied in complete parenteral nutrition depends partly on the body's requirement of essential fatty acids, and partly on the energy need which it is desired to cover by means of fat.

In a number of studies most of the energy supply was given in the form of fat. Thus Peaston (1966,1967) and Stell (1970), gave 200 g of fat (about 3 g/kg) per day, corresponding to 60-80 per cent of the total energy supply. Bergström et al, (1972) supplied about 40 per cent of the energy in the form of fat, corresponding to about 2 g of fat/kg. In view of the experience gained in connection with the intravenous supply of fat, an amount of 2 g of fat in the form of soybean egg yolk-phospholipid emulsion Intralipid per kg, has been recommended in order to cover the energy and fat requirements in adults. This quantity was previously recommended by Hallberg et al (1966), Steinbereithner (1966) and Allen and Lee (1969). To obtain the desired energy supply of about 30 kcal/kg in adults,

82

in addition to the fat given, about 2 g of carbohydrates in the form of glucose or fructose and 1 g of amino acids/kg are required. These are the quantities recommended by different investigators for an intravenous nutrition with a simultaneous supply of fat (Hallberg et al, 1966; Steinbereithner, 1966; Allen & Lee, 1969). Deitel and Kaminsky (1974) recommend for infusion in a peripheral vein a 'lipid system' consisting of 3 g of fat/kg, 1.5 g of glucose/kg and all other nutrients.

To neonates who were receiving intravenous nutrition, Rickham (1967) gave 2.5-3 g of fat/kg/day (Intralipid). Børresen and Knutrud (1969), Børresen et al (1970a,b), Grotte (1971) and Grotte et al (1974) administered 3-4 g of fat (Intralipid)/kg/day to neonates and infants with good results. The same amounts of Intralipid have been reported by many other authors. In view of this experience 4 g of fat/kg/day in the form of Intralipid can be recommended to neonates and infants.

Source of Essential Fatty Acids

An essential fatty acid deficiency in dogs on intravenous feeding was described by Meng and Early (1949). The hyperalimentation without fat, introduced by Wilmore and Dudrick (1968) might produce essential fatty acid deficiency. In 1970 Pensler et al demonstrated essential fatty acid deficiency in three children on prolonged, total parenteral alimentation. There were changes in plasma fatty acid patterns consisting in reduction of the levels of linoleic and arachidonic acids, and an increase in oleic, palmitoleic and 5,8,11-eicosatrienoic acids. These chemical abnormalities were corrected by oral intake of linoleic acid in one of the three patients. Scaly lesions of the skin were also observed. These changes were comparable to those seen in rats on essential-fatty-acid-deficient diets.

Caldwell et al (1973) reported that infants kept on a low-fat intravenous nutrition developed eczema, and this condition was readily cured by infusion of fat emulsion. A 25-week-old baby on parenteral nutrition but with no fat emulsion since its eighteenth day of life suffered from scaly skin lesions, sparse hair growth, and thrombocytopenia. Analysis of the fatty acids in the plasma phospholipids showed low levels of linoleic and arachidonic acids, and a high content of 5,8,11-eicosatrienoic acid indicating an essential fatty acid deficiency. On administration of fat emulsion (Intralipid) sufficient to provide 4 per cent of the daily energy requirement as linoleic acid, the levels of linoleic and arachidonic acid rose, and the level of 5,8,11-eicosatrienoic acid decreased, the skin lesions healed, and the thrombocytopenia was corrected. In a case of volvulus in a ten-day-old infant, 50 per cent of the bowel had to be resected. Parenteral nutrition without added fat resulted in dermatitis, insufficient growth, thrombocytopenia and a low value for essential fatty acids in serum. Wound healing was also remarkably slow. Infusion of a soybean oil-emulsion (Intralipid) with high linoleic acid content (Table III)

83

caused rapid recovery.

In infants less than six months old, on intravenous nutrition with glucose, protein hydrolysate, and no fat, a low content of essential fatty acids in the serum and dermatitis with generalised flakiness were observed (Paulsrud et al, 1972).

For a long time there was no definite evidence that the essential fatty acids were required by adults. In an adult male patient, however, maintained on intravenous nutrition without fat for 100 days, a skin rash developed, and his serum phospholipids were found to contain 10 per cent 5,8,11-eicosatrienoic acid and a low content of arachidonic acid, a biochemical sign of an essential fatty acid deficiency (Collins et al, 1971). Intralipid administered intravenously (22.8 g of linoleic acid per day) caused the serum phospholipid content of eicosatrienoic acid to fall, and the level of arachidonic acid to rise. Simultaneously, the rash disappeared.

In five of thirteen patients with severe burns it was found that the essential, polyunsaturated fatty acids, as well as phosphatidylserine and phosphatidyl-ethanolamin were much reduced in the erythrocyte membranes (Wilmore et al, 1973). The deficiency was not correlated with the degree of the burns. Stress or alcoholism was mentioned as possible additional aetiologic factors. Fat emulsion (Intralipid) given parenterally, restored the fat composition of the erythrocyte membrane.

When a patient was given intravenous nutrition without fat during a period of nine months, fatty degeneration of the hepatic tissues occurred (Jeejeebhoy et al, 1973). When 50-100 g of fat (Intralipid) were administered daily for one month, followed by 50-100 g of fat per week, the fatty degeneration of the liver diminished successively during the next period of five months. It seems that the essential fatty acids are required to prevent fatty degeneration of the liver.

DOSAGE

If the amounts of fat, amino acids and carbohydrates stated in Table V with all other essential nutrients are supplied, and the amount of energy so adjusted as to avoid loss of weight in adults and to ensure growth in infants the patient's requirement of nutrients should be amply covered. Under several conditions it may of course be necessary to increase the supply of, for example, energy, water, amino acids, carbohydrates and fat (Table VI).

In the morning following the first day's infusion of fat emulsion, a citrated blood sample is drawn. The blood sample is centrifuged at 1200-1500 rpm. If the plasma is then strongly opalescent or milky, further infusion should be postponed. In the very great majority of cases plasma is completely clear 12 hours after the conclusion of an infusion of fat. This test should be repeated at weekly intervals. It is extremely rare to find a patient who cannot eliminate the fat particles from the circulation.

TABLE V. Tentatively Recommended Daily Allowance of Energy, Water, Amino Acids, Carbohydrate and Fat for Complete Intravenous Nutrition Designed to Cover Basal Need

Group of nutrient	Nutrient	Adult Amount per kg and day	Newborns and Infants Amount per kg and day
Energy		30 kcal = 0.13 MJ	90-120 kcal = 0.38-0.50 MJ
Fluid	Water	30 ml	120-150 ml
Nutrients for synthesis of body tissue and as energy source	Amino Acids Glucose, Fructose Fat	1 g 2 g 2 g	2.5 g 12-18 g 4 g

TABLE VI. Recommended Daily Allowance of Energy, Water, Amino Acids, Carbohydrate and Fat by Complete Intravenous Nutrition in Adults when the Need is Normal or Raised

Energy and Nutrients	Amount per kg body weight and day in adults with	
	Basal or normal need	High need
Energy	25-30 kcal=0.105−0.13 MJ	50-60 kcal=0.21−0.25 MJ
Water	25-30 ml	50-60 ml
Amino acids	1 g	2 g
Carbohydrate	2 g	5 g
Fat	2 g	3 g

INFUSION TECHNIQUE

The infusion technique varies considerably. The tendency has been, and still is, to find simple infusion methods without serious side effects. Infusion via a peripheral vein is preferable to infusion via a catheter in a central vein because complications are small and easy to diagnose.

Adults

In adults on intravenous nutrition for shorter periods (7-14 days) infusion through a cannula in a peripheral vein should be applied. Preferably, the cannula should not be left in the vein for longer than 8-12 hours so as to avoid the risk of mechanical irritation leading to thrombophlebitis. Such an infusion in a peripheral vein may otherwise cause an inflammatory condition which means that the vein progressively thromboses, the infusion slows down and eventually stops. When infusions are limited to twelve hours, thrombophlebitis is rare, but the incidence rises steeply after that.

If total parenteral nutrition in adults is indicated for more than one week a central vein catheter in the superior vena cava might be necessary.

Infants and Children

In many reports of infants and children on intravenous nutrition including fat emulsion (Intralipid) the infusions have been given via peripheral veins without the use of a central vein catheter (Børresen et al, 1970a,b; Grotte et al, 1974; Coran, 1974). Scalp vein needles have been used in most cases. In older children, Coran (1974) has used the veins on the dorsum of the hand. The tip of the scalp vein needle should not be obscured, so that difficulties with the infusions can be detected early. The infusion should be discontinued at the first sign of trouble at the infusion site (viz, redness or oedema), to allow re-use at a later date. This technique has also been used by Pendray (1974), and Grotte et al (1974). The amino acid solution is mixed with glucose solution and Intralipid before entering the vein. The solutions are administered concurrently throughout the day with the aid of a 3-way connector and a constant infusion pump. Each solution may be attached to a 100 ml graduated burrette with a micro-drip. The bottles and intravenous tubing up to the junction of the scalp vein needle should be changed every 24 hours. Half the calculated requirements of each solution is given on the first day and this is gradually increased to reach the full requirements by the third day, providing the carbohydrate, fat, sodium and volume are tolerated.

INDICATIONS

In principle, complete intravenous nutrition including fat emulsion is indicated under all conditions where nutrients cannot be adequately supplied either orally or enterally. This may involve entire compensation for the inhibition of oral intake, or the intravenous administration of supplementary nutrients if oral nutrition is insufficient. Complete intravenous nutrition with all essential nutrients should always be given unless within a few days resumption of the oral intake can be counted on for certain.

ADVERSE REACTIONS AND CONTRAINDICATIONS

Acute adverse reactions have been observed only in a small percentage of patients — neonates, infants and adults — given the soybean oil-egg yolk phospholipid emulsion Intralipid. The few reactions have been febrile responses (Hartmann, 1967), chills, sensation of warmth, shivering, vomiting and pain in chest and back. Thrombophlebitis have only occasionally been observed (Hallberg et al, 1966; Hallberg et al, 1967). Adverse reactions during long-term administration of Intralipid to adults as well as infants have been rare. In all, there are only reports of a hundred cases of light or moderate reactions and seven cases of severe complications — possibly two in adults (Horisberger, 1966; Depisch, 1971) and five in infants (Chaptal et al, 1964a,b; Hanc et al, 1968).

There have been no reports of anaphylaxis in the literature after Intralipid infusions.

The 'overloading syndrome' was observed earlier following 10 to 20 infusions of cottonseed oil emulsions. This syndrome has not been reported following the infusion of Intralipid. The administration of Intralipid is contraindicated in patients with a disturbance of normal fat metabolism and in patients with severe disturbances of fat metabolism such as pathologic hyperlipaemia and lipoid nephrosis.

CLINICAL RESULTS

Adults

That it is possible to administer complete intravenous nutrition with fat for a long period in man has been demonstrated in a large number of investigations.

In a series of investigations dealing with complete intravenous nutritions Lawson (1965) gave about 3 g of fat/kg for a period varying between 8 and 36 days. Liver biopsies after 30 and 36 days showed as the only change, a pigmentation of Kupffer's cells. No appreciable changes were observed in the bromsulphthalein retention, bilirubin content in serum or serum transaminases.

Hadfield (1966) gave intravenous nutrition with Intralipid in amounts up to 12 g of fat/kg/day for 15 days to a patient with ulcerative colitis, and for 4 weeks to a patient with severe malabsorption.

Hallberg et al (1967) reported complete intravenous nutrition administered to a patient with Crohn's disease. The patient received daily 2-2.5 g of fat/kg as Intralipid, 0.4-6.2 g of glucose/kg and up to 1.2 g of amino acids/kg as Aminosol regularly during a period of more than 5 months. The total amount of fat was 15 kg.

In one case, complete intravenous nutrition was administered for 7 months and 13 days (Jacobson & Wretlind, 1970; Bergström et al, 1972). The patient was a woman of 43 years of age, who lost consciousness as a result of severe cerebral injury caused by carbon-monoxide poisoning. In that connection all the essential nutrients were supplied in adequate amounts. The amino acids were given in the form of Vamin, and fat as Intralipid 20%. Fructose and glucose were used as carbohydrates. The average, daily energy supply was about 2,000 kcal.

For 6 months, together with the fat, 408 ml of Intralipid 20% were given daily, corresponding to 816 kcal. The increase in weight during the period of intravenous nutrition was 10 kg, from 40 to 50 kg without any appreciable change in the body fluid volume. Histopathological studies were conducted by means of repeated needle biopsies of the liver (Jacobson et al, 1971). The parenchymal cells did not show significant light or electron microscopic changes during the period of intravenous nutrition. The Kupffer cells, however, showed focal proliferation, enlargement, accumulation of fat droplets and occurrence of a lipofuscin-like pigment. The evidence suggested that droplets of neutral fat in the Kupffer cells were segregated in lysosome-like bodies, which subsequently underwent structural reorganisation and transformation to lipofuscin-like granules. After cessation of the intravenous therapy there was a slow decrease in the number of lipofuscin-like bodies in the Kupffer cells during the following 1.5 years. The observed changes did not signify any liver cell damage.

Jacobson (1972a,b) administered intravenous nutrition to a 70-year-old patient during a period of 69 days after a massive resection of the small intestine and 25 cm of the ascending colon on account of acute occlusion of the superior mesenteric artery. The mean daily supply was 3.58 litres of water, 2,850 kcal, 70 g of amino acids, 405 g of carbohydrates, 100 g of fat (Intralipid) and all the other essential nutrients. After the period of intravenous nutrition the patient was able to resume oral nutrition.

Jeejeebhoy et al (1973) have a patient who since 6 October, 1970 has been exclusively nourished intravenously. The patient, who is a housewife (born 1934), stayed for the first 9 months in hospital. After that she has remained in her own home and attended to the intravenous nutrition. The infusions are made during the night through a catheter of silicone rubber inserted in the vena cava superior. An amino acid mixture has been used (Amigen), glucose, fat (500 ml of Intralipid 10%), electrolytes and vitamins. The total energy supply has been 2,000 kcal or 34 kcal/kg. Two liver biopsies were performed after fat had been supplied for 3 and 5 months respectively. They showed that the hepatic tissue was entirely normal. This case, where intravenous nutrition was continued for almost 4 years, shows that a nutritional condition can be maintained which enables the patient to perform daily work in a satisfactory manner. The study mentioned and a number of other studies on adult patients show that, by means of complete intravenous nutrition, including fat emulsions, patients can be kept in good nutritional condition for a comparatively long time.

Neonates and Infants

Complete intravenous nutrition with fat, has been thoroughly studied in neonates and infants by Børresen and Knutrud (1969), and by Børresen et al (1970a,b). By administering 3-4 g of fat per kg it was possible to avoid carbohydrate solutions which were too hypertonic. The infusions via a peripheral vein were given

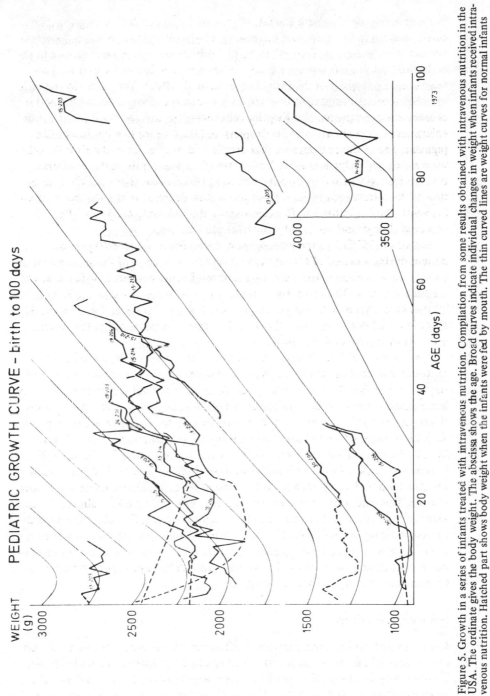

Figure 5. Growth in a series of infants treated with intravenous nutrition. Compilation from some results obtained with intravenous nutrition in the USA. The ordinate gives the body weight. The abscissa shows the age. Broad curves indicate individual changes in weight when infants received intravenous nutrition. Hatched part shows body weight when the infants were fed by mouth. The thin curved lines are weight curves for normal infants

89

for periods between 1 and 3 weeks. One report dealt with 32 neonates, who had been operated on for gastrointestinal malformations, and were subsequently treated with complete intravenous nutrition. Of these, 26 survived. In another series complete parenteral nutrition was administered to 14 infants suffering from severe surgical complications. All of these patients survived. Similar experience has been reported by Grotte (1971) and Grotte et al (1974) using a programme for *total* parenteral nutrition based on fat (Intralipid) and amino acids (Vamin) with the addition of standardised doses of electrolytes, trace minerals and vitamins.

Heird et al (1972) have reported on 107 infants who received complete intravenous nutrition with fat, after operations for severe congenital malformations. Despite the major operative intervention a positive nitrogen balance could be achieved. This was of the same magnitude as that of normal bottle-fed infants.

A survey has been made of 28 children who had been treated with intravenous nutrition in different USA hospitals. They had been given 28-69 per cent of the amount of energy supplied in the form of fat (Intralipid). The daily supply of fat was 1.1-6 g per kg. The total infusion time per child varied between 8 and 122 days. All the infusions were given via a peripheral vein. In the majority of all these severely ill children growth was satisfactory (Figure 10). According to this survey, of the 28 patients, 25 recovered. None of the three deaths could be ascribed to the intravenous nutrition of fat or any other nutrients.

Summary

Fat metabolism is of vital importance for the energy supply required both in normal and in starving situations. The serum free fatty acids derived from the adipose tissues, are the main fuel. The free fatty acids may readily be mobilised by the cascade reaction initiated by the effect of catecholamines on adenyl cyclase. The pathways for fat metabolism, during starving and stress situations are apparently not impaired. This means that fat can be given in large amounts with glucose, as a source of non-protein energy, and as part of a well balanced, complete nutrition.

Great differences in tolerance between the various fat emulsions have been reported. The fat emulsion of choice seems to be that which contains soybean oil and egg yolk phospholipids. It has been shown to be very well tolerated both in animals and man. Investigations have indicated that this fat emulsion has about the same biochemical properties as natural chylomicrons.

In a large number of experimental and clinical investigations it has been shown that an adequate, complete intravenous nutrition can be achieved by using chemically well-defined nutrients including fat.

The complete intravenous nutrition including fat emulsion can be given via a peripheral vein. This seems always to be the safest and easiest access for a parenteral feeding.

Our present knowledge of complete intravenous nutrition, including fat emulsion, is such that, it should be a matter of routine to prevent and treat malnutrition and associated complications.

References

Abbott, WE, Davies, JH, Benson, JW, Krieger, H and Levey, S (1955) *Surg. Forum, 5,* 501
Adam, DID, Hansen, AE and Wiese, HF (1958) *J. Nutr., 66,* 555
Allison, SP, Hinton, P and Chamberlain, MJ (1968) *Lancet, ii,* 113
Bergström, K, Blomstrand, R and Jacobson, S (1972) *Nutr. Metab., 14,* Suppl. 118
Bernhoff, A (1970) *Opusc. Med., 15,* 162
Birke, G, Carlson, LA and Liljedahl, S-O (1965) *Acta med. Scand., 178,* 337
Birke, G, von Euler, US, Carlson, LA, Liljedahl, S-O and Plantin, L-O (1972) *Acta chir. Scand., 138,* 321
Boberg, J, Carlson, LA and Hallberg, D (1969) *J. Atheroscl. Res., 9,* 159
Børresen, HC and Knutrud, O (1969) *Acta paediat. Scand., 58,* 420
Børresen, HC, Coran, AG and Knutrud, O (1970a) *Nord. Med., 84,* 1089
Børresen, HC, Coran, AG and Knutrud, O (1970b) In *Advances in Parenteral Nutrition. Symposium of the International Society for Parenteral Nutrition, Prague 1969.* (Ed) G Berg. Georg Thieme Verlag, Stuttgart. Page 93
Brøckner, J, Amris, CJ and Larsen, V (1965) *Acta chir. Scand., Suppl.343,* 48
Burns, TW, Langley, PE and Robison, GA (1971) *Ann. NY Acad. Sci., 185,* 115
Burr, GO and Burr, MM (1930) *J. biol. Chem., 86,* 587
Caldwell, MD, Meng, HC and Jonsson, HT (1973) *Fed. Am. Soc. Exptl. Biol., 57th Annual Meeting, NJ, April 15-20, No. 3913*
Carlson, LA and Hallberg, D (1963) *Acta physiol. Scand., 59,* 52
Carlson, LA and Liljedahl, S-O (1971) *Acta chir. Scand., 137,* 123
Carlson, LA and Rössner, S (1972) *Scand. J. clin. lab. Invest., 29,* 243
Carpentier, Y, Delepesse, G and Collett, H (1974) *Abstract. Congrès Internat. de Nutrition Parentérale. Montpellier Sept. 12-14.* Page 48
Chaptal, J, Jean, R, Crastes de Paulet, A, Guillaumot, R, Morel, G and Maurin, A (1964a) *Rev. Pract., 14,* 199
Chaptal, J, Jean, R, Crastes de Paulet, A, Guillaumot, R, Crastes de Paulet, P, Maurin-Belay, B and Morel, G (1964b) *Ann. Péd., 11,* 441
Chaptal, J, Jean, R, Crastes de Paulet, A, Pages, A, Dossa, D, Guillaumot, R, Crastes de Paulet, Mme, Robinert, Mme, Morel, G and Romen, H (1965) *Arch. Franc. Péd., 22,* 799
Collins, FD, Sinclair, AJ, Boyle, JP, Coats, DA, Maynard, AT and Leonard, RF (1971) *Nutr. Metab., 13,* 150
Coran, AG (1974) *Ann. Surg., 179,* 445
Coran, AG and Nesbakken, R (1969) *Surg., 66,* 922
Cronberg, S and Nilsson, I-M (1967) *Thromb. diath. Haemorrh., 18,* 364
Deitel, M and Kaminsky, V (1974) *CMA Journal, 111,* 152
Depisch, D (1971) *Der Anaesthesist, 20,* 437
Duckert, F and Hartmann, G (1966) *Schweiz. med. Wschr., 96,* 1205
Dudrick, SJ, Wilmore, DW, Vars, HM and Rhoads, JE (1969) *Ann. Surg., 169,* 974
Eckart, J, Tempel, G, Kaul, A and Schürnbrand, P (1973/74) *Die Infusions-*

therapie, 1, 138
Engelberg, H (1956) *J. Biol. Chem., 222,* 601
Fraser, AC (1958) *Brit. Med. Bull., 14,* 212
Fraser, R and Håkansson, I (1974) *Personal communication*
Galton, DJ (1971) *A Model for Errors in Metabolic Regulation.* Butterworth, London. Page 69
Geyer, RP, Chipman, J and Stare, FJ (1948) *J. biol. Chem., 176,* 1469
Gigon, JP, Enderlein, F and Scheidegger, S (1966) *Schweiz. med. Wschr., 96,* 71
Gilbert, C and Galton, DJ (1974) *Horm. metab. Res., 6,* 229
Greene, H, Hazlett, D, Demarre, R and Dramesi, J (1972) *Abstracts of short communication presented at the IX International Congress of Nutrition in Mexico City, September 3-9.* Page 197
Grotte, G (1971) In *Les Solutés de ubstitution et Rééquilibration Métabolique.* (Ed) G-G Nahas and P Viars. Librairie Arnette, Paris. Page 509
Grotte, G, Esscher, T, Hambraeus, L and Meurlings, S (1974) *Total Parenteral Nutrition in Pediatric Surgery. Proceedings Meeting Vancouver.* Pharmacia (Canada) Ltd, Quebec. Page 140
Gustafsson, A, Kjellmer, I, Olegard, R and Victorin, L (1972) *Acta paediat. Scand., 61,* 149
Hadfield, JIH (1966) *Clin. Med., 73,* 25
Håkansson, I (1968) *Nutr. Diet., 10,* 54
Hallberg, D (1965a) *Acta physiol. Scand., 64,* 306
Hallberg, D (1965b) *Acta physiol. Scand., 65, Suppl.,* 254
Hallberg, D, Schuberth, O and Wretlind, A (1966) *Nutr. Diet., 8,* 245
Hallberg, D, Holm, I, Obel, A-L, Schuberth, O and Wretlind, A (1967) *Postgrad. Med., 42,* A 71, A 87, A 99, A 149
Hanc, I, Klezkowska, H and Rodkiewicz, B (1968) *Ped. Polska, 43,* 1355
Hansen, AE, Wiese, HF, Boelsche, AN, Haggard, ME, Adau, DID and Davis, H (1963) *Ped., 31, Suppl.* 1
Hartmann, G (1967) *Wien. Med. Wschr., 117,* 51
Heird, WC, Driscoll, JM Jr, Schullinger, JN, Grebin, B and Winters, RW (1972) *J. Ped., 80,* 351
Horisberger, B (1966) *Schweiz. med. Wschr., 96,* 1065
Hornstra, G (1974) In *Dietary Fats and Thrombosis.* (Ed) S Renaud and A Nordøy. S Karger, Basel. Page 21
Huth, KW, Schoenborn, W and Börner, J (1967) *Med. Ernähr, 8,* 146
Jacobson, S (1972a) *Nutr. Metab., 14,* 150
Jacobson, S (1972b) *Int. Surg., 57,* 840
Jacobson, S (1974) *The postoperative utilization of crystalline amino acids given intravenously in total parenteral nutrition. Data presented at the XIX Bienniel Congress of the International College of Surgeons in Lima, Peru, March 24-28*
Jacobson, S and Wretlind, A (1970) In *Body Fluid Replacement in the Surgical Patient.* (Ed) CL Fox Jr and G-G Nahas. Grune & Stratton, New York. Page 334
Jacobson, S, Ericsson, J and Obel, A-L (1971) *Acta chir. Scand., 137,* 335
Jeejeebhoy, KN, Zohrab, WJ, Langer, B, Phillips, MJ, Kuksis, A and Andersson, GH (1973) *Gastroent., 65,* 811
Kapp, JP, Duckert, F and Hartmann, G (1971) *Nutr. Metab., 13,* 92
Lamke, L-O, Liljedahl, S-O and Wretlind, A (1974) *Ann. anesth. Franc., 15, Special II,* 27
Larsen, V and Brøckner, J (1965) *Acta chir. Scand., 343, Suppl.,* 191

92

Lawson, LJ (1965) *Brit. J. Surg., 52*, 795

Lemperle, G, Reichelt, M and Denk, S (1970) *The evaluation of phagocytic activity in men by means of a lipid-clearing-test. Abstract from 6th International Meeting of the Reticuloendothelial Society.* Page 83

Lerner, SR, Chaikoff, IL, Enteman, C and Dauben, WG (1949) *Proc. soc. exp. biol. Med., 70*, 384

MacFayden, B, Maynard, A and Dudrick, SJ (1972) *Triglyceride and free fatty acid clearances and linoleic acid repletion using 10% soybean oil emulsion in patients receiving standard parenteral hyperalimentation. Abstracts of short communication presented at the IX International Congress of Nutrition in Mexico City, September 3-9.* Page 198

Meng, HC and Early, F (1949) *J. Lab. clin. Med., 34*, 1121

Paulsrud, JR, Pensler, L, Whitten, CF, Stewart, S and Holman, RT (1972) *Amer. J. clin. Nutr., 25*, 897

Peaston, MJT (1966) *Brit. Med. J., 2*, 388

Peaston, MJT (1967) *Postgrad. Med. J., 43*, 31

Pendray, MR (1974) *Peripheral vein feeding in infants: technique, results and problems. Proceedings Meeting Vancouver.* Pharmacia (Canada) Ltd, Quebec. Page 158

Pensler, L, Whitten, C, Paulsrud, J and Holman, RT (1970) *American Pediatric Society and Society for Pediatric Research. Abstr. 177*

Reid, DJ (1967) *Brit. J. Surg., 54*, 204

Rickham, PP (1967) *Ann. Roy. Coll. Surg. Engl., 41*, 480

Rivers, JPW and Davidson, BC (1974) *Proc. Nutr. Soc., 33*, 48A

Robison, GA, Butcher, RW and Sutherland, GW (1971) In *Cyclic-AMP.* Academic Press, New York

Rodewald, G (1962) *Arch. klin. Chir., 301*, 532

Schärli, A (1965) *Int. Z. Vitaminforsch, 35*, 52

Schoefl, GI (1968) *Proc. Roy. Soc. B, 169*, 147

Scholler, KL (1968) *Z. Prakt. Anasth. Wiederbel., 3*, 193

Schultis, K and Geser, GA (1970) In *Parenteral Nutrition.* (Ed) HC Meng and DH Law. Charles C Thomas, Springfield, Illinois. Page 139

Shaw, JE and Ramwell, PW (1968) *J. biol. Chem., 243*, 1498

Sinclair, AI, Fiennes, RNT-W, Hay, AWM, Watson, G, Crawford, MA and Hart, MG (1971) *Proc. nutr. Soc., 33*, 49A

Steinbereithner, K (1966) In *Modern Trends in Anaesthesia.* (Ed) FT Evans and T Gray. Chapter 11. Butterworth, London

Stell, PM (1970) *Arch. Otolaryng., 91*, 166

Tulloch, BR, Vydelingum, N and Galton, DJ (1972) *Proc. Roy. Soc. Med., 65*, 790

Wadström, LB (1959) *Acta chir. Scand., Suppl. 238*, 1

Wadström, LR and Wiklund, PE (1964) *Acta chir. Scand., Suppl. 325*, 50

Wilmore, DW and Dudrick, SJ (1968) *JAMA, 203*, 140

Wilmore, DW, Moylan, JA, Helmkamp, GM and Pruitt, BA Jr (1973) *Ann. Surg., 78*, 503

Intermediary Energy Metabolism for the Catabolic State with Special Regard to Muscle Tissue

P FÜRST, J BERGSTRÖM, E HULTMAN and E VINNARS

St Erik's Sjukhus, Stockholm and Beckomberga Sjukhus, Bromma, Sweden

Introduction

Intermediary metabolism is often defined as the sum total of all the enzymatic reactions occurring in the cell. Metabolism is divided into catabolism and anabolism. *Catabolism* is the enzymatic degradation, largely by oxidative reactions, of relatively large molecules. Catabolism is accompanied by release of the free energy and its conservation in the form of the phosphate-bond energy of adenosine triphosphate (ATP). In general, the rate of catabolism of a cell is controlled not by the concentration of its nutrients in the environment, but rather by its second-to-second needs for energy in the form of ATP. Anabolism is the enzymatic synthesis of relatively large molecular components of cells. This synthetic process requires input of free energy, which is furnished by the phosphate-bound energy of ATP. Catabolism and anabolism take place concurrently in cells and consist of two simultaneous and interdependent processes.

Fundamental to the survival of living cells and thus of the whole body is the production of energy. The immediate source of energy in all cells is ATP. The endogenous store of ATP in cells is very small, sufficient only to meets the cells' energy needs for a few seconds or minutes. Consequently, continuous ATP resynthesis is a prerequisite for survival. The formation of ATP in the cells requires energy derived mostly from oxidation of foodstuff. This means a transfer of electrons from substrate to oxygen (aerobic metabolism) or to some other acceptor (anaerobic metabolism). Oxygen as a final acceptor is utilised by all cells with the exception of macrophages and erythrocytes which lack a suitable electron transport system (mitochondria).

ATP resynthesis can be accomplished in a number of ways. Especially in muscle and brain, the most rapid means is by transfer of active phosphate from

94

phosphoryl creatine (PC) to ADP. This reaction, however, suffers from the drawback that it itself is dependent upon a substrate (PC) which occurs only in limited quantities in the cells. Quantitatively more important means of resynthesising ATP is by way of *glycolysis* in which either glucose or glycogen is metabolised to pyruvate and lactate. Finally, ATP resynthesis occurs by *mitochondrial oxidation* of pyruvate, ketone bodies, and fatty acids. ATP may undergo loss of either an orthophosphate or a pyrophosphate group during its utilisation in biosynthetic reactions, to form ADP or AMP, respectively. AMP is rephosphorylated to ADP by the *adenylate kinase reaction,* ATP + AMP $\rightleftarrows$ 2 ADP.

In certain cells, e.g. muscle cells, all three ways of ATP resynthesis may occur simultaneously. In Table I are shown the potential energy reserves of the muscle

TABLE I

	μmol/g dry weight	Available energy as μmol $\sim$ P/g dry weight
ATP	24.6	9.8 (40%)
Phosphorylcreatine	76.8	61.4 (80%)
Glycogen	365 glucosyl units	1,060 (anaerobic)
		14,200 (aerobic)
Triglyceride	48.6	(24,520)

cells. In other tissues, e.g. red blood cells which are devoid of both a store of PC and mitochondria, ATP resynthesis is derived entirely from glycolysis with glucose as the only available substrate. The central nervous system also appears to be largely dependent upon glucose for ATP resynthesis under normal conditions. During times of hypoxia and anoxia, tissues with a normal oxidative capacity will of course become more heavily dependent upon glycolysis as their chief source of energy.

ANIMAL STUDIES

The sensitivity to anaerobiosis is very different in different tissues. The most sensitive is the brain, followed by liver and kidney (Sanders et al, 1965; Stoner & Heath, 1973). The sequence of events occurring during ischaemia in brain tissue is first a decrease in glycogen and ultimately also of ATP and the total adenine pool. The whole sequence is ended within 1–2 min (Lowry et al, 1964). In the ischaemic normothermic kidney, the ATP content falls to practically zero within 20–45 min (Collste et al, 1972). In muscle tissue, the sequence is similar to that in brain, but much slower (Threlfall & Stoner, 1957). Consequently, one of the most important questions when discussing intermediary energy metabolism under catabolic conditions is the amount of oxygen available, or the degree of tissue hypoxaemia.

Animal studies have shown pronounced changes in energy-rich phosphagens in different organs during hypoxia and following trauma (Threlfall & Stoner, 1957; Berry & Smythe, 1962; Lowry et al, 1964; Sanders et al, 1965; Collste et al, 1971). The brain of mice is depleted of glucose, phosphorylcreatine (PC), and glycogen within 30 sec of ischaemia, whereas the ATP content is decreased by 90% after 1 min. Sanders et al (1965) found in the rat a 90% decrease of ATP in brain after 1 min, in liver after 4 min, and in kidney after 60 min. Threlfall and Stoner (1957) found in ischaemic rat muscle tissue a continuous fall in PC, which was complete after 2 h. The ATP decrease was slower but was practically complete after 4 h. Simultaneously with the decrease in ATP there was an accumulation of inosine monophosphate (IMP) in the muscle tissue. Similar findings with rapid decrease in adenine nucleotides in rat brain, liver, and kidney after haemorrhagic hypoxia was reported by Bartlett (1972). He also found an increase of IMP content in the tissues. The lethal effects of the acute hypoxia were attributed to the pronounced loss of tissue ATP. He also pointed out that the regeneration of the ATP store would not only depend on rephosphorylation of AMP but also on the resynthesis of new adenine nucleotide.

In a series of experiments determinations of phosphagens and lactate were made repeatedly in surgically removed kidneys, preserved with different methods for transplantation. The kidneys were transplanted and the metabolic changes could be related to the viability of the transplants. A good correlation between the viability and the total adenine-nucleotide content (TA) was found. As observed earlier the decrease in ATP and TA was very rapid at normothermic ischaemia and much slower when the kidney was cooled to 5–8°C with an electrolyte solution with high K^+ content. Different kinds of perfusion media were tested. The best result was obtained with continuous perfusion with oxygenated plasma (Collste et al, 1971, 1972).

ENERGY METABOLISM IN HUMAN MUSCLE TISSUE

During the last forty years, there has been much study of muscle metabolism. However, the considerable progress made in *basic biochemistry* has not been adequately extended to the *clinical biochemical* field. In man only indirect evidence is available from nitrogen balance, determinations of metabolites and enzymes in blood, and catheterisation studies.

The method of obtaining samples from muscle tissue by needle biopsy in man has opened new possibilities for studying intermediary metabolism of muscle. Using the percutaneous biopsy technique of Bergström (1962) it has been possible to obtain muscle samples from man under clinical, as well as experimental conditions. Samples can be taken rapidly from the same muscle group without significant discomfort, and during the last ten years the biopsy technique has been used

96

over 12,000 times without complications. The metabolic picture in diseases, such as hypoxia, uraemia, hypercatabolism, diabetes, rheumatism, and malabsorption and under certain experimental conditions, such as dynamic and isometric exercise and different types of nutrition, is under study at the Metabolic Research Laboratory in Stockholm. The results indicate specific changes in muscle tissue and open insights into the cellular processes. The pattern of results offers evidence of energy processes both in mitochondria and in the cytoplasm of muscle.

Muscle tissue is considered to be relatively resistant to metabolic insult when

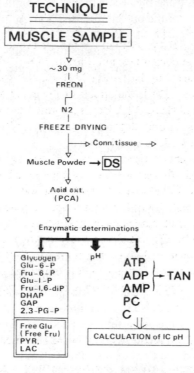

Figure 1. A schematic illustration of procedures used.
Abbreviations:

↓ (dashed)	= Processes and preparations
↓	= Direct determinations
⇓	= Calculation
DS	= Dry solids
PCA	= Perchloric acid
PC	= Phosphocreatine
Cr	= Creatine (free)
TAN	= Total adenine nucleotides

compared to the brain, liver, or kidney. Therefore, any observed changes in muscle tissue can be expected to be correlated with more severe abnormalities in other organs. It is of fundamental importance to obtain further information on the biochemical parameters of muscle during acute diseases and injury and to study the response of nutritional therapy.

Methodology

Muscle samples are taken under local anaesthesia from the lateral portion of the m. quadriceps femoris using the needle biopsy technique (Bergström, 1962). A schematic presentation of the procedures used is given in Figure 1. After having frozen the samples as quickly as possible (1–2 sec) by plunging the biopsy needle into liquid freon maintained at its melting point -150°C) the samples are moved and stored in liquid nitrogen. The frozen samples are then lyophilised by freeze drying. The samples are usually in the weight order of 30–80 mg. The dried samples are powdered and all visible connective tissue is removed. The amount of connective tissue varies from sample to sample and therefore its removal is of the greatest importance. The further preparation, the analytical technique, and normal values have previously been described (Harris et al, 1974).

Experimental Hypoxaemia

The effect of hypoxaemia in human muscle tissue was studied in normal man in which the circulation in the leg muscles was occluded by means of a tourniquet with a pressure of 250 mmHg (Harris et al, 1975a). By depleting the local muscle oxygen stores at rest, the muscle will rely only on anaerobic glycolysis and phosphagen depletion as sources of ATP supply during a subsequent contraction.

Only minor changes were detected in the levels of adenine nucleotides during the 20 min occlusion period. No significant change in TA was observed but the ATP/TA ratio slightly decreased after 6 min and was significantly below the rest value after 20 min. ADP/TA and AMP/TA were increased after 20 min. During occlusion PC decreased and Cr increased. Pyruvate + lactate concentrations increased significantly after 10 min of occlusion. The mean rate of increase over the 10–20 min period was 0.3 mmol lactate/kg dry muscle/min. The contribution to this increase by lactate from erythrocytes trapped in the muscle capillary bed was estimated to 0.01 mmol/kg dry muscle/min based on data from Levin et al (1974).

The relative changes in the phosphagens during the 20 min of occlusion are similar to the changes first observed by Bollman and Flock (1944) in ischaemic rat limb muscle and by Imai et al (1964) in rabbit muscle. However, some comparative differences do exist. For instance, in rabbit muscle the calculated average rate of PC depletion during 20 min of occlusion was more than double that in man, and this was paralleled by a much greater fall in ATP. During the 20 min

98

of occlusion some decrease in TA also occurred in rabbit muscle.

No significant change was detected in the apparent equilibrium constant of the adenylate kinase (AK) reaction ([ATP] [AMP] / [ADP^2] or K'_{AK}) during occlusion but the apparent equilibrium constant of the creatine kinase (CK) reaction ([ATP] [Cr] / [ADP] [PC] or K'_{CK}) increased progressively. Increase in K'_{CK} could be interpreted as signifying a decrease in intracellular pH (pH$_i$) (Harris et al, 1975b). Assuming 100% interavailability of the four metabolic components of the CK reaction, the change in pH$_i$ ($\triangle$pH$_i$) after occlusion can be estimated according to the formula:

$$\triangle pH_i = \log (K'_{CK} \text{ at rest} \cdot K_{CK}^{-1}) -$$
$$- \log (K'_{CK} \text{ after t min occlusion} \cdot K_{CK}^{-1}) \qquad (1)$$

in which K_{CK}^{-1} is the reciprocal of the true equilibrium constant defined as:

$$K'_{CK} = [ATP] [Cr] / [ADP] [PC] [H^+] \qquad (2)$$

The formula can be simplified to:

$$\wedge pH_i = \log (K'_{CK} \text{ at rest}) -$$
$$- \log (K'_{CK} \text{ after t min occlusion}) \qquad (3)$$

Estimates of $\triangle$pH$_i$ calculated according to formula 3 are given in Figure 2 and imply a fall of up to 0.30 pH units after 20 min of occlusion. However, these calculations were not in agreement with the direct determinations made in the

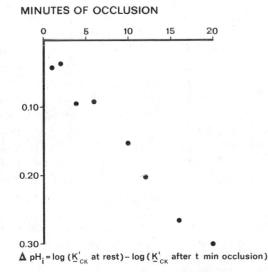

MINUTES OF OCCLUSION

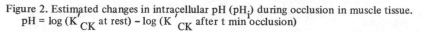

Δ pH$_i$ = log ($\underline{K}'_{CK}$ at rest) − log ($\underline{K}'_{CK}$ after t min occlusion)

Figure 2. Estimated changes in intracellular pH (pH$_i$) during occlusion in muscle tissue. pH = log (K'_{CK} at rest) − log (K'_{CK} after t min occlusion)

99

same biopsy specimens (Sahlin et al, 1975). A linear relationship between muscle pH and the apparent equilibrium constant of the creatine kinase reaction was obtained. The decrease in muscle pH was also linearly related to accumulation of lactate + pyruvate. The changes were more pronounced when occlusion was followed by isometric contraction.

Changes in Muscle Energy Metabolism in Severely Ill Patients in Catabolic State

We have also studied high energy phosphates and glycolytic intermediates in muscle tissue from 18 patients treated in the Intensive Care Unit at the St Eriks Hospital. The patients have been grouped into two series, each comprising 9 patients (Hultman et al, 1972; Bergström et al, to be published).

The first group comprised 9 patients who were admitted with acute circulatory or respiratory insufficiency. Of these 9 patients 7 died within one day to two weeks. Muscle biopsies were taken within a few hours to a few days after admission. The second group of 9 had a longer history before the biopsy was taken. Two survived after 3 months of intensive treatment, but the other 7 patients died after 3 weeks to 2 months. In the first group most of the patients

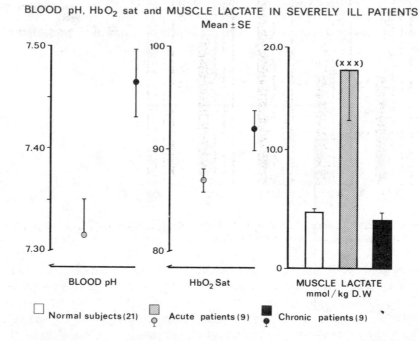

Figure 3. Blood oxygen saturation (HbO_2), blood pH, and lactate in muscle in severely ill patients

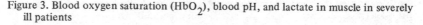

100

had a decreased oxygenation of the blood and some a decreased blood pH. An increase in muscle lactate content was found, which could be related to an increased anaerobic glycolysis in the muscle. An increased anaerobic glycolysis is logical to the decreased HbO_2 saturation in these patients. In the second group the mean oxygen saturation was decreased, but no acidosis was seen. Muscle lactate content was normal (Figure 3). In the first group the changes in active phosphates were small. A slight decrease in ATP and in total adenine nucleotides were found compared with normals.

The mean PC was slightly decreased and the mean Cr was increased but there were significant changes in only a few patients. ADP and AMP were not altered significantly. In the second group the largest change was seen in ATP and total adenine nucleotide contents which were decreased to about half the normal

ENERGY RICH PHOSPHATES AND FREE CREATINE IN MUSCLE TISSUE

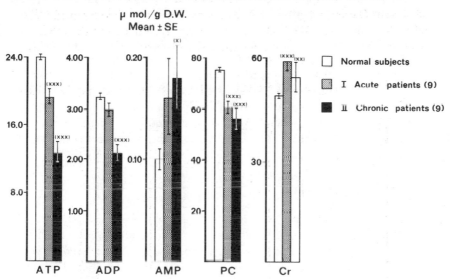

Figure 4. Adenine nucleotides (ATP, ADP, AMP), phosphocreatine (PC), and free creatine (CR) in muscle tissue in severely ill patients

values. Also the PC and ADP contents were decreased, but in contrast to the first group the free Cr was unchanged (Figure 4). The equilibrium constant for the ATP : creatinephosphotransferase reaction; $H^+ + PC + ADP \rightleftarrows Cr + ATP$ was expressed in formula 2. The apparent equilibrium constant (K'_{CK}) is dependent on pH and can under certain conditions be used as an indicator of intracellular pH. A significant increase was found in group 1. As could be expected, the largest increases were seen in patients with an increased lactic acid content in muscle tissue. The apparent constant for the creatine kinase equilibrium was only slightly changed in the second group.

Similar results were found in acute cardiogenic shock with pronounced increases in blood and muscle lactate and with PC values approaching zero in muscle tissue. At this stage a decrease of ATP was also seen (Karlsson et al, 1975). In group 2 there was no sign of anaerobic metabolism in the muscle due to hypoxia but still these patients showed very pronounced changes in the ATP content and in the TA content. The normal balance between excretion and production of adenine and adenine nucleotides seems to have been disturbed in these patients due to either a decreased production or an increased excretion. It is known that de novo synthesis of purines, which occurs predominantly in the liver (Murray et al, 1970) requires a vast expenditure of energy (6 moles of ATP per mole of AMP synthetised). In patients showing a low energy status and/or liver damage the net result may well be a decreased rate of purine synthesis. Alternatively, the low adenine nucleotide content could be explained by an increased rate of deamination of AMP and/or enhanced complete degradation and excretion.

There is evidence that short-term total anoxia results in deamination of AMP to IMP and decreases in the TA pool (Lowry et al, 1964; Sanders et al, 1965; Bartlett, 1972). This effect of anoxia is deleterious, primarily to organs such as brain, liver, and kidney, whereas muscle is relatively resistant. In group 2 prolonged hypoxia, low energy state, and possibly liver damage could be the reason for a decreased de novo synthesis of adenine nucleotides. Similar lowering of the adenine pool has been observed in a series of patients with malnutrition and liver damage due to severe bowel disease (Fürst et al, to be published).

Malnutrition – Malabsorption

In muscle tissue, very low ATP, slightly decreased PC, normal ADP, increased Cr, and slightly increased AMP contents were found at admission to the hospital. The ratios ATP/ADP and PC/Cr were clearly decreased. Muscle glycogen was decreased and muscle free glucose was elevated. Increased blood lactate and slightly decreased blood pyruvate concentrations were observed. In spite of intensive therapy with complete parenteral nutrition (Intramin forte®, carbohydrates, and Intralipid® corresponding to 17 g amino acid nitrogen and 3,000 kcal/day) one of the patients died after 4 days of treatment. After one week on parenteral nutrition, the other two patients were kept on an elementary synthetic oral diet (Vivonex® corresponding to 8 g amino acid nitrogen and 2,400 kcal/day) during two weeks and were then put on a protein-calorie rich hospital diet (150 g protein and 2,500 kcal/day). The muscle biopsy was repeated 30 days after the hospitalisation. All biochemical changes that initially showed a severely abnormal pattern were normal (Figure 5).

The adenine pool was also depleted in obese patients operated upon for ileo-

102

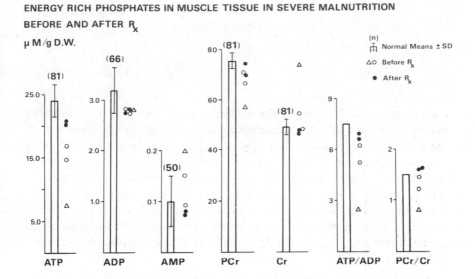

Figure 5. Adenine nucleotides (ATP, ADP, AMP), phosphocreatine (PC), and free creatine in muscle tissue in three patients with severe malnutrition before and after treatment. Patient indicated by △ died after 4 days of intensive therapy.

ENERGY RICH PHOSPHATES AND FREE CREATINE IN MUSCLE TISSUE IN PATIENTS OPERATED UPON MORBID OBESITAS

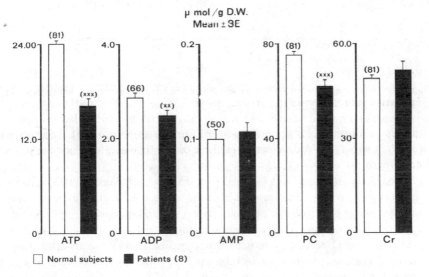

Figure 6. Adenine nucleotides (ATP, ADP, AMP) and phosphocreatine (PC) in muscle tissue in patients operated upon with jejuno-ileal by-pass for morbid obesitas

103

jejunal shunt (Figure 6) [Fürst, Hultman & Moberg, to be published). Three months after the operation the patients exhibited signs of protein malabsorption. Plasma amino acid pattern typical for protein malabsorption was observed with low concentrations of valine, isoleucine, and leucine, increased ratio of glycine to valine and decreased ratio for the essential to non-essential amino acids. These abnormalities had occurred within three months after the operation and were

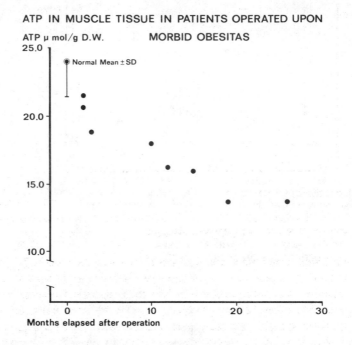

Figure 7. Correlation between ATP in muscle tissue and the elapsed time after operation in patients operated upon with jejuno-ileal by-pass

not changed during the observation period (Fürst & Moberg, 1975). The decrease of ATP, however, showed a clear correlation to the time elapsed since the operation (Figure 7).

It was shown by Sandberg et al (1953) and Walker and Walker (1959) that Cr is produced in liver and pancreas and brought to the muscle via the blood. The Cr in the muscle has a half-life of about 30 days (Fitch & Shields, 1966) and is very resistant to changes. Only after prolonged protein starvation are decreases seen in the total Cr content in muscle. During isometric exercise and also during prolonged exercise, pronounced decreases in PC are observed but TCr is not changed (Bergström et al, 1971; Ahlborg et al, 1972). Thus, it is reasonable that in the acute cases in group 1, the TCr should not be changed in the muscle. There was no significant mean decrease in TCr.

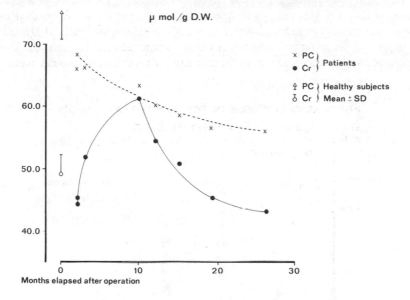

PHOSPHOCREATINE AND FREE CREATINE CHANGES IN MUSCLE TISSUE
RELATED TO TIME ELAPSED AFTER OPERATION IN MORBID OBESITAS

Figure 8. Correlation between PC, Cr in muscle tissue, and the elapsed time after operation in patients operated upon with jejuno-ileal by-pass

In group 2 with a prolonged severe illness there was a decrease in TCr which can be attributed to a prolonged disturbance of the liver metabolism or to an increased amount of connective tissue in the muscle samples. However, most of the patients had a long history of illness involving the intestinal tract. In patients operated upon for morbid obesity continuously decreasing PC content was found when it was correlated to elapsed time after operation. During the first year the results also indicated unchanged TCr due to increasing free Cr content. However, one year after operation a sudden fall of the free Cr content in muscle tissue was observed. This means a concomitant and consequent decline of the TCr content (Figure 8). These results indicate, as mentioned above, severe protein starvation in these patients.

Rheumatoid Arthritis

Muscle biopsies were also taken from patients with rheumatoid arthritis (RA) and analysed for energy rich phosphates and a number of glycolytic intermediates (Nordemar et al, 1974). The results were compared with corresponding values from normal healthy subjects and from a group of patients with connective tissue diseases (other than RA). In patients suffering from RA negative nitrogen balance has been reported (Bayles, 1964; Wilkinson et al, 1965). Muscle atrophy and

105

muscular weakness are early and obvious signs in patients with RA. No significant differences in the muscle content of glycolytic intermediates were detected between the three groups of subjects, with the exception of Glu-6-P and lactate which were significantly lower in the RA patients compared with the healthy subjects but of the same order as found in the other patients, probably reflecting immobilisation due to inactivity in these patient groups.

Muscle cell ATP and ADP were significantly lower in the RA patients than in the healthy subjects, whereas AMP was the same. The levels of ATP, ADP, and

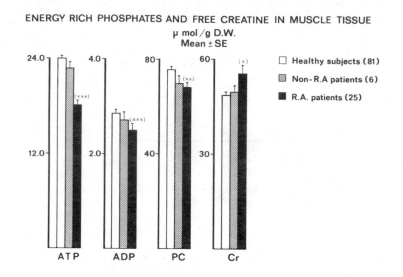

ENERGY RICH PHOSPHATES AND FREE CREATINE IN MUSCLE TISSUE
µ mol / g D.W.
Mean ± SE

□ Healthy subjects (81)
▩ Non-R.A patients (6)
■ R.A. patients (25)

Figure 9. Adenine nucleotides (ATP, AMP, ADP), phosphocreatine (PC) and free creatine (Cr) in muscle tissue in patients with rheumatoid arthritis (RA) compared with normal healthy subjects and with a group of patients with connective tissue diseases (non-RA)

AMP in the non-RA patients were not significantly different from those in the healthy subjects. ATP differed significantly between the two groups of patients (Figure 9). The proportion of ATP of the total adenosine phosphate pool (TA), i.e. ATP/TA, in the RA patients (mean $0.868 \pm SD\ 0.023$) was the same as in the normals (mean $0.877 \pm SD\ 0.017$). Also the mean value for the apparent equilibrium constant of adenylate kinase, i.e. $[ATP]\ [AMP] / [ADP^2]$ (RA patients $0.29 \pm SD\ 0.19$ and normals $0.25 \pm SD\ 0.12$) was the same in patients and normals. These results indicate a normal interrelationship of ATP to the total adenine pool in contrast to the findings in severely ill patients and patients suffering from malnutrition and protein malabsorption.

A significantly lower PC and a significantly higher Cr were found in the RA patients, when compared with the healthy subjects, but not when compared with the non-RA patients. Total creatine (TCr) was the same in the three groups.

PC/TCr in the RA patients averaged 0.563 ± SD 0.065 and was significantly lower than that of the healthy subjects (mean 0.613 ± SD 0.033) but not of the other patient group. The mean value of the apparent equilibrium constant of creatine kinase, i.e. [Cr] [ATP] / [PC] [ADP] in the RA patients (5.71 ± SD 1.91) did not differ significantly from that of the healthy subjects (4.83 ± SD 1.25). From the absence of any significant change in the mean value of the apparent equilibrium constant of creatine kinase between RA patients and the healthy subjects it would appear that the changes in the relative levels of PC and Cr in the RA patients were responsible for changes in ATP and ADP.

A weak but significant correlation ($r = 0.44$, $p < 0.05$) was obtained when the muscle ATP content of the RA patients was related to the duration of the

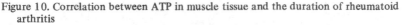

Correlation between duration and ATP Concentration in muscle

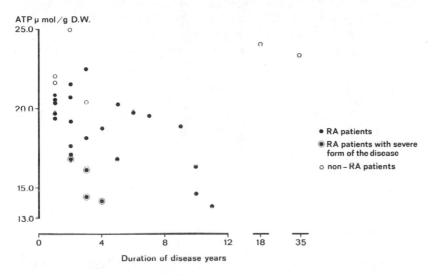

Figure 10. Correlation between ATP in muscle tissue and the duration of rheumatoid arthritis

disease suggesting that the degree of the severity also may influence the muscle ATP level (Figure 10). The observed low muscle ATP content in RA patients is probably not due to interference with resynthesis by the drugs given, which is indicated by the fact that in several patients, to whom no drugs were administered, the low ATP concentration was of the same order as in the others.

The range of age covered by the healthy group (range 18–30 years) differed from that of the patient group. No trend, however, with age towards high or low values of muscle ATP was found within either patient groups, indicating that age may not be an important factor.

General Conclusions

The reported results indicate that the ATP resynthesis under pathological conditions, as in severe catabolism or in protein malnutrition—malabsorption, is dependent on the rate of energy expenditure in the muscle cells. The active carbohydrate stores in muscle and liver are very limited and consequently during prolonged malnutrition the decreased adenine pool probably is a result of adaptive changes in the enzymatic system responsible for ATP resynthesis.

Another possibility is that the decrease is limited to the same specific pool, e.g. the sarcoplasmic or mitochondrial pool. It remains also to be determined whether the diminished adenine pool is a result of a decreased capacity to resynthesise ATP or secondary to other cell changes, e.g. a result of a lower mitochondrial number.

The probability of a metabolic factor being the most likely cause of the change in the adenine nucleotide content is also supported by the findings in a diabetic patient with severe ketoacidosis, with normal HbO_2 saturation, and with normal blood pressure (Figures 11 & 12). He showed a very large decrease in ATP and in TA but these abnormalities as well as his acidosis could be corrected within one day by insulin treatment. Prior to treatment this patient could

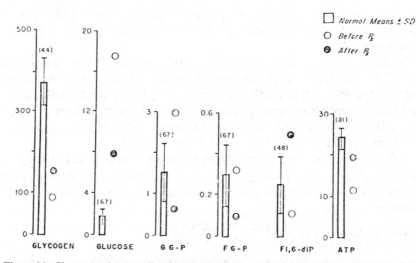

GLYCOGEN, GLUCOSE, INTERMEDIATES AND ATP IN MUSCLE TISSUE
DIABETIC COMA – BEFORE & AFTER R_x

$\mu M/g\,DW$

Figure 11. Glycogen, glucose, glycolytic intermediates, and ATP in muscle tissue in a patient with severe diabetic coma and ketoacidosis (O) and after one day of treatment with insulin and bicarbonate (●)

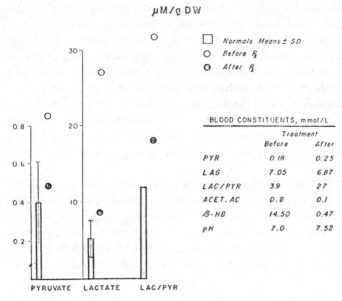

PYRUVATE, LACTATE AND LACTATE/PURUVATE RATIO IN MUSCLE TISSUE
DIABETIC COMA–BEFORE & AFTER Rx
μM/g DW

□ Normals Means ± SD
○ Before Rx
◑ After Rx

BLOOD CONSTITUENTS, mmol/l

	Treatment Before	After
PYR	0.18	0.25
LAC	7.05	6.87
LAC/PYR	39	27
ACET. AC	0.8	0.1
β-HB	14.50	0.47
pH	7.0	7.52

PYRUVATE   LACTATE   LAC/PYR

Figure 12. Pyruvate, lactate, and the lactate/pyruvate ratio in muscle tissue in the patient described in Figure 11

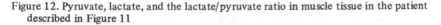

have had a decreased content of phosphoribosyl pyrophosphate (PRPP) due to his diabetic state. A lack of PRPP would decrease the activity in the 'purine salvage system'.

In discussing the regulation of glycolysis and respiration, as mentioned before, the relative concentrations of ADP and ATP in the cell are the most important controlling elements. When ATP is utilised in many biosynthetic reactions, it undergoes pyrophosphate cleavage to yield AMP, whereas in muscular contraction, ADP is the primary product of ATP utilisation. At any given moment, a living cell contains not only ATP and ADP but also AMP.

Atkinson and Walton (1967) proposed the *energy charge* concept for the adenylate pool. The energy charge of the ATP–ADP–AMP system can easily be calculated for any given set of concentrations of ATP, ADP, and AMP by the equation:

$$\text{energy charge} = \frac{1}{2}\left(\frac{[ADP] + 2\,[ATP]}{[AMP] + [ADP] + [ATP]}\right)$$

Because many regulatory enzymes in both catabolic and anabolic pathways are responsive to AMP, ADP, or ATP as modulators, Atkinson (1968) has suggested that the regulation of pathways, that produce and utilise high-energy phosphate

109

bonds, is a function of the energy charge of the ATP—ADP—AMP system, which runs optimally in a steady state and strongly resists any deviations from it. Several enzymes that catalyse reactions in glycolysis or the citric acid cycle are either inhibited by ATP or stimulated by AMP. These enzyme reactions are thus activated at a low energy charge in the adenylate pool. Other reactions utilising ATP for biosynthesis or production of storage compounds will be enhanced at high energy charge but inhibited at low.

In severely ill patients and in patients with untreated malnutrition, especially in series 2, we found low energy charge (Figure 13).

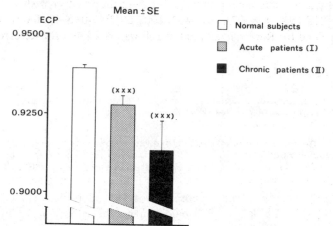

Figure 13. Energy charge potential (ECP) in muscle tissue in severely ill patients

$$ECP = \frac{1}{2}\left(\frac{[ADP] + 2\,[ATP]}{[AMP] + [ADP] + [ATP]}\right)$$

This would mean that these patients had a decreased capacity for biosynthetic reactions and for production of storage compounds. Such a situation is often referred to as a catabolic state and it has been repeatedly found that in the post-operative or post-traumatic situation most patients are 'catabolic'. Possibly the low energy charge seen here is the cellular expression for this 'catabolic state'. It is interesting to note that the lowest energy charge was seen in the diabetic patient, who in spite of a very low muscle glycogen content had a high intracellular lactate. When the energy charge potential was increased after treatment with insulin and bicarbonate, the lactate decreased in the muscle in spite of ample amounts of blood glucose and muscle glycogen. Similar alterations were observed in patients with severe malnutrition in connection with the treatment (Figure 5).

Kinney has suggested (personal communication) that the required amount of ATP from a given amount of substrate oxidation may not be synthesised during periods of surgical hypermetabolism. There is increasing evidence that the coupling of oxidation and phosphorylation in the mitochondria is seriously disturbed in hypermetabolism. The extent to which mitochondrial coupling can be reduced and still recover, has not been determined. The important question must be asked whether prolonged surgical hypermetabolism in the absence of shock may be associated with a decreased coupling efficiency, producing a situation where the patient has increased demands for oxidative substrate, gas exchange, and heat loss, while producing relatively less ATP for tissue and organ work.

Acknowledgment

This investigation was supported by grants from the Swedish Medical Research Council (B75-19X-2647-07A, B74-19X-1002-09, B75-03X-4210-02), Tore Nilsson's Fund for Research, and Eaton Laboratories Fund for Research.

References

Ahlborg, B, Bergström, J, Guarnieri, G, Harris, RC, Hultman, E and Nordesjö,L-O (1972) *J. appl. Physiol., 33,* 224
Atkinson, DE (1968) *Biochemistry, 7,* 4030
Atkinson, DE and Walton, GM (1967) *J. biol. Chem., 242,* 3239
Bartlett, GR (1972) *Scand. J. clin. lab. Invest., 29, Suppl.126,* 5
Bayles, TB (1964) In *Modern Nutrition in Health and Disease Dietotherapy.*
    (Ed) MG Wohl and RS Goodhart. Lea & Febiger, Philadelphia. Page 982
Bergström, J (1962) *Scand. J. clin. lab. Invest., 14, Suppl.68*
Bergström; J (1971) In *Advances in Experimental Medicine and Biology, Vol.11.*
    (Ed) B Pernow and B Saltin. Plenum Press, New York. Page 341
Berry, LJ and Smythe, DS (1962) *Amer. J. Physiol., 203,* 155
Bollman, JL and Flock, EV (1944) *Amer. J. Physiol., 142,* 290
Collste, H, Bergström, J, Hultman, E and Melin, B (1971) *Life Sci., 10,* 1201
Collste, H, Bergström, J, Groth, CG, Melin, B and Hultman, E (1972) *Acta chir. Scand., Suppl.425,* 31
Fitch, CD and Shields, RP (1966) *J. biol. Chem., 241,* 3611
Fürst, P and Moberg, S (1975) Submitted to *Amer. J. clin. Nutr.*
Harris, RC, Hultman, E and Nordesjö, L-O (1974) *Scand. J. clin. lab. Invest., 33,* 109
Harris, RC, Hultman, E and Sahlin, K (1975b) Submitted to *Scand. J. clin. lab. Invest.*
Hultman, E, Bergström, J, Boström, H, Fürst, P, Harris, R, Melin, B and Vinnars, E (1972) *Scand. J. clin. lab. Invest., 29, Suppl.126,* 5.2
Imai, E, Riley, AL and Berne, RM (1964) *Circ. Res., 15,* 443
Karlsson, J, Willerson, JR, Leshin, SJ, Mullins, CB and Mitchell, JH (1975) *Scand. J. clin. lab. Invest., 35,* 73
Lehninger, AL (1970) *Biochemistry.* Worth Publishers Inc., New York
Levin, K, Fürst, P, Harris, R and Hultman, E (1974) *Scand. J. clin. lab. Invest., 34,* 141

Lowry, OH, Passonneau, JV, Hasselberger, FX and Schulz, DW (1964) *J. biol. Chem., 239,* 18

Murray, AW, Elliot, DC and Atkinson, MR (1970) *Prog. nucleic acid res. mol. Biol., 10,* 87

Nordemar, R, Löfgren, O, Fürst, P, Harris, RC and Hultman, E (1974) *Scand. J. clin. lab. Invest., 34,* 185

Sanders, AP, Hale, DM and Miller, AT (1965) *Amer. J. Physiol., 209,* 438

Sandberg, AA, Hecht, HH and Tyler, EH (1953) *Metabolism, 2,* 22

Stoner, HB and Heath, DF (1973) *Brit. J. Anaesth., 45,* 244

Threlfall, CJ and Stoner, HB (1957) *Brit. J. exp. Pathol., 38,* 24

Walker, JB and Walker, MS (1959) *Proc. soc. exp. biol. Med., 101,* 807

Wilkinson, P, Jeremy, R, Brooks, FP and Hollander, JL (1965) *Ann. intern. Med., 63,* 109

The Importance of Energy Source and the Significance of Insulin in Counteracting the Catabolic Response to Injury

S P ALLISON, PAMELA HINTON*, A WOOLFSON† and
R V C HEATLEY

General Hospital, Nottingham; Accident Hospital, Birmingham*, City Hospital, Nottingham†, England

Introduction

The original work of Sir David Cutherbertson (1930, 1932) which demonstrated increased oxygen consumption and protein catabolism after injury has provided the broad cloth upon which each of us has embroidered his own contribution. In particular, Professor Kinney has shown that the increase in net protein breakdown after injury is related to the requirement for essential new glucose rather than for calories, and that raising the blood glucose artificially, after injury, fails to switch off hepatic gluconeogenesis. The only other condition in which this happens is diabetes mellitus.

STUDIES ON PATIENTS UNDERGOING SURGERY

I had become concerned about some of the arrhythmias which arose in patients at the end of cardio-pulmonary bypass procedures. Many of these arrhythmias, in patients who had been receiving digoxin were of the type caused by digitalis toxicity and were reversible by the administration of potassium. Our measurements showed that a fall in serum potassium occurred at this time and that this could be correlated with changes in blood glucose. A large volume of 5% glucose solution was used in priming the by-pass pump. It was found that this sudden load of 75–100 g of glucose caused a rise in blood glucose which was maintained during the period of bypass. Towards the end of the operation the blood glucose fell and it was assumed that the passage of glucose into cells took potassium with it, causing an abrupt fall in extracellular potassium concentration and precipitating

113

digitalis toxicity. Further observations showed that insulin secretion was suppressed during the operative procedure but recovered after surgery was complete. This seemed to explain the changes in both blood glucose and serum potassium (Allison et al, 1967, 1971).

In view of the complexity of the situation during cardiac surgery we extended our studies to general surgical patients, and found similar results (Allison et al, 1969). A standard 25 g intravenous glucose tolerance test (Samols & Marks, 1965) was performed before and repeated during operation. Blood samples were taken in the basal condition and again at 2, 5, 10, 20, 30, 40, 50 and 60 minutes after glucose injection. Preoperatively, glucose tolerance, insulin secretion and fatty acid levels were normal but during the operation insulin secretion was suppressed. After the injection of glucose, there was no net removal of glucose from the peripheral blood during the hour of study. Fatty acid levels instead of falling as they normally do after glucose administration continued to rise, presumably under the unopposed action of catecholamines. Further studies showed that the anaesthetics employed in these patients, halothane and nitrous oxide had no significant effect upon the metabolic changes observed (Allison et al, 1969). However, it was felt desirable to study patients who had undergone trauma in the absence of anaesthesia.

STUDIES OF BURNED PATIENTS

I was privileged to be allowed to work in the Burns Unit of the Birmingham Accident Hospital in association with the late Dr Pamela Hinton whose premature death was a great sadness to me and a great loss to the study of the metabolic response to injury. We studied patients during the first twelve hours after injury and again, seven to ten days later. The same intravenous glucose tolerance test was employed and similar changes observed as in our previous studies (Allison et al, 1968). During the acute phase of injury there was failure of insulin secretion, glucose intolerance and high fatty acid levels. These changes were found to be proportional to the severity of injury and to last up to 72 hours after burning. Recent studies have shown that these changes may recur during episodes of septicaemia or similar intercurrent complications (Woolfson et al, unpublished). After the shock phase, glucose intolerance may persist in the presence of high endogenous insulin levels. We proposed that failure of insulin secretion during the acute phase of injury followed by a period of insulin resistance was a non-specific effect of injury, proportional to its severity but not its type. It seemed likely that suppression of insulin secretion was related to adrenergic activity in view of the work of Coore and Randle (1964) who showed the suppressive effect of adrenaline on pancreatic tissue slices and of Porte et al (1966) who showed that insulin response to glucose could be suppressed by adrenaline infusion in normal man. Recent work from Czechoslovakia (Vigas — personal communication) has shown that in rats after the removal of the adrenal medulla insulin secretion is not suppressed by injury. The insulin resistance which occurs after injury has not been explained. The data of Ross et al (1966) suggests that hormonal antagonists are not the only factors involved.

ENDOCRINE AND METABOLIC CHANGES

Other workers have shown that the secretion of catecholamines, cortisol, glucagon and growth hormone is increased after injury (Birke et al, 1957; Browne et al, 1944; Cope et al, 1943; Ross et al, 1966; Wilmore et al, 1974). In the light of our own findings of changes in insulin secretion and activity after injury, we proposed that many of the metabolic changes might occur as a result of an alteration in balance between the anabolic hormone insulin and the catabolic hormones listed above. The synthesis of glycogen from glucose and the oxidation of glucose are enhanced by insulin, whereas glycogenolysis is stimulated by adrenaline and glucagon, and glucose oxidation is inhibited by cortisol. This is in keeping with the known rapid exhaustion of glycogen stores after injury and, in the ebb phase, the inhibition of glucose oxidation (Stoner, 1970). The passage of amino acids into cells and their incorporation into protein is enhanced by insulin whereas protein breakdown for gluconeogenesis with an increase in urea synthesis from the redundant amino groups is enhanced by cortisol and glucagon. This is in keeping with the findings of Kinney (1970). Triglyceride is synthesised from glucose under the influence of insulin whereas lipolysis is enhanced by catecholamines. Considering intermediary metabolism in a rather simplified form, the sites of metabolic control are exerted largely at 'irreversible' reactions. These require a different enzyme for the forward reaction to that which catalyses the reverse process. In the flow of substrate down the glycolytic pathway into the Krebs cycle, these 'irreversible' reactions occur at the levels of hexokinase, phosphofructokinase, pyruvate kinase and pyruvate dehydrogenase. Intrinsic control mechanisms act at these points. A fall in ATP and a rise in ADP, for example, stimulate phosphofructokinase activity. This may be the mechanism of the Pasteur effect whereby anoxia stimulates glycolysis.

The work of Randle and others has shown that, particularly in heart muscle, there is a reciprocal relationship between fat and glucose oxidation. Increased lipolysis causes a rise in plasma levels and hence of cellular uptake and oxidation of free fatty acids. The consequent rise in citrate inhibits phosphofructokinase and the rise in acetyl CoA causes product inhibition of pyruvate dehydrogenase. Thus, in situations such as fasting and injury, where lipolysis is increased, glucose oxidation is inhibited. After a meal, however, the exogenous glucose supply causes a rise in insulin levels, inhibition of lipolysis and a switch back to predominantly glucose oxidation. Although these control sites may be affected by such intrinsic metabolic controls, hormones act in an over-riding capacity, a fact which may have important therapeutic implications. On the gluconeogenic pathway, a different route has to be taken from pyruvate to oxaloacetate and thence to phospho-

115

enolypyruvate. Phosphatases allow the flow of carbon to pass back up to the glycolytic pathway. According to Ashmore and Weber (1968) glycolytic enzymes are not only activated directly or indirectly by insulin but may also be induced. Cortisol has the reverse effect on glycolysis and both enhances and induces glyconeogenic enzymes. We therefore have a picture of the 'two lane highway' of glycolysis and gluconeogenesis. The relative rates of carbon flow along the two pathways are affected by fasting, by feeding, by injury and by specific diseases of hormone deficiency or excess such as diabetes mellitus and Cushing's syndrome. The relationship of these pathways to protein and fat metabolism and the relative rates of anabolism and catabolism of these substances is similarly affected.

THERAPEUTIC IMPLICATIONS

It was this line of reasoning that led us to the use of insulin and glucose in an attempt to reduce the excessive protein breakdown of burned patients (Hinton et al, 1971). Attempts to use fructose on the grounds that its initial passage into cells and phosphorylation are insulin independent failed. This was due to the fact that no metabolite is insulin independent once it has entered the main pathways. Since hypercatabolic patients have a high rate of gluconeogenesis, it was found that the administration of fructose to burned patients merely resulted in a high blood glucose so that insulin had to be administered.

Insulin and Glucose Regime

The insulin and glucose regime was originally given as 50% glucose at a rate of 50 ml per hour. Sufficient insulin was added to each bottle of glucose to maintain the blood glucose in the range 100—180 mg/100 ml. It was found that hyper-catabolic patients sometimes required as much as 800 units of soluble insulin per litre of 50% glucose, whereas non-catabolic patients could only tolerate 100 to 120 units of insulin per litre. More recently we have adopted the practice of delivering the insulin via a separate line by constant infusion pump. This results in less insulin being absorbed onto bottles and tubing and hence rather lower doses being required. It has been found easy to titrate each patient's insulin requirements using Clinitest estimations on the urine to ensure 0—¼% glycosuria and Dextrostix estimations of blood glucose using the Ames Reflectance Meter to maintain a normal blood glucose. The insulin requirements of individual patients tend to remain fairly stable, although they may fall as the patient's condition improves. Nearly all patients were treated in an intensive care or high dependency area. No severe hypoglycaemic reactions have been seen during the eight years we have been employing this method. Sufficient potassium chloride was given to maintain normokalaemia. This has varied from 50 to 300mM of potassium per day according to the clinical situation. It should be emphasised that all patients were receiving a high nitrogen intake in the form of protein by mouth or amino acids intravenously. Insulin and glucose have been used to minimise nitrogen losses and are not a substitute for an adequate nitrogen intake. We have used the urea production rate as an index of protein catabolism. Moore has shown that four-fifths of waste nitrogen after injury is excreted as urea. An estimate of urea production rate may be obtained by measurement of the 24 hour urinary urea excretion with a correction for changes in body urea calculated from the change in blood urea multiplied by total body water (approximately 60% of body weight). Lee (1974) has shown that a clinically useful measurement of protein balance may be obtained as follows:

Protein catabolism = 24 hour urinary urea x 28/60 (28 = atomic weight of 2 molecules of nitrogen in urea; 60 = molecular weight of urea) x 5/4 (correction for total urinary nitrogen) x 6.25 (factor to convert g of nitrogen to g of protein = 24 hour urinary urea [g]) x 3.6. A correction is made for change in blood urea (g/litre) x total body water x 28/60 x 6.25.

Nitrogen and associated potassium losses were markedly less during the period of treatment, falling to a level at which it was possible to give sufficient protein to achieve a positive nitrogen balance. This is particularly important when we consider Professor Kinney's reminder that seriously ill patients can tolerate only up to 30% loss of body weight before death occurs on a nutritional basis. In burned patients this state may be reached within weeks, since metabolic rate and protein catabolism may be increased by 100%.

In a further study of the insulin and glucose regime we compared two groups of nine patients in each. The two groups were comparable in terms of age, weight, area of burn, blood transfused, diet and potassium supplements. The treated group however received insulin and glucose during the first fourteen days after injury and showed significantly lower urinary urea and potassium losses over this period. These studies did not distinguish the effect of insulin per se from the effect of glucose administration. It could be argued however that we would not have been able to give so much glucose in such severely ill patients without giving insulin as well. Without insulin, a severe hyperosmolar state would have been created. In order to divorce the effect of giving insulin from that of administering calories, my colleagues Dr Woolfson and Dr Heatley have compared two intravenous feeding regimes. Nitrogen intake was kept constant (1 litre Vamin daily = 9 g N) and the calorie source was alternated every three days between sorbitol and Intralipid in regime II and 50% glucose with insulin in regime I. A highly significant advantage was found for the insulin and glucose regime. It may be argued that this demonstrates the superiority of carbohydrate over fat as a protein sparing calorie source. On the other hand the content of carbohydrate in regime II was high, 400 g, including 300 g of sorbitol, 50 g of glucose, and 50 g of glycerol in the Intralipid. We have been attemping the experiment of administering enough glucose to keep the blood glucose at about 200 mg/

100 ml and comparing the protein sparing effect of this with the same amount of glucose with sufficient insulin to maintain the blood glucose at 60–80 mg/100 ml. Early results suggest that insulin does confer an additional advantage, but final conclusions must await completion of the study.

ELECTROLYTE CHANGES AFTER INJURY

A piece of serendipity was the observation of the effects of insulin on electrolyte chemistry (Hinton et al, 1971, 1973). Wilkinson et al (1949, 1950) and also Moore (1959) have described the sodium and water retention which occur after injury. At the same time there is an increase in potassium excretion owing chiefly to the release of potassium from cells as protein is broken down. With recovery, these situations are reversed and a sodium diuresis occurs. However, should complications arise, the sodium retention phase persists.

Our own observations on changes in the red cell sodium of injured patients are in keeping with those found in muscle cells by Flear (1970) and Bergström (1969). Following uncomplicated surgery red cell sodium was no different from the normal range. When identifiable complications, such as wound or chest infection occurred, red cell sodium was elevated but returned to normal as recovery took place. Raised levels were also found in burned patients. Some unpublished observations by Dr Hinton showed that insulin and glucose administration caused red cell sodium levels to fall to normal within twelve hours. Incubation of abnormal red cells in vitro with insulin and glucose failed to produce any change in red cell sodium concentration over four hours (Allison, unpublished).

It seems unlikely that the 'sick-cell' syndrome plays an important part in the majority of surgical patients with hyponatraemia. The dilutional effect of hypotonic fluid administration is more often the major cause of this phenomenon. When two litres of 0.18 per cent saline in 5% dextrose are given daily by the intravenous route, in spite of a persistent fall in plasma osmolality, the urine concentration remains high, because of the inability of injured patients to excrete a water load. Antidiuretic hormone secretion is elevated after surgery, although it is uncertain whether this is the sole cause of water retention after injury.

Sodium retention after injury may have several causes. Aldosterone secretion is increased (Zimmerman, 1955) and this may be exacerbated by any fall in renal perfusion due to fluid deficits. Changes in glomerular filtration and in distribution of blood flow within the kidney may, however, be more important. The importance of renal under-perfusion as a cause of sodium retention is illustrated by the effect of blood transfusion in promoting a sodium diuresis. These results are taken from a study (Hinton et al, 1972, 1973) on burned patients after the shock phase, in some cases many weeks after injury. Many such patients continually drift back into an underperfused state due not only to red cell deficits, but largely because of their inability to maintain compensatory expansion of plasma volume. In some patients glucose and insulin alone produced a sodium diuresis. In others who were hypovolaemic, blood transfusion had the same effect. In a third group insulin and glucose produced an additional effect only when blood volume had been expanded.

Summary and Conclusion

Following injury, insulin secretion is initially suppressed. This is followed by a period of insulin resistance. An alteration in balance between the anabolic hormone insulin and the catabolic hormones, catecholamines, cortisol and glucagon may be responsible for some of the metabolic changes after injury, in particular the high rate of gluconeogenesis from protein. Insulin administration may help to reverse these metabolic changes. This effect is additional to the provision of adequate carbohydrate calories. The reduction in protein catabolism and urea production rate is particularly striking and has been used to advantage in hypercatabolic states such as burns and acute renal failure. Insulin may also help to reverse the 'sick-cell' syndrome by restoring the sodium pump mechanism. The resulting sodium and water diuresis has been used to advantage in cases of burn injury, congestive heart failure, acute renal failure and malnutrition with fever.

References

Allison, SP (1971) Br. J. Anaesth., 43, 138
Allison, SP (1974) Brit. J. Hosp. Med., 11, 860
Allison, SP, Prowse, K and Chamberlain, MJ (1967) Lancet, i, 478
Allison, SP, Hinton, P and Chamberlain, MJ (1968) Lancet, ii, 1113
Allison, SP, Tomlin, PJ and Chamberlain, MJ (1969) Br. J. Anaesth., 41, 588
Allison, SP, Morley, CJ and Burns-Cox, CJ (1972) Br. Med. J., 3, 675
Ashmore, J and Weber, G (1968) In Carbohydrate Metabolism and its Disorders, Volume 1. (Ed) Dickens, Randle and Whelan. Academic Press, London and New York. Page 336
Bergström, J (1969) In Biological Basis of Medicine. (Ed) EE Bittar and N Bittar. Academic Press, London and New York. Volume 6, page 495
Birke, G, Duner, H, Liljedahl, S-O, Pernow, B, Plantin, LO and Troell, L (1957) Acta Chir. Scand., 114, 87
Browne, JSL, Schenker, V and Stevenson, JAF (1944) J.Clin. Invest., 23, 932
Coore, HG and Randle, PJ (1964) Biochem.J., 93, 66
Cope, C, Nathanson, IT, Rourke, GM and Wilson, H (1943) Ann.Surg., 117, 937
Cuthbertson, DP (1930) Biochem.J., 24, 2, 1244
Cuthbertson, DP (1932) Quart.J.Med., 25 (1,New Series), 233
Cuthbertson, DP (1942) Lancet, i, 433
Flear, CTG (1970) J.Clin.Path., 23, Suppl.4, 16
Hinton, P, Allison, SP, Littlejohn, S and Lloyd, J (1971) Lancet, i, 767
Hinton, P, Allison, SP, Farrow, S, Littlejohn, S and Lloyd, J (1972) Lancet, i, 913
Hinton, P, Allison, SP, Littlejohn, S and Lloyd, J (1973) Lancet, ii, 218
Kinney, JM, Duke, JH, Long, CL and Gump, FE (1970) J.Clin.Path, 23, Suppl.4, 65
Lee, HAA (1974) In Parenteral Nutrition in Acute Metabolic Illness. (Ed) HAA Lee. Academic Press, London and New York.

Majid, PA, Sharma, B, Meeran, MKN and Taylor, SH (1972) *Lancet, ii*, 937
Moore, FD (1959) In *The Metabolic Care of the Surgical Patient*. Saunders,
   Philadelphia
Porte, D, Graber, AL, Kurzuya, T and Williams, RH (1966) *J.Clin.Invest., 45*, 228
Ross, H, Johnston, IDA, Welborn, TA and Wright, AD (1966) *Lancet, ii*, 563
Samols, E and Marks, V (1965) *Lancet, i*, 462
Stoner, HB (1970) *J.Clin.Path., 23, Suppl.4*, 47
Wilkinson, AW (1973) In *Body Fluids in Surgery*. Churchill Livingstone,
   Edinburgh and London
Wilkinson, AW, Billing, BH, Nagy, G and Stewart, CP (1949) *Lancet, i*, 640
Wilkinson, AW, Billing, BH, Nagy, G and Stewart, CP (1950) *Lancet, ii*, 135
Wilmore, DW, Lindsey, CA, Moylan, JA, Faloona, GR, Pruitt, BA and Unger, RH
   (1974) *Lancet, i*, 73
Zimmerman, B, Casey. JH, Bloch, HS, Bickel, EY and Covrik, K (1955)
   Surg.Forum, 6, 3

Surgical Diagnosis, Patterns of Energy, Weight and Tissue Change

J M KINNEY

Department of Surgery, Columbia University College of Physicians and Surgeons, New York, USA

The metabolic response to major trauma and infection has traditionally been associated with weight loss, fatigue, weakness and variable degrees of starvation. Cuthbertson (1942) separated this response into the initial, or 'ebb' phase, lasting 24 to 48 hours, and the following 'flow' phase, lasting days to weeks. He suggested that the initial phase was one of depressed vitality, associated with efforts to stabilise cardiopulmonary function and to mobilise emergency supplies of tissue fuel. Survival was associated with the flow or catabolic phase where the weight loss and associated tissue depletion developed. Since these pioneering observations, the metabolic response to injury and infection has become accepted during the flow or catabolic phase as being one of resting hypermetabolism, increased nitrogen loss, glucose intolerance and increased fat mobilisation. This discussion will be devoted to a consideration of weight loss and its relationship to energy expenditure, protein breakdown, fat oxidation and the resultant tissue composition of weight loss. Measured increases in resting metabolism will be considered in the light of possible alterations in the overall energy flow of the patient with major injury or infection.

WEIGHT LOSS

Keys and co-workers (1950) conducted an extensive study of partial starvation during World War II, utilising young, adult males who served as volunteers. These subjects were placed on diets which provided approximately half of the predicted normal caloric needs and 50 g per day of low quality protein, in order to study the effects of partial starvation on wartime populations. The subjects lost 25% of their body weight and decreased their BMR an average of 40% over a 24-week

121

BASAL METABOLISM AND WEIGHT LOSS
IN PARTIAL STARVATION

(DAILY INTAKE = APPROXMATELY 1500 CALORIES WITH 50 GRAMS PROTEIN)

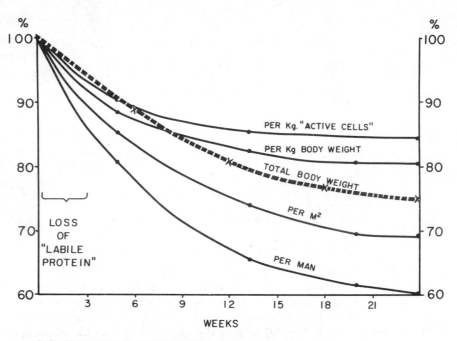

DATA FROM: BIOLOGY OF HUMAN STARVATION; KEYS AND OTHERS 1950

Figure 1. The basal metabolic rate (on the vertical scale) is shown over 24 weeks of partial starvation, when represented in four different ways. The loss of body weight is shown in a superimposed heavy dashed line (from Keys et al, 1950)

period (Figure 1). This study resulted in a two volume publication comparing the results obtained with information from over 2900 references on starvation in the world literature. The chapter on weight loss includes figures for estimated weight loss over three, six and twelve month intervals for individuals whose dietary intake is limited to various fractions of the caloric intake needed for equilibrium. These estimates are shown in Figure 2 as an important reference for considering the weight loss of surgical patients.

Routine loss of body weight can be thought of as the small losses of the intercurrent infection with temporary fever and anorexia, or the somewhat greater weight loss, commonly associated with uncomplicated surgical operation. The former might represent 2 to 4% of body weight, while the postoperative patient will commonly lose 4 to 8% of body weight (Kinney et al, 1968). There seems

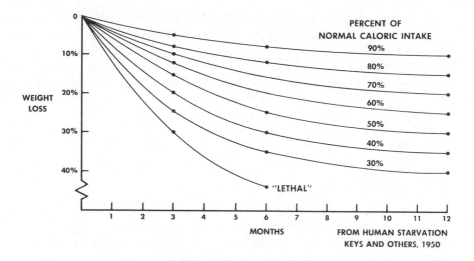

Figure 2. The estimated general magnitude of weight losses, as percentage of original body weight, resulting from subsistence on limited diets with caloric values expressed as per cent of intake needed for maintenance of normal weight (from Keys et al, 1950. Page 129)

to be a general acceptance among physicians of the idea that loss of up to 10% of body weight can be sustained without jeopardising convalescence. However, there is increasing evidence that the nitrogen loss, following injury and infection, is largely due to the breakdown of skeletal muscle protein. It is not surprising, therefore, that the last thing to return to normal in surgical convalescence is the ability to work a full day without fatigue. The weight loss and associated nitrogen deficit are usually complete within 10 to 14 days after operation. However, normal work capacity may not be restored for two months or longer, despite the weight loss being considered to be common and appropriate for the clinical problem. At the other extreme from these small and 'unimportant' ranges of weight loss are the most extreme losses which the human body can withstand before death from tissue depletion occurs, usually with lethal complications such as pulmonary infection, hepatic failure or upper GI haemorrhage. Reports from survivors with experiences in concentration camps includes various cases of 40 to 50% loss of body weight, usually developing over a period of eight months or longer (Keys et al, 1950). The civilian counterpart of this is anorexia nervosa. In this condition, three factors are thought to contribute to the extreme degree of weight loss which may reach 45 to 55% of normal body weight (Berkman et al, 1947). These factors are a gradual reduction in food intake with previously normal organ function; no major catabolic stimulus which would limit the adaptation to starvation; and limitation on water intake, as well as food intake, which might restrict the development of nutritional oedema. Therefore, the range of weight loss that is of the greatest surgical importance is between 10 to 40%.

123

It is our impression that weight loss can be serious, both because of its ultimate extent and because of the rapid rate of development seen in major catabolic states. Therefore, it seems reasonable to expect that the extent of weight loss which can be tolerated in major catabolism will be less than that which can be tolerated from partial starvation, without injury or sepsis. The most rapid rates of weight loss are seen in the young, heavily muscled male with good previous nutrition. Conversely, lesser degrees of weight loss are seen in the female, the elderly and the poorly nourished. Studley (1936) was among the first to attempt to correlate the degree of pre-operative weight loss, with post-operative mortality. He studied 46 patients undergoing operation for chronic ulcer disease and noted that the patients, with less than 20% of weight loss, had a post-operative mortality of 3.5% and that this was increased to 33% in the patients who had lost over 20% of their body weight. Loss of body weight beyond 30 to 35% may be considered precachexia. This degree of weight loss in a concentration camp would be followed by increasing trouble from weakness, decubitus ulcers and joint contractures. An equivalent degree of protein and fat depletion may occur in surgical patients without recognition of the severity of the problem because of the extracellular water retention which accompanies prolonged clinical care.

A project is under way in our department to examine the tissue composition of weight loss during periods of severe catabolic depletion. The weight loss of four previously healthy, young adult males is shown in Figure 3. They lost between 14 and 18% of their body weight in 3 weeks as a result of major injury and/or infection. The four severely catabolic patients showed an average loss of 0.8% of

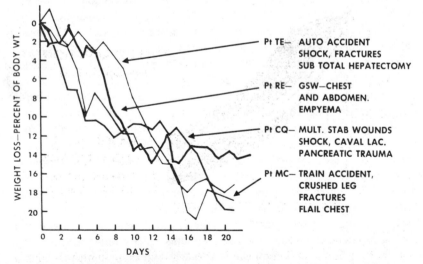

Figure 3. The weight loss of four previously healthy, young adult males as a result of severe injury and/or infection, while receiving calorie intake which averaged 40 to 60% of their caloric expenditure

124

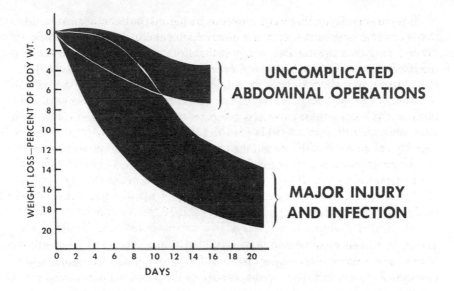

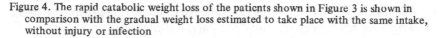

Figure 4. The rapid catabolic weight loss of the patients shown in Figure 3 is shown in comparison with the gradual weight loss estimated to take place with the same intake, without injury or infection

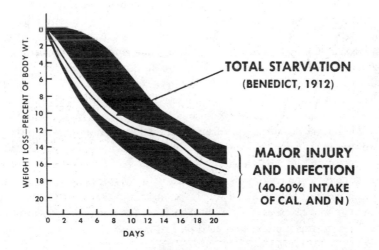

Figure 5. The weight in total starvation (Benedict, 1915) is shown to be in the same general range as the four severely catabolic patients shown in Figure 2, despite the latter patients receiving food intake amounting to 40 to 60% of their caloric expenditure during the weight loss

body weight per day (670 g/day) despite receiving a daily caloric intake which averaged between 40 and 60% of the measured expenditure over the 3 week period. Figure 4 compares their weight loss with that estimated by Keys et al (1950) for that level of partial starvation alone. It can be seen that the weight loss of these catabolic patients is roughly curvilinear as is that of partial starvation, but is approximately five-fold faster. The comparison of the range of catabolic weight loss for these patients is compared with the weight loss observed in Benedict's starvation study (1915) [Figure 5]. The similar weight loss in the partially fed catabolic patients and the totally starving subject prompted comparison of the protein composition of the weight loss in each case, which will be discussed later.

NITROGEN METABOLISM

The clinical impressions of muscle loss after injury were placed on a quantitative basis by the work of Cuthbertson (1931, 1932), who reported the increase in resting metabolism and the excretion of nitrogen, sulphur, phosphorus and creatine following long-bone fracture in man. These observations were extended by subsequent metabolic balance studies, which emphasised a negative nitrogen balance as the hallmark of the response to injury and infection. The work of Howard (1944), Browne (1944), Moore (1952) and their co-workers confirmed that the increased nitrogen excretion seemed to occur in proportion to the severity of the clinical problem. Efforts made by various investigators to improve the nutrition of acute surgical patients produced conflicting results (Moore, 1958). One opinion was that it was impossible to expect nitrogen utilisation at the height of the catabolic response, while others reported that the majority of the post-operative nitrogen loss was due to starvation (Abbott et al, 1959), rather than being the result of obligatory neuroendocrine responses. Only later was it established that a positive nitrogen balance could be approached and sometimes achieved in severe catabolic states with increasing nitrogen intake, though the increased nitrogen loss was not diminished by the nitrogen intake (Dudrick et al, 1970). Therefore, the advantage of nitrogen intake was in improving nitrogen balance, not in reducing the rate of protein breakdown, with its associated amino acid deamination and urea synthesis.

The large nitrogen excretions, associated with acute infection, were observed by various workers before World War I. Extensive nitrogen loss was particularly severe in typhoid fever, as reported by Shaffer (1908), who emphasised the extremely high nitrogen intake needed if one attempted to offset a large excretion rate. Peters (1948) reviewed this 'toxic destruction of protein' with infection and reported that there was no increase, and sometimes a decrease, in the levels of circulating amino acids at the time that nitrogen excretion was elevated. Biesel and co-workers (1967) performed detailed balance studies in experimental infections in man. They demonstrated a fall in circulating amino acids, following exposure to the typhoid organism, which occurred in advance of the febrile response. The significance of the protein breakdown after injury was initially thought to be associated with local protein destruction in the area of injury. Since this seemed to be an unlikely explanation for the increases which were largely in the form of urea, various workers suggested that protein breakdown occurred in response to the large increase in caloric expenditure. This also seemed unlikely because the amount of tissue fuel available from protein breakdown remained relatively small, while 80 to 90% of the total calorie needs were met from the oxidation of fat (Duke et al, 1970). Therefore, the suggestion was made that increased nitrogen loss was primarily to provide a supply of carbohydrate intermediates for various synthetic functions, which fatty acids could not supply in mammalian tissue (Kinney et al, 1970).

ENERGY EXPENDITURE

The original observations of Cuthbertson (1932) on long-bone fractures revealed a mild increase in resting oxygen consumption, which seemed to parallel the increase in daily nitrogen excretion. This work has been extended by the use of indirect calorimetry to establish a daily resting calorie balance in a variety of surgical conditions (Kinney et al, 1970a). These data have indicated that uncomplicated, elective operation does not produce any increase beyond approximately 10% of the pre-operative value; major fracture is followed by 15 to 30% increases for periods of 2 to 3 weeks; major sepsis, such as peritonitis, causes increases of 20 to 50%, and major third degree burns cause sustained increases of up to twice normal.

Dubois and co-workers (1924) conducted historic studies in the calorimetry of various clinical infections. From this work came the commonly quoted '7% rule', which states that the resting energy expenditure is increased 7% for each degree F rise in body temperature. Studies of the caloric equivalent of fever in surgical patients (Kinney & Roe, 1962; Roe & Kinney, 1965), revealed a considerable variation from the 7% rule (which was only an average value in the infection patients that were studied by DuBois). Depleted and elderly surgical patients demonstrated fever, with minimal increases in caloric expenditure, similar to the behaviour of chronic infection, such as pulmonary tuberculosis. These cases were in contrast to the extreme catabolism of infections, such as typhoid fever, where the increase in resting metabolism was higher than predicted by the 7% rule and appeared to be similar to the surgical catabolism of major peritonitis.

The major third degree burn represents an extreme example of sustained resting hypermetabolism. During the 1960s it was discovered that thermal damage to the skin removed the vapour barrier properties of the dermis and that a large insensible water loss could be demonstrated in burn patients. It was assumed that this major, uncontrolled route of evaporative cooling caused a stimulus to heat producing mechanisms in order to sustain a normal body heat content.

127

Evidence then appeared which indicated that abolishing the large evaporative heat loss from a burn by wrapping it with an impermeable plastic did not abolish the resting hypermetabolism (Zawacki et al, 1970). Other data showed a disassociation between a large insensible water loss and the increased metabolic rate during the first week following a major burn (Gump & Kinney, 1970b). Wilmore et al (1975) have utilised a special chamber for heat studies in burn patients and concluded that these burn patients behave much more as though they had too much interior heat, rather than responding to a surface which is too cold. These same workers have extended their studies to document the significantly higher ambient comfort temperature in the burn patient.

TISSUE COMPOSITION OF WEIGHT LOSS

The composition of weight loss can be studied by serial measurements of body composition or by cumulative balance studies. The latter approach indicates that total starvation in Benedict's subject (1915) caused a loss of 17% body weight in three weeks, with protein accounting for 12% of the weight loss. Iampetro et al (1961) studied partial and total starvation in soldiers exposed to cold

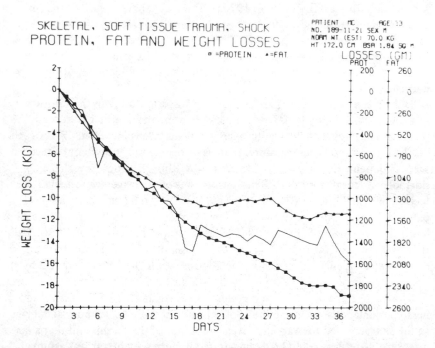

Figure 6. The losses of body weight, protein and fat of one of the patients shown in Figure 2, obtained by performing measurements of daily nitrogen and resting calorie balance

128

weather and found that in such cases the protein accounted for 10% of the weight loss over a 2-week period.

Each of the severely catabolic patients in Figure 2 received only isotonic peripheral glucose infusions until oral intake was begun, as tolerated, on the 3rd to 5th day after injury. Measurements of the daily resting calorie balance and nitrogen balance allowed calculation of the protein and fat content of the weight loss. Such data for one patient (M.C.), a 33-year old healthy male who sustained multiple fractures in a train accident, is presented in Figure 6.

Average values for the weight loss in 3 weeks of severe surgical catabolism were as follows: protein 12%, fat 13% and water, by difference, was 74% (Figure 7).

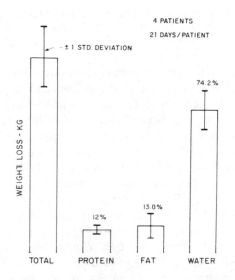

Figure 7. The contribution of protein and fat to the weight loss of the four severely catabolic patients, presented in Figure 2. The difference between the sum of the protein and fat loss and total weight loss is assumed to represent loss of body water

It is of particular interest that total starvation for this period resulted in the same range of weight loss, as the catabolic patients, with protein contributing 12.5% of the loss. However, the fat loss in total starvation contributed 33% of the weight loss, in contrast to 13% in the severely catabolic patients, receiving 40 to 60% caloric intake. Thus, it appears that the food intake which the catabolic, surgical patients received did more to protect their body fat, than their protein stores.

POSSIBLE FACTORS IN SURGICAL HYPERMETABOLISM

The evidence for increased energy metabolism with injury or infection, is based on the sustained increase in oxygen consumption and CO_2 production of the

129

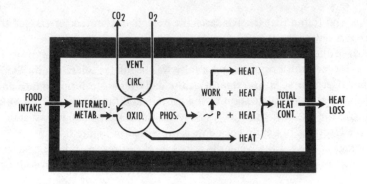

Figure 8. The human body can be represented in schematic fashion, as an energy exchange device. The overall energy flow can be increased because of primary alterations in successive steps in this sequence. See text for details

resting patient. Such increases are not possible (except for temporary and limited changes in body gas stores), unless there is increased oxidation of foodstuffs. Overall energy exchange is obviously a series of interlocking states, beginning with the intake of energy in chemical bonds of foodstuffs (Figure 8). This intake is intermixed with other organic molecules in the pathways of intermediary metabolism. The net result of these interconversions is the contribution of each foodstuff to a final fuel mixture which is oxidised in the TCA cycle. This oxidation produces high energy phosphate bonds, the 'energy currency' of the body, as well as considerable heat. The high energy phosphate bonds are then available for various kinds of tissue and organ work. All of this work except for mechanical work done on the environment, is then realised as an addition to body heat, whenever a steady state exists. It has been assumed that body heat content should remain unchanged. It is worthwhile to consider the various ways in which alterations in the energy sequence might result in resting hypermetabolism.

The hypermetabolism of surgical catabolic states might be considered to arise because of alterations in any of the following categories:

1) Intermediary metabolism:	Protein turnover
	Specific dynamic action
	Gluconeogenesis
	Triglyceride turnover
2) Utilisation of high energy bonds:	Increased demand for work
	Reduced work efficiency
3) Heat metabolism:	Fever
	Increased heat losses

4) Abnormal 'setting' of hypothalamic centre

Alterations in intermediary metabolism could theoretically be associated with increased rates of oxidation without a corresponding increase in high energy bond production. Evidence for these changes will be discussed in another article, parti-

130

cularly in association with nitrogen metabolism. There is extensive qualitative evidence to suspect both an increase in absolute demand for organ work (such as an increase in minute ventilation and cardiac output) or decreased organ efficiency (such as increased dead space ventilation or increased 'shunting' of blood flow) in major catabolic states. Unfortunately, the quantitative significance of these changes remains uncertain. The increased metabolism of fever is well accepted but whether this represents a general stimulus to many chemical reactions or whether it is linked to certain reactions which may be depressed selectively with weight loss, remains to be studied. Evidence from Wilmore et al (1975a) is turning attention from the role of heat loss through the burned skin to the possibility of hypothalamic centres being reset in a way that may be stimulating hypermetabolism secondarily in each of the categories mentioned above.

Future studies of hypermetabolic patients, aimed at elucidating which steps in energy exchange have undergone primary changes, will be needed to guide rational therapy.

NITROGEN INTAKE AND NITROGEN BALANCE

The relationships between energy expenditure and nitrogen metabolism are poorly understood, hence the proper calorie intake to achieve nitrogen balance on a given nitrogen intake remains indefinite. However, the goal of acute surgical nutrition is the protection or restoration of the body cell mass, which must

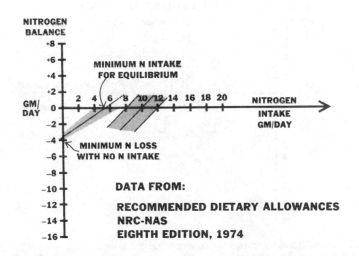

Figure 9. The influence of nitrogen intake on nitrogen balance is shown as the minimum nitrogen intake for equilibrium and as the minimum nitrogen loss with zero intake. The range of average dietary intake is presented for comparison

131

start by seeking the nitrogen balance which is considered optimal for a given condition. Figure 9 shows the minimum nitrogen loss to be expected on a zero intake and the minimum nitrogen intake needed for equilibrium in the average normal adult male. Data from Soroff et al (1961) is summarised in Figure 10 to illustrate the extremely high intakes of nitrogen found by these workers to be

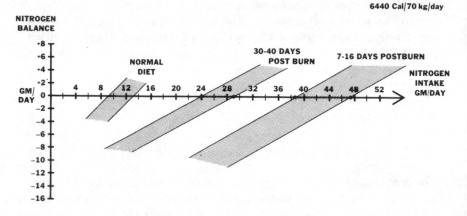

Figure 10. The extreme alterations caused by a major burn on the relation of nitrogen intake to nitrogen balance (Data from Soroff et al, 1961)

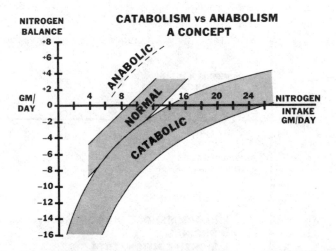

Figure 11. The diagram represents the concept that the catabolic influence of injury and infection causes the influence of nitrogen intake on nitrogen balance to be shifted to the right in a curvilinear fashion. The suggestion is made that the depleted patient may show an anabolic curve in the opposite direction from normal. (Redrawn from Trémolières, 1970)

needed for nitrogen equilibrium during the acute post-burn phase. Each burn patient received high caloric intakes (3500 Cal/m²/day) throughout the study. Trémolières (1970) has presented a modified concept of catabolic nitrogen loss which is shown in Figure 11. In this concept the catabolic nitrogen loss on varying intake is moved to higher levels of intake for a given nitrogen balance, but the relationship is considered to be curvilinear. If this is supported in future studies, it would lend support to the concept of using peripheral amino acids alone as proposed by Blackburn et al (1973). Thus the moderate intake of amino acids which is possible by peripheral vein would achieve a higher proportion of nitrogen retention than would be predicted if the relationship of intake to balance were a linear one.

Summary

The clinical response to major injury and infection commonly includes weight loss, fatigue, weakness and varying degrees of starvation. The associated metabolic response in the 'flow' or catabolic phase involves resting hypermetabolism, increased nitrogen loss, glucose intolerance and increased fat mobilisation. Analysis of sustained weight loss in such patients has revealed that protein loss accounts for 10-12% of the weight loss. Evidence is presented to suggest that the proportion of protein in weight loss is similar in total starvation and in patients with major injury and infection who are receiving 40 to 60% of the calories and nitrogen which they appear to be metabolising. Factors which may contribute to the resting hypermetabolism of injury and infection, need to be separated for future study into alterations in intermediary metabolism, energy use for organ and tissue work, and alterations in heat metabolism and body temperature.

References

Abbott, EE, Levey, S and Kreiger, H (1959) *Metabolism, 8,* 847
Beisel, WR, Sawyer, WD, Ryll, ED and Crozier, D (1967) *Ann. intern. Med., 67,* 744
Benedict, FG (1915) *Washington Publ. No. 203,* 521
Berkman, JM, Weir, JF and Kepler, EJ (1947) *Gastroenterol., 9,* 357
Blackburn, GL, Flatt, JP, Clowes, GHA and O'Donnell, TE (1973) *Amer. J. Surg., 125,* 447
Browne, JSL, Schenker, V and Stevenson, JAF (1944) *J. Clin. Invest., 23,* 932
Cuthbertson, DP (1931) *Biochem. J., 251,* 245
Cuthbertson, DP (1942) *Lancet, i,* 443
DuBois, EF (1924) *Basal Metabolism in Health and Disease.* Lea & Febiger, Philadelphia and New York
Dudrick, SJ, Steiger, E, Long, JM and Rhoads, JE (1970) *Surg. Clin. N. America, 50,* 1031
Duke, JH, Jørgensen, SB, Broell, JR, Long, CL and Kinney, JM (1970) *Surgery, 68,* 168

Gump, FE and Kinney, JM (1970) *Surg. Clin. N. America, 50,* 1235

Howard, JE, Parson, W, Stein, KE, Eisenberg, H and Reidt, V (1944) *Johns Hopk. Hosp. Bull., 75,* 156

Iampietro, PF, Goldman, RF, Mager, M and Bass, DE (1961) *J. Appl. Physiol., 76,* 624

Keys, A, Brozek, J, Henschel, A, Mickelson, O and Taylor, HL (1950) *The Biology of Human Starvation, Vol.I.* University of Minnesota, North Central Publishing Co

Kinney, JM and Roe, CF (1962) *Ann. Surg., 156,* 610

Kinney, JM, Long, CL, Gump, FE and Duke, JH (1968) *Ann. Surg., 168,* 459

Kinney, JM, Long, CL and Duke, JH (1970) In *Energy Metabolism in Trauma.* (Ed) R Porter and J Knight. J & A Churchill, London

Kinney, JM, Duke, JH, Long, CL and Gump, FE (1970) *J. Clin. Pathol., 23 Suppl. (Royal College of Pathology),* 4

Moore, FD and Ball, MR (1952) *The Metabolic Response to Surgery.* Charles C Thomas, Springfield, Illinois

Moore, FD (1958) *Canadian Med. Ass. J., 788,* 85

Peters, JP (1948) *Amer. J. Med., 5,* 100

Roe, CF and Kinney, JM (1965) *Ann. Surg., 161,* 140

Shaffer, PA (1908) *JAMA, L I,* 12

Soroff, HS, Pearson, E, Arney, GK and Artz, CP (1961) *Surg., Gynec., Obstet., 112,* 425

Studley, HO (1936) *JAMA, 106,* 458

Trémolières, J (1970) Quoted in *Parenteral Nutrition.* (Ed) HC Meng and HL David. Charles C Thomas, Springfield, Illinois

Wilmore, DW, Mason, AD, Johnson, DW et al (1975) *J. Appl. Physiol., 38,* 593

Wilmore, DW, Orcutt, TW, Mason, AD and Pruitt, BA (1975a) *J. Trauma, 15,* 697

Zawacki, BE, Spitzer, KW, Mason, AD et al (1970) *Ann. Surg., 171,* 236

Weight Loss and Calorimetry Studies Following Injury

J R RICHARDS, J K DRURY and R G BESSENT

University Department of Surgery, Royal Infirmary; Institute of
Physiology, University of Glasgow and WSHB Department of Clinical
Physics and BioEngineering, Glasgow, Scotland

Introduction

The views of Cairnie et al (1957) on the importance of post-injury protein catabolism were challenged by Caldwell (1970), who examined the effect of bilateral
femur fracture in rats using a gradient layer calorimeter. Caldwell found that the
increased rate of urinary nitrogen excretion in his rats could not account for
more than 35% of the increase in rate of heat production on the second day after
fracture, and less than that on the other days. Direct comparison of these studies
was impossible because of differences in experimental design. Cairnie et al made
continuous calorimetry and urinary nitrogen studies on a group of nine rats,
housed individually but put together in the chamber at 19°C. In Caldwell's experiments rats housed individually at 25°C were studied individually in a calorimeter at 28°C for two 30-minute periods daily and estimates made of how closely
this represented true resting metabolic energy. Under these conditions bilateral
femur fracture resulted in 10-20% increases in heat production due to increased
sensible heat loss. In the rat, the significance of protein catabolism after injury
still remained unsettled, although studies by Caldwell alone (1962), and with
others (1959, 1966), on rats with 30% body surface area full thickness burns
had shown that protein catabolism by itself could not provide the increased
energy required after burning.

It was left to the human studies of Kinney (1959) and Kinney et al (1968,
1970a, 1970b) and others (Duke et al, 1970) to establish beyond doubt that
nitrogen loss after injury occurred for reasons other than to supply extra calories
directly. Kinney and his group concentrated on the notion that any metabolic
behaviour thought to occur after injury must account for the extent of the weight

loss which is commonly observed. Using an indirect calorimetry system Kinney et al (1964) measured the increased calorie requirements after injury in man, and the contribution to them made by protein breakdown. Pre-operative studies in patients undergoing elective surgery indicated that 15% of their total caloric expenditure was derived from protein. Post-operatively, protein (or amino acids) contributed only 12-22% of the caloric expenditure, even in severe injury when the nitrogen excretion per day was significantly increased. Kinney noted, in common with many other investigators, that the rate of post-injury weight loss was parallel to the extent of the negative nitrogen losses. He pointed out that fat is anhydrous, supplies 9 kcal g^{-1} and is a high energy fuel source, whereas protein in its hydrated state in lean body tissue supplies only 1 kcal g^{-1} and is a relatively low energy fuel source. Therefore, although sizeable weights of lean body tissue might be lost after injury, the calorie contribution from this low energy source remained a small proportion of the total energy balance. Kinney felt that the extreme weight loss of injury was not due to substantial needs for fuel, but that the body was meeting a proportion of the increase in energy demands with a relatively low energy, high weight fuel, protein, and most of the calorie deficit was being met by oxidation of fat. This would appear at first sight to be a wasteful and inefficient method of meeting the energy challenge of injury both in evolutionary terms and in terms of the available energy reserves. Explanation of the nitrogen loss after injury must be sought in alterations of intermediary metabolic pathways, other than in the final fuel mixture for oxidation.

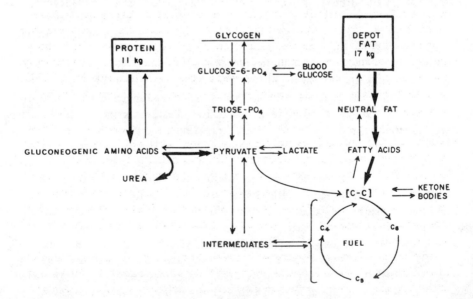

Figure 1. Metabolic fuel pathways

136

In a 70 kg man, the body fat store (shown in Figure 1 as 24% of the total weight) is the largest available energy supply. Protein stores are smaller and are intimately associated with the body cell mass, a large loss of which would seriously impair the ability to withstand the effects of injury. Total carbohydrate stores are small, providing less than 1,500 kcal, and amount to less than 1% of body weight.

The metabolic pathways in Figure 1 have been simplified to illustrate that most amino acids yield carbohydrate intermediates, or are 'glucogenic' on deamination. Kinney et al (1970b) stated that in the metabolic fuel 'mixture' of lower mammals and injured man there is a continuous requirement for carbohydrate intermediates for synthetic purposes, for which deamination of amino acids is the primary endogenous source. While two-carbon units are readily available from adipose tissue and are utilised as the major energy source in most tissues after injury, fatty acids cannot be used directly to yield a net gain of carbohydrate intermediates, glucose or glycogen (Coleman, 1969). Therefore, after injury, body fat can be utilised to provide the bulk of additional caloric needs, but protein is the only significant supply of carbohydrate intermediates.

Studies of metabolism after injury in man are further complicated by the effects of the starvation to which injured patients have been subjected in the past. In starvation, Cahill (1970) has shown that gluconeogenesis from amino acids is progressively reduced to conserve body protein for long-term survival, in sharp contrast to the changes observed after injury. The factors leading to this pattern of metabolic alteration after injury can be understood only when accurate quantitative analysis of bodily substrate changes can be made and related to overall alterations in heat production, nitrogen losses, oxygen consumption and other readily measured parameters. For such studies we selected the rat as a useful analogue for man. Because of conflicting evidence from the early rat studies of Cuthbertson et al (1939) and his co-workers (Cairnie et al, 1957), and the later findings of Caldwell (1970), the original rat data was reviewed in the light of Kinney's patient studies.

Cutherbertson found that in 9 days after fracture of the femur, 17 g of body weight was lost. The urinary nitrogen output was increased by 0.425 g compared with the basal value and if all the weight lost was entirely protein it would account for 0.522 g nitrogen (Figure 2). These observations led Cuthbertson to conclude that the source of post-injury weight loss during the first 9 days was mainly accounted for by loss of protein. This is inconsistent with Kinney's later data on man (Kinney et al, 1970b), which indicates that fat is the major factor in body weight loss.

We report a further rat injury study carried out in our laboratory to investigate the reason for this apparent discrepancy between rat and man. In relating urine nitrogen losses to protein metabolism, the following simple premise was used:

137

Urine N + Faecal N = Dietary N + (Catabolism − Anabolism)
Hence −

$\triangle$ Urine N = $\triangle$ Protein Catabolism − $\triangle$ Protein Anabolism + $\triangle$ Dietary N
    − $\triangle$ Faecal N.

Changes in urine nitrogen will therefore reflect changes in protein turnover rate only if diet and faecal losses remain constant (Waterlow & Alleyne, 1971).

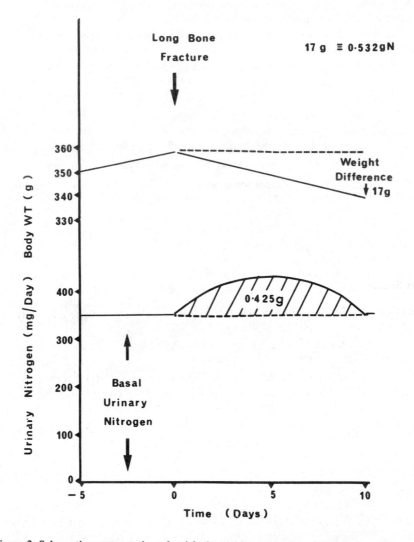

Figure 2. Schematic representation of weight loss and excess urinary nitrogen excretion following long bone fracture in rats (Cuthbertson et al, 1939)

EXPERIMENTAL

Methods (A)

A purpose-built animal and laboratory unit was created within the Institute of Physiology, University of Glasgow. Unwanted experimental variation was minimised wherever possible (Richards & Drury, 1976).

1. Inbred closed colony young adult male Wistar rats were used exclusively.
2. The rats were maintained in single cages housed within a soundproof environmental chamber kept at $20°C \pm 0.5°C$.
3. Special handling techniques were developed to lessen rat psychological and physical stresses.
4. A standard injury was devised, viz, a 25% body surface area (BSA) whole-skin thickness burn of the dorsum of the rat which enabled the reproduction of a uniform burn from rat to rat. Controls were subjected to the same anaesthetic procedures as the burned animals.
5. Rats were fed only an ultra low residue 19% protein diet to decrease faecal bulk and hence faccal nitrogen losses.
6. Almost constant intake of food and hence nitrogen was achieved by using an ad libitum −6% feeding regime.

Routine biochemical analyses were performed in the Department of Pathological Biochemistry at Glasgow Royal Infirmary. Nitrogen was estimated using a modification of Fleck's (1967) method. Carcase analysis was performed in the Department of Biochemistry, Western Infirmary, Glasgow, using a modification of Shaw's (1973) method.

Results (A)

The effect of a 25% whole thickness dorsal burn on the food intake and body weight of rats kept in our controlled environment is shown in Figure 3.

The data represent the mean ± standard deviation of 5 burn rats and 5 controls. Food intake is little affected by the burn, except for a two-day reduction in the immediate post-burn period. Thereafter the use of an ad libitum −6% regime has resulted in an almost constant nitrogen intake for both burn and control rats. Rate of weight gain in the controls was unaffected by this slight restriction in nitrogen intake save for the weight loss associated with the two-day post-burn period, during which controls were pair-fed with the burn group.

The burned rats by contrast displayed a marked fall in body weight despite a constant nitrogen intake over the post-burn period. The rate of weight loss was not constant. There was an initial rapid phase of weight loss followed by a more prolonged interval during which rat body weight remained steady. This was terminated around the 15th to the 17th post-burn day by another phase of more rapid weight loss which persisted to the end of the experimental period. Nitrogen balance studies were carried out also in both groups. The results for daily urinary

139

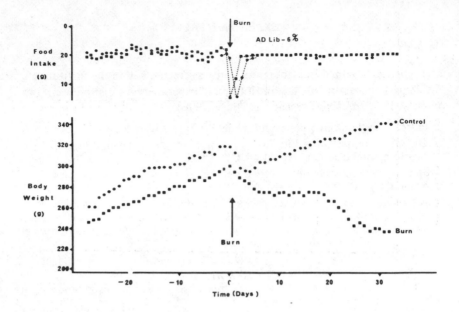

Figure 3. Daily dietary intake and body weight changes for rats subjected to 25% BSA burn and for pair-fed controls

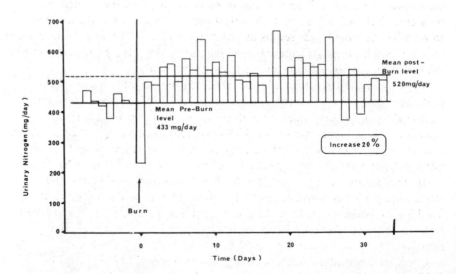

Figure 4. Daily urinary nitrogen excretion for rats subjected to 25% BSA burn

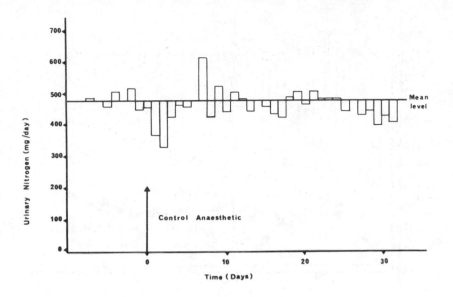

Figure 5. Daily urinary nitrogen excretion for pair-fed control rats anaesthetised only

nitrogen losses are shown in Figures 4 and 5, and enable ready comparison with the findings of Cuthbertson et al (1939).

After injury there was an increase of 20% in mean daily urinary nitrogen losses but there was no significant increase in nitrogen losses in the control group. If these results are related directly to loss of body weight, then the burned rats apparently lost 24.7 ± 2.6 g of body weight per g of excess urine nitrogen loss above basal. Calculating the results of Cuthbertson et al (1939) in a similar manner revealed that, in their rats with unilateral femur fracture, 30.2 ± g of body weight were shed per g of excess urine nitrogen lost above basal.

These figures apparently clearly indicated that the weight loss after injury could be accounted for entirely on the basis of protein breakdown. However, carcase analysis was performed on both groups in our study and the results equally clearly indicate that at least 30-40 g of body fat are lost in the burn group over the experimental period. The nitrogen data were re-examined and partial nitrogen balances (daily dietary intake — urine losses) plotted (Figure 6). Previous experiments indicated that with the low residue diet used in our study faecal nitrogen losses remained relatively constant before and after injury at 5 ± 3% of the total losses. In contrast to the findings in humans, nitrogen balance remained positive after burn injury in the rat, even after allowing for slightly restricted food intake and the addition of estimated likely faecal losses.

Confirmation of this finding was sought by examining data published by Caldwell in 1962 on a similar burn study in rats kept at 20°C ambient temperature.

141

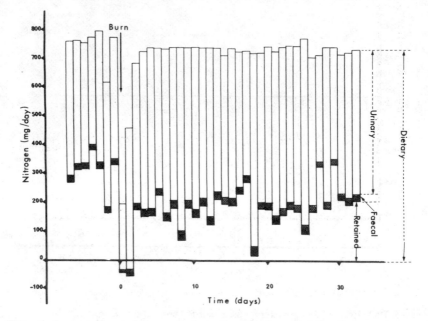

Figure 6. Average nitrogen balances for burned group of rats, showing dietary, urinary and estimated faecal contributions

Despite a statement in the conclusion of his paper to the contrary, Caldwell's published results indicated that his burned rats also remained in overall positive nitrogen balance, even after suffering a 30% BSA dorsal burn, and being supplied with a restricted dietary intake. This then represented a major point of difference in response to injury between the laboratory rat and man, in whom significant negative nitrogen balance has been documented following similar injuries.

Further, the relationship between excess urinary nitrogen excretion above basal and the post-injury weight loss, gave a good estimation of protein losses in man but was misleading in the injured rat, since it failed completely to account for the large quantities of body fat lost by the rat. The rat, unlike man, never reaches a definitive adult size, but continues to grow throughout its life and continues to retain nitrogen and remain in strongly positive nitrogen balance (Elder, 1975). In this way the rat is probably equivalent in this respect to the growing human child. In the rat basal urine nitrogen losses are not good indicators of nitrogen balance. In the analysis of weight lost after injury in a growing rat, one must account for not only the difference in weight between the pre- and post-injury weights, but also for the weight not gained as a result of failure to grow, as compared with the weight gain of the identically fed control rats.

Thus, the problem remained of relating changes in body weight, food and hence nitrogen intake and urinary nitrogen losses after injury in a way which was consistent with the experimental observations in our own and in other laboratories.

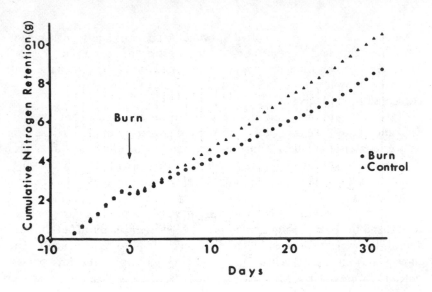

Figure 7. Cumulative nitrogen retention. Mean values for burned and control group of rats

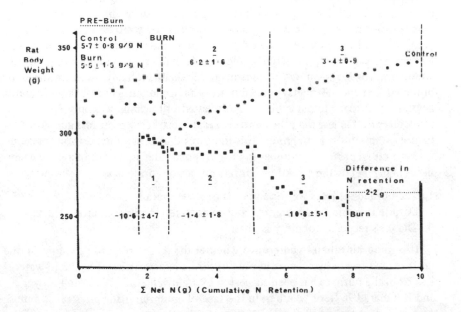

Figure 8. Weight change versus cumulative nitrogen retention for burned and control rats, showing mean values of weight increase per gram of retained nitrogen for each phase

143

Initially the data were re-plotted showing the effect of injury on cumulative nitrogen retention (dietary nitrogen — urinary nitrogen) against time (Figure 7). This indicated that, while the burned rats retained less nitrogen than the controls, the difference was not marked. This was in contrast to the marked body weight changes shown in Figure 3.

If the rat is growing normally, it retains nitrogen and puts on body weight. The ratio between weight gain and nitrogen retention is a measure of the efficiency of conversion of dietary nitrogen into body tissue which should not change if the animal's metabolism is normal. An indication of changed metabolism is, therefore given by plotting body weight against cumulative nitrogen retention, as shown in Figure 8.

In the pre-burn phase, all the animals gain weight steadily as nitrogen is retained, and the control animals continue to do so after the burn, but the burned animals lose weight consistently while still retaining nitrogen (Figure 8). The three phases which are labelled correspond in time course to the three phases noted in Figure 3. Phase I is a period of rapid weight loss. Phase II is characterised by very slow weight change, and Phase III by return to a much more rapid rate of body weight loss at around the 15th to the 17th post-burn day. It is important to note that for each of these post-burn phases, nitrogen retention continues. Hence, in the pre-burn period, controls gained 5.7 ± 0.8 g of body weight per g of nitrogen retained and this continued after the anaesthetic. Burned rats gained 5.5 ± 1.5 g of body weight per g of nitrogen retained. In Phase I post-burn, burned rats lost 10.6 ± 4.7 g of body weight per g nitrogen retained. In Phases II and III burned rats lost 1.4 ± 1.8 g and 10.8 ± 5.1 g of body weight per g of nitrogen retained, respectively.The slight fall in rate of growth per g of retained nitrogen shown by the controls in Phase III probably indicates the effect of the ad libitum -6% dietary restriction used. In the burned rats, the cumulative amount of nitrogen retained by the 35th day after burning, was only 2.2 g of nitrogen (or 20%) less than the controls despite marked weight loss and growth failure overall in the burn group. This indicates that protein deposition (presumably structural protein) continues in the burned rat, the bulk of its increased energy needs being met by the breakdown of fat and carbohydrate stores. In summary —

1. The burned rat loses weight and fails to grow overall.
2. Despite this, the rat apparently continues to retain nitrogen after injury.
3. The rat's response to injury is phasic.

It is important then to determine whether the phasic response to injury in the rat is related to phasic changes in the physical characteristics of heat and water loss from the burn, as has been suggested by Caldwell et al (1959) and Moyer and Butcher (1967), or whether, in the face of an unremitting physical stimulus such as a burn wound, the phasic changes in the rat's response are related to endogenous alterations in the metabolic fuel mixture or energy substrate stores available to the rat, as has been suggested by Kinney et al (1970b).

144

Methods (B)

Small animal calorimetry was performed on a parallel group of experimental rats to those described in the previous section. As far as possible, all rats were similar, both in phenotype at the onset of the experiment, and in methods of handling and other experimental details. The design, construction and use of the calorimetry system is fully described elsewhere (Carter et al, 1975; Carter et al, 1976).

Only calorimetric or energetic values based on direct measurements are reported. No assumptions have been introduced regarding the caloric value of oxygen consumed.

Results (B)

Figure 9 clearly shows that the burned rats lose significantly more total heat per day than do the control animals. In addition to increased sensible heat losses in the burned animals their rate of insensible (or evaporative) heat loss was increased compared with controls.

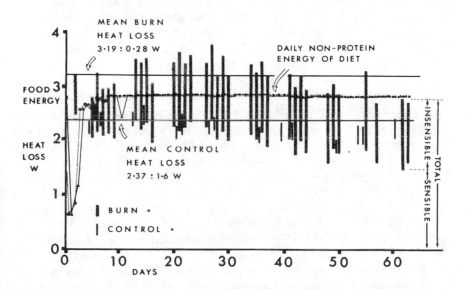

Figure 9. Mean values of sensible and insensible heat losses for burned and control groups of rats, together with daily non-protein energy of diet

Insensible Heat Losses

Burn Group	1.18 ± 0.19 W
Control Group	0.28 ± 0.05 W

145

The source of this increased evaporative loss is due to breakdown of the epidermal keratin water barrier in the burned skin area (Moyer & Butcher, 1967). The heat loss pattern which results as a consequence of suffering a 25% (whole skin thickness) burn is a sustained and unremitting increase in losses, mainly evaporative, which extends well beyond the 35th post-burn day (shown in Figure 9).

There are no phasic increases, as described after a similar rat burn experiment by Caldwell et al (1959). The phasic changes in rat body weight previously noted in Figure 3 must therefore be due to alterations in substrate availability within the burned animal in order to meet the sustained increase in heat loss after a burn.

Discussion

The daily non-protein energy of the diet of burned and control groups is also shown in Figure 9. Burned rats are consistently in negative heat balance, whilst controls remain in positive heat balance. As the burned rats must maintain body temperature, the heat deficit must be met from the energy released by catabolising the animals' tissue stores. Conversely, the heat surplus of the control animals must represent that heat required to bring about synthesis of new tissues (or more simply, growth) which is essentially an endothermic reaction. Relating the positive heat balance of the control animals to their daily weight gain shows average energy requirements of 3.7 kcal per g of weight gain.

A good indication of the nature of the tissue which is consumed to make up the dietary heat deficit in the burned animals may be obtained from its calorific content. The daily heat deficit of each animal is obtained directly from the calorimetry and dietary data. However, some care is needed in defining the corresponding body weight loss of the burned animals. As pointed out earlier, the control rats, after a sharp drop in weight for two days post-burn, due to pair-feeding, continued to gain weight steadily. It is therefore clearly incorrect to compare weight at any given point post-burn directly with the animal's weight immediately pre-burn, and some attempt must be made to include weight not put on by the burned animal as well as weight actually lost. The estimate is made from the nitrogen data of the control animals. The average rate of weight gain per g of retained nitrogen (total dietary nitrogen − total urinary nitrogen) is calculated for the control animals in the 'post-burn' period. After the burn, the burned animals continue to retain nitrogen (though at a lower daily rate than the controls). We suggest that this retained nitrogen is converted into structural tissue despite the effects of the injury. We also assume that the ratio between nitrogen retention and increase in weight of structural tissue is the same as for the control animals. Thus, for each burned animal the total retained nitrogen is calculated for each post-burn phase. These values, when multiplied by the factor obtained from the control animals, give the weights of structural tissue put on in

146

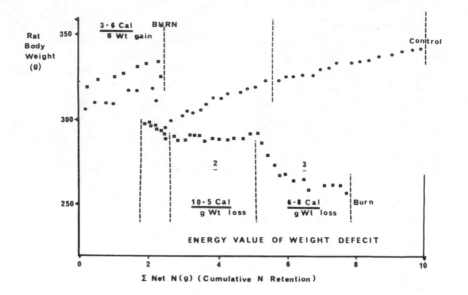

Figure 10. Weight changes versus cumulative nitrogen retention for burned and control rats, showing mean calculated caloric equivalents of weight lost or gained in each phase

each phase. Since the burned animal's weight actually fell, this amount is more than compensated for by the loss of some other tissue. Thus, the total weight loss of this other tissue is equal to the actual body weight loss plus the calculated gain in structural tissue weight for each phase. The calorific value of tissue consumed in each phase is calculated from these results, and the total dietary heat deficit for each phase (Figure 10).

The high energy value and relatively low weight of the tissue catabolised during Phase II post-burn is consistent with combustion of mainly fat stores, whereas the lower energy value and relatively greater weight of tissue lost during the third post-burn phase is in keeping with breakdown of increasing amounts of protein.

Partial carcase analysis was carried out to confirm or refute the above hypothesis. The following results were obtained:

Controls (mean of 4 rats)		35 Days Post-Burn (mean of 5 rats)
Pelt weight	60.6 ± 10.1 g	29.5 ± 2.2 g
Perinephric fat	6.2 ± 1.9 g	0.7 ± 0.2 g
	66.8 ± 11.8 g	30.0 ± 2.2 g

More detailed carcase analysis showed that most of the lost pelt weight was due to loss of fat.

The burned rat therefore appears to utilise only body fat as an energy source

147

during the early phase of its metabolic response to burning, while continuing to conserve body protein. The increase in urinary nitrogen losses which is seen during the early phase of the rat's burn response results from the provision of two-carbon intermediates from the Kreb's cycle by breakdown of small amounts of protein. Only when fat tissue stores are nearing total depletion is protein utilised as an energy source more directly to meet the burned rat's continuing heat deficit.

It was anticipated that the continuing energy deficit noted in the burned animals would ultimately result in death when their tissue energy stores were exhausted. Energy balance studies were accordingly continued beyond the 35th post-burn day in order to assess the extent of the burned animals' tissue reserves. A number of rats continued to lose body weight daily and died between the 40th and 50th post-burn days. Unexpectedly, a number of animals showed no further

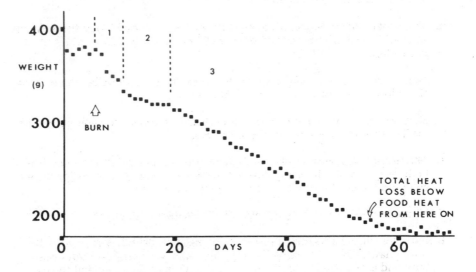

Figure 11. Long term weight loss of burned rat

body weight loss after the 50th post-burn day, and survived beyond the 65th post-burn day, at which point the experiment was ended (Figure 11). Total heat losses in the burned animals fell after the 35th post-burn day due to a decrease in sensible heat losses because of the reduction in the metabolic cell mass or body size of the animal. Insensible heat losses continued unabated. By the 50th post-burn day, total heat losses in the burned animals were less than the non-protein food heat available to the animal, and there was no further weight loss.

It is interesting to note that whilst further weight loss ceased when the burned animal was in heat balance, growth or weight gain did not take place, and presumably would not do so until the rat was in significant positive heat balance.

148

This is clearly seen in Figure 10 where the energy required to ensure weight gain is 3.8 kcal of energy supplied per gram of weight fained.

Summary

1. The experimental rat on ad libitum food is a continually growing animal in significantly positive nitrogen balance. At a body weight of 250-300 g it gains 5.6 g body weight for each g of nitrogen retained. The energy required for normal growth is 3.7 kcal per g of body weight gained. Failure to grow as well as actual weight loss must be considered in assessing the results of injury.

2. Following a 25% BSA full thickness burn, the insensible heat loss of the rat at 20°C increases by over 300%. Largely due to this, the total heat losses amount to more than can be supplied by a low-residue diet of 6% less than ad lib for the unburned animal.

3. To maintain body temperature, the animal must catabolise body tissue simply to provide heat. This manifests itself as a loss of body weight in which three phases may be identified.

4. From partial carcase analysis and estimates of the calorific value, the primary tissue lost is identified as fat rather than protein.

5. However, some protein breakdown is necessary to provide carbohydrate intermediates for the operation of the Krebs cycle.

6. The relationship between the resulting increase in urinary nitrogen and loss of body weight which appears to identify the tissue lost as protein is fortuitous and does not exist if point 1 above is taken into account.

7. Nitrogen continues to be retained even after severe burn injury.

8. Fat is lost during the second post-burn phase and weight loss is small. The third phase of much more rapid weight loss supervenes at 15-17 days post-burn and is tentatively identified with exhaustion of fat stores and the catabolism of an increasing proportion of lean body protein.

9. If the animal survives this greater weight loss, its body cell mass can fall sufficiently to reduce the total heat loss to less than that supplied by the diet, by reduction of the sensible heat loss. Weight loss then ceases.

Application to Man

Improvement of prognosis following a burn can be achieved by:
1. Reduction of insensible heat loss from the wound
2. Reduction of sensible heat loss by raised environmental temperature
3. Increase of readily available calorific content of diet or intravenous alimentation
4. Provision of carbohydrate intermediates.

References

Cahill, GF (1970) *New Eng. J. Med., 282,* 668

Cairnie, AB, Campbell, RM, Pullar, JD and Cuthbertson, DP (1957) *Brit. J. exp. Path., 38,* 504

Caldwell, FT (1962) *Ann. Surg., 155,* 119

Caldwell, FT (1970) *Energy Metabolism in Trauma. Ciba Foundation Symposium.* (Ed) R Porter and J Knight. Churchill, London. Page 23

Caldwell, FT, Hammel, HT and Dolan, F (1966) *J. appl. Physiol., 21,* 1665

Caldwell, FT, Osterholm, JL, Sower, ND and Moyer, CA (1959) *Ann. Surg., 150,* 976

Carter, KB, Richards, JR, Shaw, A, Boyd, IA and Harland, WA (1975) *J. med. Biol. Eng., 13,* 551

Carter, KB, Drury, JK and Richards, JR (1976) *J. med. Biol. Eng.* (In press)

Coleman, JE (1969) *Duncan's Diseases of Metabolism. Vol. 1 Genetics and Metabolism, 6th Edition.* (Ed) PK Bondy and LE Rosenberg. Saunders, Philadelphia. Page 89

Cuthbertson, DP, McGirr, JL and Robertson, JSM (1939) *Quart. J. exp. Physiol., 29,* 13

Duke, JH, Jørgensen, SB, Broell, JR, Long, CL and Kinney, JM (1970) *Surgery, 68,* 168

Elder, HY (1975) Personal communication

Fleck, A (1967) *Proc. Assn. clinical Biochemists, 4,* 212

Kinney, JM (1959) *Metabolism, 8,* 809

Kinney, JM, Morgan, AP, Domingues, FJ and Gildner, K (1964) *Metabolism, 13,* 205

Kinney, JM, Long, CL, Gump, FE and Duke, JH (1968) *Ann. Surg., 168,* 459

Kinney, JM, Duke, JH, Long, CL and Gump, FE (1970a) *J. clin. Path. 23, Suppl. (Roy. Coll. Path.), 4,* 65

Kinney, JM, Long, CL and Duke, JH (1970b) *Energy Metabolism in Trauma. Ciba Foundation Symposium.* (Ed) R Porter and J Knight. Churchill, London. Page 103

Moore, FD (1959) *Metabolic Care of the Surgical Patient, Chapter 17.* Saunders, Philadelphia

Moyer, CA and Butcher, HR (1967) *Burns, Shock and Plasma Volume Regulation, Chapter 5.* CV Mosby Co., St Louis

Richard, JR and Drury, JK (1976) — In press

Waterlow, JC and Alleyne, GAO (1971) *Adv. prot. Chem., 25,* 117

Shaw, W (1973) Personal communication

Nutritional Aspects of the use of Amino Acids for Intravenous Nutrition

ARVID WRETLIND

Nutrition Unit, Medical Faculty, Karolinska Institutet, Stockholm, Sweden

Introduction

Protein may be supplied to the body intravenously in the form of blood, erythrocytes, plasma, albumin and amino acid mixtures. Five hundred millilitres of *blood* contain 90 grams of proteins. The average length of life for erythrocytes is about 120 days; only at the end of this period is all the erythrocyte protein broken down into amino acids which can be used by the body for the synthesis of other body proteins. Haemoglobin does not contain isoleucine. Harper (1958) has shown that it is not possible to obtain a positive nitrogen balance by means of haemoglobin or globin. The supply of large quantities of blood also incurs the risk of overloading the vascular system, of infections (hepatitis, lues), of immunisation, of haemosiderosis and of inhibition of the bone marrow (Jordal, 1965). Consequently, blood should only be given to replace lost blood.

One litre of *plasma* contains about 70 grams of protein. Experiments on young dogs by Allen et al (1956) have shown that plasma protein can be utilised as the sole protein source in parenteral alimentation. Because of the osmotic effect of plasma, there is, however, a danger of overloading the vascular system if an attempt is made to meet protein needs with plasma. The conversion rate of plasma protein is low, about one two-thousandth of that of amino acids (Jordal, 1965). A positive nitrogen balance following infusions of plasma is misleading, since this does not involve the formation of new body protein, only a depositing of the plasma proteins. Plasma protein has low contents of isoleucine and tryptophan.

Infused albumin is distributed in the vascular system and intercellular space in the proportions of 30 per cent and 70 per cent respectively (Artz, 1959). The turn-over rate of albumin is 8-12 per cent per day. Consequently, albumin should be used only when treating patients suffering from hypoalbuminaemia.

Only with *amino acid mixtures,* is it possible to provide a *physiological, intravenous protein* alimentation. In this way — if the amino acid composition is correct — the amino acid pool may receive the same supply of amino acids as through absorption of amino acids from the intestinal tract.

METABOLISM OF AMINO ACIDS

The Role of the Digestive Tract

The foods consumed are degraded by the digestive enzymes. The split products of the proteins, the amino acids, are absorbed by the mucosal cells of the intestine. In the mucosal cells, some of the glutamic and aspartic acids participates in a transamination reaction with pyruvic acid to produce alanine. This enteral transformation is one of the first steps in amino acid metabolism. A substantial part of the glutamic acid absorbed from the intestinal villi, however, enters into the general circulation. After oral administration of sodium glutamate (50 mg/kg), Belanger et al (1972) found an increase in the venous plasma glutamic acid level from about 50 to 90 μmoles/litre. Most of the amino acids absorbed in the intestine are conveyed intact by the portal vein to the liver. There is also a substantial synthesis of protein in the intestinal mucosa (Lang, 1972).

The Role of the Liver

In the liver, amino acids are metabolised in several different ways. Elwyn (1970) found that in rats, after a meal rich in protein, 57 per cent of the ingested amino acids were oxidised to urea, 23 per cent passed into the general circulation, 6 per cent were used for synthesis of plasma proteins and 14 per cent were retained temporarily as liver protein (the labile liver protein). It must be pointed out that Elwyn's results refer to a *large* intake of protein.

Stegink and Baker (1971) found 0.48 mmol/litre of glutamate in the portal vein of newborn pigs and only 0.08 mmol/litre in the periphery, showing the rapidity of the utilisation. The regulating action of the liver limits the plasma amino acid concentration to 0.3–0.4 mmol/litre (= 4–5 mg per cent).

An abundance of amino acid entering the liver causes an increase in the amount of transforming enzymes. Thus, increased concentrations of threonine-serine dehydratase (Harper, 1968) and glutamic acid-oxaloacetate aminotransferase (Stegink & Baker, 1971) have been reported. Tyrosine aminotransaminase is also stimulated, as shown by Fishman et al (1969). The enzyme induction seems to be a very fundamental biological reaction, well known to microbiologists, as it occurs readily in unicellular organisms. The complicated interaction of multiple transaminases in cells and mitochondria is very well reviewed by Munro (1970). A diurnal variation in tyrosine-aminotransferase (Fishman et al, 1969; Wurtman, 1970) is an expression of an amino acid-induced activity. After ingestion of a complete amino acid mixture protein synthesis is caused by a larger number of polysomes in the liver cells (Munro, 1972). If the amino acid mixture is deficient in tryptophan, the protein synthesis is arrested by a disaggregation of polysomes, resulting in an accumulation of inactive monosomes in the cells (Fleck et al, 1965).

The amino acid metabolism in the liver is very selective. Leucine, isoleucine and valine pass into general circulation to be metabolised mainly in muscles and kidney (Miller, 1962). The liver seems to serve as a buffer to protect other organs from the effect of excessive concentrations of amino acids. Hallberg (1974) has reported that amino acids dilate the splanchnic vessels. In this way more blood is carried to the portal circulation during digestion. During parenteral nutrition an increased portal blood flow supports the metabolic processes just described.

Blood Amino Acid Levels

Zimmermann and Scott (1965) fed chickens with amino acid mixtures which contained too little lysine to support growth. When lysine was added growth was proportional to the lysine content up to 0.8 per cent. When more lysine was added no further increase in weight occurred, but the level of lysine in the serum then started to increase. Valine and arginine produced similar effects. Young et al (1971) found that when more than 3 mg tryptophan per kg body weight was added to the food of children, there was a steep rise in the tryptophan content of the serum. More than 5 mg/kg caused a rise in the liver tryptophan pyrrolase activity, limiting the serum tryptophan to a constant level. These results are in good agreement with other investigations which show that about 3 mg of tryptophan per kg body weight and day is optimal for man. Studies of serum amino acids have been used by Young et al (1971) to determine the requirement of amino acids.

The regulating power of the liver keeps the serum concentration of the amino acids at a constant level. If the level falls, amino acids from the liver protein are mobilised to cover the need. The amino acid concentration in serum is also regulated by hormones such as insulin, glucagon, growth hormone and glucocorticoids. By a feedback system, these hormones are partly controlled by the amino acid content in the serum (Munro, 1970). In principle, insulin release is stimulated by the branched amino acids, and glucagon by the non-essential amino acids (Cahill, 1972).

Amino Acids and Protein Synthesis

Besides the supply of free amino acids from the intestine and liver, there is also a contribution from the body proteins which undergo constant breakdown and renewal. Food protein is digested in the alimentary tract to form amino acids which after absorption are mixed with the free amino acids in the amino acid pool of the body (Figure 1). The total amino acid pool in man contains about 70g of amino

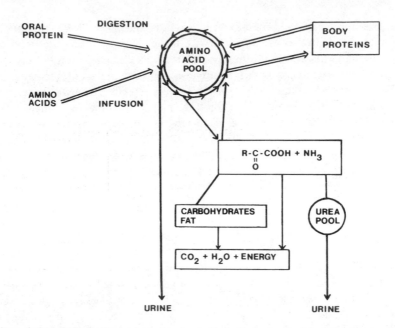

Figure 1. Metabolism of protein and amino acids in the body. Protein taken by mouth is digested in the gastrointestinal tract and converted into amino acids which enter the body's amino acid pool. From this depot, tissue protein, hormones and enzymes are formed. There is a dynamic equilibrium between synthesis and breakdown of protein. Some amino acids are excreted via the urine and others are metabolised into carbohydrates, lipids, carbon dioxide, urea etc. After intravenous administration, the amino acids go directly to the amino acid pool where they are metabolised in the same way as amino acids taken orally. When blood proteins are given, these must be broken down into amino acids before they can be used for synthesis of other proteins in the body

acids and its turnover rate is very high. It is from this pool that amino acids are drawn for the synthesis of blood and tissue proteins, while at the same time amino acids, formed through a breakdown of the body proteins, are returned to the pool. The 'transport fraction', i.e. the amino acid content of the plasma is 1 g (Lang, 1972). Under normal conditions there is a dynamic equilibrium between the synthesis of body proteins on the one hand, and the breakdown of proteins on the other. Some of the amino acids are deaminated and then metabolised to carbohydrates, fat, carbon dioxide, water, urea, and energy. Another, smaller part is excreted in the urine. When amino acids are administered intravenously, they enter directly the body's amino acid pool and are then metabolised in the normal physiological way (Figure 2). If proteins in the form of blood, plasma or albumin are supplied intravenously, they have first to be broken down into amino acids before the infused proteins can be used for the synthesis of other body proteins, or to cover the metabolic requirements of amino acids.

The mechanism of protein synthesis starts with the desoxyribonucleic acid sending a 'messenger'-ribonucleic acid, m-RNA, to the protein synthetising

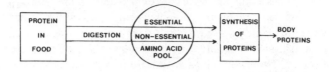

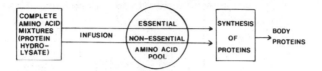

III. WITH ESSENTIAL AMINO ACIDS AND NON-SPECIFIC NITROGEN

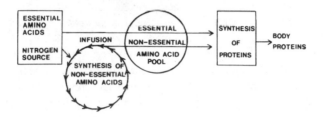

Figure 2. Amino acid nutrition. In the upper two examples, the protein in food and the complete amino acid mixture contain both essential and non-essential amino acids, which directly enter the amino acid pool, and are then used for the synthesis of body proteins. When a mixture of essential amino acids and a non-specific nitrogen source are given (lowest part of the diagram), a synthesis of non-essential amino acids has first to take place before the body proteins can be synthetised

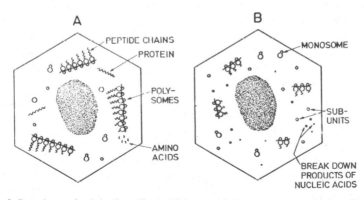

Figure 3. Protein synthesis in the cell. A. This part of the figure shows a body cell with the normal supply of all necessary amino acids. Protein chains, free or under formation in polysomes, are also illustrated. B. In a cell given an amino acid mixture deficient in tryptophan, there are few and small incomplete polysomes with an abundant number of monosomes and breakdown products of nucleic acids

155

ribosomes in the cell (Figure 3). Each m-RNA is attached to two points in one ribosome and serves as the template for the production of one kind of protein. The sequence of the components, the nucleotides, in m-RNA determines the order in which the amino acids are combined in the growing peptide chain. The purpose of nutrition is to supply the ribosomes with a sufficient pool of amino acids and energy. The capacity of the tiny ribosomes is enormous, three hundred amino acids may be combined by covalent bonds in ten seconds by one ribosome. There are some hundred thousand ribosomes per cell. It is evidently of paramount importance that the ribosomes are surrounded by an amino acid pool containing all the amino acids in sufficient concentration to keep protein synthesis functioning satisfactorily.

AMINO ACID IMBALANCE, ANTAGONISM AND TOXICITY

Amino acids show many very complex interrelationships. An amino acid mixture has an ideal amino acid pattern where all undesirable interactions are reduced to a minimum. These interactions are *amino acid imbalance, amino acid antagonism* and *amino acid toxicity* (Harper & Rogers, 1965).

Amino acid imbalance has been studied in experimental animals, especially in rats. There is every reason, however, to predict that the same condition could exist in human pathophysiology. If rats are given a mixture of amino acids which causes less weight increase than that produced by an optimal mixture, they will suffer from amino acid imbalance. It is natural that imbalance can occur if the diet contains too little or none of one or more essential amino acids. But imbalance will also result when amino acids are *added* to an optimal diet because of an impairment of the nutritional value of some essential amino acids, and this type of imbalance can be compensated by the addition of the limiting amino acid (Harper & Rogers, 1965). Harper (1970) found that the rapid loss of appetite, that is so evident in amino acid imbalance, can also be reproduced by intravenous injection of the imbalanced mixture. This observation was followed up by Rogers and Leung (1973), who injected an amino acid solution into the carotid artery, and showed that it was the low plasma content of one amino acid that caused the depressed food intake.

Amino acid antagonism is different from imbalance (Harper & Rogers, 1965). It is compensated by addition of an amino acid not 'limiting', but chemically related to the amino acid added in excess.

Large amounts of single amino acids added to diets induce various *toxic reactions* including depression of growth. Large amounts of tyrosine lead to damage in paws and eyes of rats; methionine causes pathological changes in several organs.

Doolan et al (1965) noted that a human subject receiving a 5 per cent solution of glycine intravenously at a mean rate of 0.67 milligrams of amino nitrogen per kilogram per minute (about 15 g of glycine per hour) suffered a severe toxic reaction reminiscent of ammonia intoxication. Harper et al (1956) followed this up with a study of the blood ammonia and urea levels in dogs receiving infusions of glycine and of an isonitrogenous casein hydrolysate separately. The data showed that the infusion of glycine produced a marked rise in the blood ammonia levels with no corresponding increase in urea. This suggested to the authors that certain amino acids in the mixture decrease blood ammonia levels by enhancing urea production. The protective effect of casein hydrolysate against the toxicity of glycine had already been shown by Handler et al (1949). Najarian and Harper (1956) found that, when arginine was given concomitantly with glycine there was no significant rise in the blood ammonia levels. An appreciable increase in urea was recorded, indicating that the urea was probably formed from the ammonia. Because of this glycine toxicity, it seems that an excess of glycine, in any amino acid preparation for intravenous use, should be avoided.

AMINO ACID REQUIREMENTS

Total Amino Acid Requirement

The basal requirements of amino acids in the form of mixtures with high biological values have been determined by studies of complete parenteral nutrition in man, and partly by calculations from nitrogen losses. In one case, a patient who received complete parenteral nutrition with a mixture of 18 amino acids in a crystalline form (Vamin) for more than 7 months (Jacobson & Wretlind, 1970; Bergström et al, 1972), a minimum daily quantity for nitrogen balance was found to be 4.1 g of nitrogen, equivalent to 80 mg of N or 0.6 g of amino acids/kg body weight/day.

The requirements of amino acids can be calculated from known nitrogen losses. The endogenous nitrogen loss via the urine is estimated at 2 mg of N/basal kcal (Hegsted, 1964; FAO/WHO, 1965; Recommended Dietary Allowances, 1968; Recommended Intakes of Nutrients for the United Kingdom, 1969). The minimum loss through faeces has been indicated as 0.57 mg of N/basal kcal (Recommended Intakes of Nutrients for the United Kingdom, 1969). This is the average of the values indicated by FAO/WHO (1965). The loss through sweat, skin, hair and nails has been estimated at 0.08 mg of N/basal kcal (Sirbu et al, 1967). This estimate appears in 'Recommended Intakes of Nutrients for the United Kingdom' (1969) and also corresponds to the results reported by Darke (1960) and by Ashworth and Harrower (1967). The losses thus amount to a total of 2.65 mg of N/basal kcal, equivalent to 17 mg (2.65 x 6.25) of a protein with a biological value of 100, or 20 mg (2.65 x 7.5) of an adequate amino acid mixture per basal kcal. This means that 56–66 mg of N (2.65 x 21 kcal – 2.65 x 25 kcal) of an adequate amino acid mixture/kg/day cover the minimum requirement of protein in adults. The standard error of the required nitrogen quantity for balance is probably between 10 (Garrow, 1969) and 15 per cent (Calloway & Margen, 1967;

Hussein et al, 1968) of the nitrogen quantity consumed. A supply of 73–86 mg of N (0.55–0.65 g of amino acids) per kg, which is 30 per cent above the average minimum requirements, would thus cover the basal requirement of protein in almost all adults (Recommended Dietary Allowances, 1968). After compensating a loss of amino acids through the urine of up to 10 per cent, one can expect to require 80–95 mg of N (0.60–0.71 g of amino acids)/kg/day to cover the basal needs. The quantity calculated in this way equals that which, in the above mentioned case (Jacobson & Wretlind, 1970; Bergström et al, 1972), was sufficient to obtain nitrogen balance.

On the basis of various results and calculations, a daily amino acid allowance of about 95 mg of N, or 0.7 g of amino acids/kg would correspond to the basal requirements of adults. This quantity exceeds somewhat the protein supply (calculated as protein with an NPU value of 100) in a British or Swedish average national diet with an energy supply of 1,500–2,000 kcal/day. For basal conditions, Allen and Lee (1969) have recommended a supply of 0.11–0.13 g of N or 0.8–1 g of amino acids/kg. Hallberg et al (1966) and Steinbereithner (1966) has recommended a quantity of 1 g of amino acids/kg/day for adults.

Børresen and Knutrud (1969) and Dudrick et al (1969) have given to neonate and infant 0.40–0.53 g of N, or 3–4 g of amino acids/kg body weight/day. With this amino acid supply, satisfactory growth and a positive nitrogen balance were obtained. The requirement of protein in neonates and infants up to the age of 12 months has been calculated at 1.2–2.2 g/kg/day (Fomon, 1967). This corresponds to 1.5–2.7 g of amino acid mixture. According to these findings an amount of about 330 mg of nitrogen, or 2.5 g of amino acid mixture/kg/day is recommended for neonates and infants on total intravenous nutrition.

Requirements of Individual Essential and Non-essential Amino Acids

The protein-synthesising system in the body cells needs eighteen to twenty amino acids in order to produce the various proteins of the body. Eight of the amino acids cannot be synthesised by the adult body. Consequently, they have to be supplied to the body in food, or in some other way. These eight so-called essential amino acids are isoleucine, leucine, lysine, methionine (or the sulphur-containing amino acids, methionine and cysteine-cystine), phenylalanine (or the aromatic amino acids which include phenylalanine and tyrosine), threonine, tryptophan and valine. For infants histidine has also been found to be an essential amino acid (Holt & Snyderman, 1961). Kofranyi et al (1969) have indicated that histidine prevents liver derangement in men. Investigations by Bergström et al (1970) have indicated that histidine also seems to be necessary for an optimal utilisation of amino acid mixtures in patients with uraemia. The capacity of the body to synthesise arginine is limited. Thus, arginine must be included in amino acid mixtures for intravenous nutrition in order to obtain optimal utilisation of the other amino acids supplied. Moreover, the arginine counteracts the toxic effects which are produced when glycine is used in larger amounts.

Cystine is, according to Sturman et al (1970), an essential amino acid for the fetus and immature human. This was indicated by the lack of cystathionase activity in the liver of the fetus and immature infant. In these cases there was also an increased level of cystathionine in the liver. The results show that the synthesis of cystine or cysteine from methionine must be blocked. Stegink and den Besten (1972) administered amino acid solutions free from cysteine to eight healthy men through catheters in the superior vena cava and through nagogastric tubes. When the solutions were given intravenously, the plasma cystine concentration dropped markedly. When feeding was switched to the enteral route, the concentration rose, but returned to base line only when a cystine-containing diet was fed. These studies indicate that the synthesis of cysteine from methionine is limited, even in the adult subject.

The phenylalanine hydroxylase system is not fully developed in prematures. This means that phenylalanine cannot be converted into tyrosine. An intravenous supply of an amino acid mixture with phenylalanine, but without tyrosine, results in a decrease of the tyrosine concentration in serum. Thus, amino acid solutions for intravenous nutrition of prematures and infants should contain tyrosine as well as phenylalanine (Jürgens & Dolif, 1972; Sturman et al, 1970; Panteliadis et al, 1975). This applies also to two per cent of adults (Munro, 1972).

Jürgens and Dolif (1968) and Dolif and Jürgens (1969) have shown that the utilisation of intravenous amino acid preparations is higher if alanine, proline and glutamic acid are also included in the amino acid mixture. In this connection, it may be of interest to consider the report of Schlappner et al (1972), that the use of an amino acid mixture lacking cysteine, tyrosine and glutamic acid produced acute papulopustular acne in three male patients on intravenous nutrition for two to four weeks. Glycine is, according to Panteliadis et al (1975), necessary in small amounts (0.2 g/kg) for neonates on parenteral nutrition to maintain normal levels of glycine and serine in serum.

Hitherto there have been no investigations of the specific effects of aspartic acid and serine on the utilisation of an intravenous amino acid mixture. They may, however, be used as a source of non-specific nitrogen. The nutritional value of the various amino acids is summarised in Table I.

Absence of the non-essential amino acids from the food can partly be compensated for by providing a suitable source of nitrogen, which will permit the synthesis, by the body, of the amino acids in question. This synthesis by the organism must take place in such a way that, at all times, the enzyme systems are always supplied with sufficient quantities of both essential and non-essential amino acids. As mentioned in the previous paragraph, the capacity of the body for synthesis of some non-essential amino acids is limited, and not sufficient for an optimal utilisation of the essential amino acids.

An amino acid mixture for intravenous nutrition involves two components; the essential amino acids, and the non-essential amino acids or nitrogen sources

TABLE I. Nutritional Value of Amino Acids for Intravenous Alimentation

Isoleucine Leucine Lysine Methionine Phenylalanine Threonine Tryptophan Valine	Essential in all conditions[1]
Arginine	Necessary for optimal utilisation of amino acid mixtures and for detoxification (2)
Cystein-cystine	Essential for the fetus, and necessary for the maintenance of normal plasma level of cystine in adults (3)
Glycine	Necessary for neonates[4]
Histidine	Essential for infants and in uraemia[5] Necessary to prevent liver derangement[6]
Tyrosine	Essential for neonates[4,7]
Alanine Glutamic acid Proline	Necessary for optimal utilisation of amino acid mixtures (8)
Aspartic acid Serine	Source of non-specific nitrogen

(1)   Rose (1957)
(2)   Najarian and Harper (1956); Malvy et al (1961)
(3)   Sturman et al (1970); Stegink and den Besten (1972)
(4)   Panteliadis et al (1975)
(5)   Holt and Snyderman (1961); Bergström et al (1970)
(6)   Kofranyi et al (1969)
(7)   Jürgens and Dolif (1972)
(8)   Jürgens and Dolif (1968); Dolif and Jürgens (1969)

for the synthesis of these. The proportion of the essential amino acids, and the total nitrogen, are of great importance from the nutritional point of view.

The essential amino acid requirements have been investigated in various connections. Previously, research workers have usually adopted the recommendations given by Rose in 1957. Rose determined the requirements experimentally in rats and men. According to Rose the minimum daily requirements for the adult male are 0.7 g of isoleucine, 1.1 g of leucine, 0.8 g of lysine, 1.1 g of methionine, 1.1 g of phenylalanine (Rose et al, 1948), and cystine or cysteine up to 30 per cent of methionine (Womack & Rose, 1941). More recently a number of other studies have been carried out to determine the requirements at various ages and in various conditions (Inoue et al, 1971; Hegsted, 1963). Watts et al (1964) and Tuttle et al (1968) found that elderly persons need about twice as much methionine and lysine as younger ones. Munro (1972) has summarised the results obtained by various investigators for the requirements of the individual essential amino acids. It is obvious (Munro, 1972) that a healthy growing infant needs a relatively high content of essential amino acids (35–40 per cent) in the protein or amino acid mixture. In healthy adults it seems possible to maintain a positive nitrogen balance, for a short period of time, with an amino acid mixture having a lower content of essential amino acids (Hegsted, 1963; Inoue et al, 1971; Fürst et al, 1970). In cases where intravenous nutrition is indicated in the adult patient, it is usually desirable to replete the body proteins. Thus, it would seem reasonable to require an amino acid mixture with the same high content of essential amino acids as occurs in body proteins or other proteins with an high biological value (about 45–50 per cent essential amino acids). Expressed in another way, we could say that the amino acid mixture optimal for the growing infant should be the most suitable.

A reference pattern of the essential amino acids is given by the FAO/WHO Expert Group (1965) in terms of the relations of each essential amino acid to the *total essential amino acids*. The Group concluded that its data justified adoption, for reference, of the essential amino acid pattern of either *egg or human milk protein*. The optimal pattern of non-essential amino acids is not yet known. Some of the amino acids appear to be interchangeable as nitrogen sources. This was to be expected from the rapidity of transamination reactions in the body. It seems, therefore, that within wide limits, the body is indifferent to the composition of the non-essential nitrogen component, but single amino acids may, if fed in excess, produce toxic effects. The most effective is a mixture of all the non-essential amino acids (Swenseid et al, 1959). Then come the following in terms of decreasing effectivity; glutamic acid, alanine, aspartic acid, asparagine, proline, glutamine, glycine, serine and an excess of essential amino acids (Reissigl, 1957; Frost, 1959; Frost & Sandy, 1949).

TIME FACTOR IN UTILISATION OF AMINO ACIDS

For the optimal utilisation of an amino acid mixture, it is of great importance that all essential amino acids are given simultaneously, whether administration is intravenous or oral (Elman, 1939; Cannon et al, 1947; Geiger, 1951). As early as 1939 Elman showed that the simultaneous infusion of an acid casein hydrolysate (containing no tryptophan) and tryptophan could produce a positive nitrogen balance. If the acid casein hydrolysate and the tryptophan were administered at separate times, they caused a negative nitrogen balance (Cox et al, 1942).

The time factor is important not only in the administration of the single amino acids, but also when amino acid mixtures are given in combination with other nutrients, such as carbohydrates or fat. Intravenous infusions in man have shown that the best effect of glucose on nitrogen balance was recorded when glucose was given prior to casein hydrolysate (Christensen et al, 1955). In many other investigations on intravenous nutrition the best metabolic results were obtained when the amino acids and the sources of energy were supplied at the same time (Larson & Chaikoff, 1937; McNair et al, 1954; Lawson, 1965).

When amino acids are given with fat emulsions and other nutrients to patients on total intravenous nutrition, the daily infusions may be given either during the day or at night time for 10–14 hours (Hallberg et al, 1966; Jacobson & Wretlind, 1970) or for 24 hours (Liljedahl, 1972). No difference in utilisation or in the nitrogen balance have been recorded or indicated. Amino acids in combination with glucose as the only source of energy should always be administered slowly; the daily infusions have to be continued for 24 hours (Dudrick et al, 1972). This is because of the high osmotic pressure of the amino-acid-glucose solutions used in this kind of intravenous nutrition.

EFFECT OF ENERGY INTAKE ON UTILISATION OF AMINO ACIDS

Calloway and Spector (1954) showed that the nitrogen loss in persons who were not given any protein was slightly reduced by an increase in the energy supply up to 750 kcal. When more energy was supplied — 2,300 kcal — no further reduction in the nitrogen loss was observed. When protein was administered in amounts equivalent to seven or eight grams of nitrogen and in increasing supply of energy, there was a decreasing loss of the nitrogen. With a supply of more than 3,000 kcal a positive nitrogen balance was obtained.

In a patient suffering from malnutrition it is possible, with a moderate supply of amino acid nitrogen, to obtain a positive nitrogen balance with 800–1,000 kcal per 24 hours. Thus, the worse the patient's nutritional condition, the better the utilisation of the dietary protein or amino acids. The explanation seems to be that, in a poor state of nutrition the protein metabolism shifts towards anabolism. In this poor nutritional state, an exogenous supply of energy in the form of carbohydrates or fat, has also a more marked effect in reducing protein breakdown than in a healthy person.

Fat and glucose seem to be of equal value in supporting amino acid utilisation.

162

Broviac (1974) made a double blind investigation in surgical patients with short bowel syndrome. When glucose was the sole source of non-protein energy, the average nitrogen balance was + 1.8 ± 0.2 g of N/day, and the change in body weight was + 0.06 ± 0.03 g/day. When a fat emulsion (Intralipid) was substituted for part of the glucose energy (1.6 g of fat/kg/day) and comprised 35 per cent of the total energy input, the nitrogen balance averaged + 1.3 ± 0.4 g of N/day, and the change in body weight was + 0.06 ± 0.04 g/day.

The optimal utilisation of an amino acid mixture occurs when the ratio of energy to nitrogen as calories per g of N in the amino acids is 150 : 1 as recommended by Moore (1959) and Lawson (1965) or 200 : 1 as applied by Johnston et al (1972).

Physical activity is a factor in improving the retention of amino acid nitrogen in the body. Early mobilisation of patients after herniotomy has thus been shown to produce a much more positive nitrogen balance than could be obtained by an increased supply of energy and protein (Jordal, 1965).

COMPARISON OF ENTERAL AND INTRAVENOUS SUPPLY OF AMINO ACIDS

The alimentary tract and the liver may protect the organism from too high concentrations of amino acids from food. Consequently, it is most likely that amino acid solutions for parenteral use should have a different composition from the aminogram of the dietary proteins. The discovery by Miller (1962) that branched amino acids (isoleucine, leucine and valine) pass the liver with only slight transformation makes it likely that they have to be enriched in parenteral solutions compared with the other five essential amino acids.

Peaston (1967) observed the same positive nitrogen balance during intravenous and oral feeding with equal amino acid mixtures. Johnston and Spivey (1970) reported investigations which indicated that the intravenous route was as effective as the alimentary in maintaining nitrogen balance. Investigations by Fürst et al (1970) on nitrogen balance also showed that the need of total nitrogen and of essential amino acids is the same whether they are given by mouth or intravenously. Their results have been confirmed by Bässler (1971). The most likely explanation of the evident success of parenteral nutrition seems to be that the liver receives a substantial part of the total blood circulation and, consequently, all the infused amino acids will soon reach the liver.

NUTRITIONAL EFFECTS OF AMINO ACIDS SUPPLIED INTRAVENOUSLY

The utilisation by the body of amino acid mixtures supplied intravenously has been confirmed by the effect on nitrogen balance and body weight.

The *nitrogen balance* technique has been used to show that mixtures of the amino acids are utilised as expected. It has also been used to determine the biological value of an amino acid mixture (Lidström & Wretlind, 1952). Several investigations have shown that it is possible to maintain a positive nitrogen balance for several months in adults. Bergström et al (1972) reported that in one case the average daily nitrogen balance was positive during total intravenous nutrition for 7 months and 13 days. Dudrick et al (1969) obtained positive nitrogen balance in adults on total intravenous nutrition during periods from 7 to 210 days. Many other investigators have also obtained a positive nitrogen balance in adults (Peaston, 1967; Jürgens & Dolif, 1972; Josephson et al, 1972; Halmagyi & Kilbinger, 1972).

Body weight has been increased or maintained during periods of several months in adult patients on intravenous nutrition. Bergström et al (1972) showed a pronounced weight increase in a patient who was totally fed intravenously for more than 7 months. Hallberg et al (1967) have reported complete intravenous nutrition for more than 5 months in a patient suffering from Crohn's disease. Jacobson (1972) has administered complete intravenous nutrition to a 70-year old male patient after massive resection of the small intestine. During the 69 days of intravenous nutrition, the body weight was maintained.

In infants on intravenous nutrition positive nitrogen balance and body growth have been reported by Dudrick et al (1969), Filler et al (1969), Das et al (1970) Børresen and Knutrud (1969), Børresen and Knutrud (1972) and Grotte (1971).

AMINO ACID PREPARATIONS

The two types of amino acid preparations for intravenous nutrition are *protein hydrolysates* and *mixtures of crystalline amino acids*. Tables IIa and b show the composition of some commercial amino acid preparations for intravenous nutrition, as well as the aminogram of egg protein.

Protein Hydrolysates

Woodyatt et al in 1915 and Rose in 1934 suggested the parenteral use of amino acids, but it was not until 1937 that Elman initiated the modern use of such intravenous, amino-acid alimentation. Both an acid protein hydrolysate, fortified with tryptophan and cystine, and an enzymatic protein hydrolysate were employed.

An enzymatic casein hydrolysate widely used in Europe, is *Aminosol Vitrum*. The preparation is produced by a special method, which includes dialysis, and in this way all the high-molecular peptides and other substances which might cause allergic reactions are removed. It contains about 67 per cent of free amino acids and 33 per cent of low-molecular peptides (Wretlind, 1947). Lidström and Wretlind (1952) have shown that this dialysed, enzymatic casein hydrolysate has in man a biological value of about 90. The dialysed, protein hydrolysate does not produce hyperpetidaemia, which might occur when using non-dialysed hydro-

164

TABLE IIa. Amino acid content of egg protein and some commercial amino acid preparations. The amino acid values are given in grams per 16 g of Total Nitrogen (T) of the protein or of the amino-acid mixtures

L-AMINO ACIDS	Amount of amino acid in 16 g of total nitrogen					
	Egg protein	Artirosol[1]	Aminofusin[2]	Aminofusin L-Reihe[3]	Aminonorm[4]	Aminoplasmal L 5[4]
Isoleucine	6.6	6.5	2.5	3.3	2.6	5.1
Leucine	8.8	11.4	4.4	4.6	4.5	8.9
Lysine	6.4	10.1	3.6	4.2	7.2	5.6
Aromatic amino acids	10.0	7.5	4.0	4.6	4.7	6.4
Phenylalanine	5.8	6.4		4.6	4.2	5.1
Tyrosine	4.2	1.1		–	0.3	1.3
Sulphur-containing amino acids	5.5	5.5	4.4	4.4	4.5	4.3
Methionine	3.1	3.7	4.4	4.4	4.4	3.8
Cysteine-cystine	2.4	1.8			0.1	0.5
Threonine	5.1	5.0	1.8	2.1	4.1	4.1
Tryptophan	1.6	1.3	0.9	1.0	2.4	1.8
Valine	7.3	8.7	2.9	3.2	5.9	4.8
E = total amount of Essential Amino Acids per 16 g of N	51.3	55.0	25.4	27.4	35.8	41.0
Alanine	7.4	4.1	23.6	12.6	9.4	13.7
Arginine	6.1	4.3	11.8	8.4	5.0	9.2
Asparagine	–	–	–	–	2.6	3.3
Aspartic acid	9.0	8.6	–	–	0.8	1.3
Glutamic acid	16.0	27.6	22.7	19.0	4.3	4.6
Glutamine	–	–	–	–	19.6	–
Glycine	3.6	2.4	2.7	21.1	4.9	7.9
Histidine	2.4	3.2	–	2.1	4.4	5.2
Ornithine	–	–	–	–	2.4	3.2
Proline	8.1	13.4	5.5	14.7	5.2	8.9
Serine	8.5	5.6	–	–	2.0	2.4
E/T ratio	3.2	3.5	1.6	1.7	2.24	2.6
E in percent of total amino acids	46	45	28	26	37	41

1) Vitrum, Stockholm, Sweden
2) Earlier composition from J. Pfrimmer, Erlangen, Germany
3) Present preparation from J. Pfrimmer, Erlangen, Germany
4) B. Braun, Melsungen, Germany

165

TABLE IIb. Amino acid content of some commercial amino acid preparations. The amino acid values are given in grams per 16 g of Total Nitrogen (T) of the protein or of the amino-acid mixtures

L-AMINO ACIDS	Amount of amino acid in 16 g of total nitrogen.					
	Intramin[1]	Intramin novum[1]	Intramin forte[1]	Sohamin[2]	Trophysan[3]	Vamin[4]
Isoleucine	2.5	4.0	4.6	8.1	1.6	6.6
Leucine	4.0	6.2	7.2	12.2	2.6	9.0
Lysine	2.9	4.5	5.3	18.7	5.8	6.6
Aromatic amino acids	4.0	6.5	7.2	11.7	2.2	10.2
Phenylalanine						9.4
Tyrosine	-	-	-	-	-	0.8
Sulphur-containing amino acids	4.0	6.2	7.2	8.3	2.6	5.6
Methionine						3.2
Cysteine-cystine	-	-	-	-	-	2.4
Threonine	1.8	2.8	3.3	8.6	1.6	5.1
Tryptophan	0.9	1.4	1.7	3.7	1.0	1.7
Valine	2.9	4.5	5.3	7.8	2.2	7.3
E = total amount of Essential Amino Acids per 16 g of N	23.0	35.8	41.8	79.1	19.6	52.1
Alanine	4.0	-	15.0	11.0	1.8	5.1
Arginine	-	6.2	9.4	-	-	5.6
Asparagine	-	-	-	-	-	-
Aspartic acid	-	-	8.2	-	-	7.0
Glutamic acid	-	-	-	-	-	15.3
Glutamine	-	-	-	-	-	-
Glycine	61.7	48.1	9.4	7.3	59.8	3.6
Histidine	2.0	3.1	5.6	4.2	-	4.1
Ornithine	-	-	-	-	-	-
Proline	-	-	9.4	-	-	13.8
Serine	-	-	4.7	-	-	12.8
E/T ratio	1.44	2.2	2.6	4.9	1.23	3.2
E in percent of total amino acids	25	38	40	78		44

1) Astra, Södertälje, Sweden
2) Tanabe, Seijaku Co, Osaka, Japan
3) Egic, Montargis, France
4) Vitrum, Stockholm, Sweden

166

lysates (Lidström & Wretlind, 1952). Lidström and Wretlind (1952) found that
4.3 per cent of the quantity of free, and 21 per cent of the peptide-bound α-
amino nitrogen supplied, were excreted via the urine in man. The total excretion
of α-amino nitrogen was 9.8 per cent. The total urinary excretion of amino acids
and peptides was 8.9 per cent after intraportal infusion of this dialysed, enzymatic casein hydrolysate in man (Lidström, 1954). Schärli (1965) found no difficulty
in obtaining a positive nitrogen balance with this preparation when an adequate
amount of energy was given.

Another protein hydrolysate – *Aminosol Abbott* – is prepared by enzymatic
hydrolysis of fibrin. In a large number of investigations it has been shown that
this hydrolysate is also well utilised and Dudrick et al (1968) obtained normal
growth in both infants and puppies with it. Dudrick et al (1969) and Kaplan et
al (1969) have shown that casein and fibrin hydrolysate produce about the same
growth in infants on total intravenous nutrition.

The amino acid preparations in the form of protein hydrolysate have now been
on the market for more than thirty years. Hyperammonaemia was found by
Johnston et al (1972) in seven infants who were receiving casein or fibrin hydrolysate intravenously and suggested that the concentration of ammonium ion in
the protein hydrolysates may have contributed to the hyperammonaemia. It
would thus seem significant to develop an amino acid mixture free from ammonium ion.

Crystalline Amino Acid Preparations

Mixtures of crystalline amino acids offer the advantages of flexibility in composition. Their relatively high cost, however, has limited their practical use. In
1940, Shohl and Blackfan first used a complete mixture of crystalline amino
acids for parenteral nutrition. Nitrogen balance in infants was promoted equally
well by this mixture as by a commercial protein hydrolysate. Since then numerous investigations into intravenous alimentation with mixtures of crystalline
amino acids have been carried out.

Examples of amino acid preparations containing crystalline essential amino
acids are Aminofusin, Aminonorm, Intramin forte and Vamin (Tables IIa and b),
all of which contain the L-forms of the amino acids. In older preparations some
of the essential amino acids were present in DL-forms. Very little of the D-amino
acids is utilised for the synthesis of body proteins (Bansi et al, 1964) in experiments where mixtures containing D-amino acids were given parenterally to human
beings. D-amino acids are poorly reabsorbed in the kidney tubules and a large
part of the D-amino acids was excreted via the urine; this may cause osmotic
diuresis.

Mixtures of amino acids with a high content of glycine have been used by
several investigators. In general, few side effects have been reported, but Malvey
et al (1961) noticed that a commercial amino acid preparation, with DL-amino

167

acid and a high glycine content, produced ammonia coma in humans, perhaps because of the tendency of glycine to produce ammonia. Heird et al (1972a) also observed hyperammonaemia in three infants who were receiving total parenteral nutrition, including a crystalline amino acid preparation with a relatively high content of glycine. The hyperammonaemia and the associated clinical signs were corrected by the administration of arginine-glutamate, or arginine. This suggests that the preparation used may be deficient in arginine (Heird et al, 1972b). These findings appear to indicate that an excess of glycine should be avoided.

The relation between the various essential amino acids in the amino acid mixtures (Tables IIa and b) follows more or less the amino acid pattern found in egg protein. It is also similar to the relation between the requirements of the essential amino acids found by Rose (1957) when investigating nitrogen balance in man.

Many investigations have demonstrated that crystalline amino acid mixtures are well utilised for the synthesis of body protein when the requirement of essential amino acids is covered, and the amino acid mixtures are well balanced. The best results have been obtained in humans when the preparations were complete, and contained all the essential, and ten to twelve non-essential, amino acids (Mayer et al, 1969; Deckner et al, 1970; Jacobson & Wretlind, 1970). Studies on dogs also showed better utilisation, and a more positive nitrogen balance, when a complete crystalline amino acid mixture, containing the essential, and ten non-essential, amino acids was used, as compared with incomplete mixtures containing essential amino acids, arginine, histidine and a high concentration of glycine.

EFFECT OF VARIOUS AMINO ACID PREPARATIONS ON NITROGEN BALANCE AND BODY WEIGHT

In Animals

The various amino acid preparations for intravenous nutrition produce a quite different growth effect when fed orally to rats (PER-values) [Levin, 1973]. These results indicate that many of the preparations are not well balanced. One amino acid preparation with an optimal oral growth effect was given intravenously (Roos, 1973) and showed a biological value of about 100 (Figure 4). An amino acid preparation with reduced growth on oral feeding tested intravenously in this way showed a biological value of only 57 (Figure 4).

Dudrick et al (1970) have shown that growth and positive nitrogen balance can be obtained in dogs by using enzymatic protein hydrolysate as part of total intravenous nutrition. Holm et al (1975a) compared the utilisation in dogs on total intravenous nutrition of amino acid solutions, Aminonorm, Intramin, Intramin Novum, Sohamin and Vamin during periods of seven days (Figure 5). The nitrogen balance was positive and approximately the same with Vamin as with Aminonorm. These solutions contain both the essential and non-essential amino acids present in proteins with high biological value. A pronounced positive

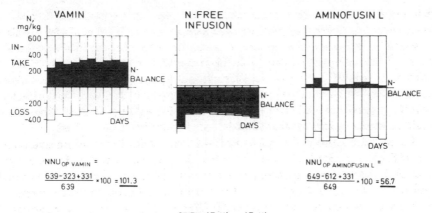

$$NNU_{OP} = \frac{GIVEN - (F+U)_{AA} - (F+U)_0}{GIVEN} \times 100$$

Figure 4. Urinary nitrogen and nitrogen balances in rats on total intravenous nutrition without, and with amino acid supply. Each test lasted ten days and was performed with four rats weighing 150–200 g. One complete amino acid preparation (Vamin, Table IIb) and one amino acid containing low amount of essential amino acids and only a few non-essential amino acids (Aminofusin L = Aminofusin, earlier composition, Table IIa) were tested. When the complete amino acid preparation (left diagram) was added, there was no increase in the urinary nitrogen compared to the test without amino acids (diagram in the centre). A pronounced positive nitrogen balance and a high Net Nitrogen Utilisation (NNU) were obtained. With the 'unbalanced' amino acid preparation (right diagram), there were increases of urinary nitrogen and only a small positive nitrogen balance with low NNU-value.

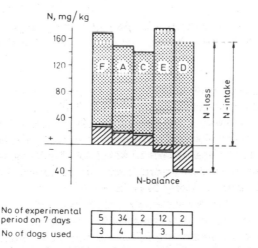

Figure 5. Effect of various amino acid preparations on nitrogen balance in dogs on complete intravenous nutrition. Each test period covered one week. The figure shows the average daily nitrogen intakes and nitrogen balances. A=Vamin, C=Aminonorm, D=Intramin, E=Intramin novum, F=Sohamin (Tables IIa and b). The given amounts of nitrogen are indicated by the height of the columns in the diagram. The nitrogen losses via urine and faeces are marked from the upper part of the columns downwards. The horizontal heavy lines represent the nitrogen balances. The number of test periods for each amino acid preparation is given in the lowest part of the diagram

169

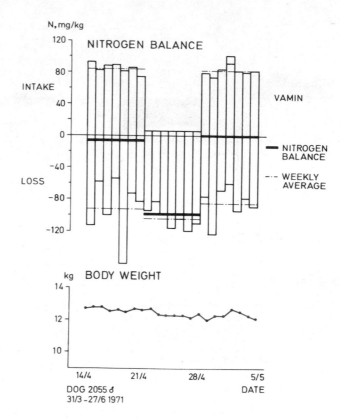

Figure 6. Urinary nitrogen and nitrogen balances in a dog on total intravenous nutrition, with and without a complete amino acid preparation (Vamin, Table IIb). The urinary nitrogen loss decreased during the seven-day period with the amino acid preparation. This indicates a biological value of about 100

nitrogen balance was also obtained with Sohamin, which mainly contains essential amino acids. Intramin and Intramin Novum gave a negative nitrogen balance. The explanation of the observed difference in the utilisation between the various types of amino acid solutions may be that certain of the non-essential amino acids were not present in some of the solutions. Holm et al (1975b) have shown that a complete amino acid preparation with good utilisation in rat both on oral and intravenous supply is very well utilised in dog (Figure 6). The test indicates a biological value of about 100.

The degree of utilisation of amino acid preparations may depend on variations in the concentration of the essential amino acids in the various amino acid mixtures. This can be measured as the ratio of essential amino acids (E) to total nitrogen (T) in the mixture. In growing subjects the best results seem to be obtained when the E : T ratio is about the same as in body protein. Young and Zamora (1968) found maximum growth in rats when the E : T ratio was about 3 to 4.7.

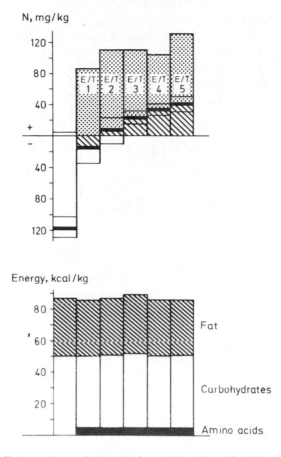

Figure 7. The effect on nitrogen balance in dogs with amino acid solutions of various E : T ratios. The investigations were performed on dogs (Beagles) receiving exclusively complete intravenous feeding. Each period covered one week. During the first week the dogs received no amino acids. In the following periods amino acid solutions with an E : T ratio of 1, 2, 3, 4 or 5 were given. Three series with different orders of the E : T ratio were performed. The diagram is a summary of all investigations arranged with increasing E : T ratio. The solutions were prepared by mixing a solution of only the essential amino acids with a solution of only the non-essential amino acids. The solution of essential amino acids contained, per 100 ml, 240 mg of L–histidine, 390 mg of L–isoleucine, 525 mg of L–leucine, 385 mg of L–lysine, 545 mg of L–phenylalanine, 300 mg of L–threonine, 100 mg of L–tryptophan and 425 mg of L–valine. The solution of non-essential amino acids contained, per 100 ml, 300 mg L–alanine, 330 mg of L–arginine, 405 mg of L–aspartic acid, 140 mg of L–cysteine, 900 mg of L–glutamic acid, 210 mg of glycine, 810 mg of L–proline, 750 mg of L–serine and 50 mg of L–tyrosine. The given amount of nitrogen is indicated by the height of the column in the diagrams of the nitrogen balances. From the upper part of the columns downwards the nitrogen losses via urine and faeces are marked. The horizontal heavy lines represent the nitrogen balances, and the interrupted thin lines indicate the daily variation of nitrogen balances during the period. In the lower part of the diagrams the given amounts of energy in the form of fat, carbohydrate and amino acids are indicated

In dogs on complete intravenous nutrition Holm et al (1975a) used amino acid mixtures with E : T ratio of 1, 2, 3, 4 and 5 (14, 27, 44, 53 and 66 per cent essential amino acids of the total amount of amino acids). They found that the most positive nitrogen balance was observed with amino acid mixtures which had a ratio of 3 to 5, containing 44 to 66 per cent essential amino acids (Figure 7).

In Adult Patients

Schärli (1964, 1965) was readily able to obtain a positive nitrogen balance in man by using an enzymatic casein hydrolysate (Aminosol) in combination with an energy supply of about 2,000 kcal per 24 hours from glucose and soybean oil emulsion Intralipid. Hallberg et al (1967) have reported complete intravenous nutrition for more than 5 months in a patient suffering from Crohn's disease. The body weight was maintained. The patient received up to 1.2 g of amino acids as an enzymatic casein hydrolysate (Aminosol), 0.4–6.2 g of glucose and 2–2.5 g of fat (Intralipid) per kg and day. Peaston (1967) has, in a series of investigations, performed complete parenteral nutrition in adult patients. The daily supply was, on the average, 100 g of amino acids as an enzymatic casein hydrolysate (Aminosol), 225 g of carbohydrates as glucose and fructose, 200 g of fat (Intralipid) amounting to 3,100 kcal.

Abbott and Albertsen (1963), Larsen and Brøckner (1965) and other investigators have shown that in the post-operative period complete parenteral nutrition reduces nitrogen and weight losses. Hallberg et al (1967) studied the effect on cumulative nitrogen balance in the post-operative period after gastrectomies. One group of patients received only 4 g of glucose or 16 kcal per kg which resulted in a cumulative nitrogen loss of about 32 g. By adding 1.5 g of amino acids as enzymatic casein hydrolysate (Aminosol) per kg the loss of nitrogen became less. When 2 g of fat (Intralipid) per kg were given, together with the amino acids and glucose, supplying 36 kcal, the total cumulative nitrogen loss was only about 8 g.

The above mentioned and other investigations have demonstrated that, with enzymatic protein hydrolysate administered intravenously, together with an energy source, such as carbohydrates or carbohydrates and fat in quantities calculated to meet the energy need, a positive nitrogen balance was obtained.

EFFECT OF AMINO ACID SOLUTIONS ON ACID-BASE BALANCE

In parenteral nutrition, all nutrients have to be given in such proportions that a dietary acidosis or alkalosis is not produced. In general, there is a greater risk of acidosis than alkalosis. One reason for this is that the sulphur in the methionine and cystine produces sulphate ion and large amounts of acid may be formed (Wretlind, 1972) [Table III]. Chan (1972) found that sulphate production was lower with casein hydrolysate than with a synthetic amino acid mixture. The

TABLE III. Acid Formation from some Amino Acid Preparations

Infusions solutions	Acid formation in excess of base	
	mEq/l	mEq/g amino acid
Aminosol 3.3%	14	0.42
Aminosol 10%	26	0.26
Aminofusin 10%*	- 26	- 0.26
Intramin forte†	103	0.94
Vamin††	28	0.41

* Containing electrolytes with an excess of cations
† 11 per cent of amino acids without any electrolytes
†† 7 per cent of amino acids, 10 per cent of carbohydrates and electrolytes

high titratable acidity of amino acid solutions was suggested by Chan et al (1972a) as an explanation of the severe metabolic acidosis encountered in total intravenous feeding (Kaplan et al, 1969; Heird et al, 1972a,b; Chan et al, 1972b). The high titratable acidity represents organic acids metabolisable to carbon dioxide and eliminated via the lungs. Heird et al (1972a) have shown that patients receiving protein hydrolysates did not become acidotic. This is because protein hydrolysates contain alkali salts of anionic amino acids (glutamic and aspartic acid), which are metabolised in the body. This causes a reduction of the anions, resulting in a better balance between the inorganic anions (SO_4^{--}, Cl^-) and the cations (Na^+, K^+). In some crystalline amino acid preparations, there is no glutamic and aspartic acid. This must cause an excess of inorganic anions — 'a cation gap' — resulting in an acidosis (Heird et al, 1972a).

If the amino acid mixtures have an excess of non-metabolisable anions, or anions produced by the metabolism of (SO_4^{--}), sodium acetate or lactate, and potassium bicarbonate should be used instead of sodium chloride and potassium chloride solutions; there should always be an equilibrium between the inorganic cations given, and the inorganic anions supplied and those produced by metabolism.

AMINO ACIDS AND CARBOHYDRATES

When solutions of amino acids and carbohydrates, such as glucose and fructose, are heated or stored, a reaction may occur between the two substances. This so-called Maillard reaction was comprehensively described by Hodges et al (1963). The large number of heterocyclic compounds produced by the reaction has been studied by Johnson et al (1966). The conditions under which the reaction takes place have been investigated by El'Ode et al (1966). During a series of reactions, the free amino groups diminished in number, especially those belonging to the

173

basic and sulphur-containing amino acids. Strecker degradations, the formation of Schiff bases and carbonyl compounds are the dominant final products (Rooney et al, 1967). From the nutritional point of view the extensive destruction of lysine is of paramount importance (Ehle & Jansen, 1965).

The Maillard reaction depends on the pH of the solution. In a series of experiments, the solutions containing 18 amino acids at a total concentration of 10 per cent, and 10 per cent fructose were heated to temperatures of 80 and $100°C$ for periods of 1, 2, 3 and 4 hours respectively. The pH, of the various solutions were 5, 6, 7, 8 and 9. The intensity of the Maillard reaction was measured by the absorption of the solution at 300 nm. No Maillard reaction was observed in solutions with a pH of less than 6.

Studies have been made in dogs to see whether nitrogen balance was affected by the administration of amino acid solutions containing fructose stored at different temperatures. The solutions had a pH of 4.40–5.20. There was no difference between solutions freshly prepared compared with those which had been stored for two years at room temperature, nor when an amino-acid-fructose solution was prepared immediately before the investigation and another was stored for 7 days at a temperature of $70°C$.

The Maillard reaction may be avoided by sterilising the amino acids and carbohydrates separately, or by sterile filtration of an amino-acid-carbohydrate mixture with a pH lower than 5.5. An alternative is to use sorbitol instead of glucose or fructose. According to Bansi (1963), however, between 9 and 16 per cent of the sorbitol is lost in the urine. From a physiological standpoint, the natural carbohydrates are to be preferred to sorbitol.

Summary

An adequate, intravenous protein nutrition can be obtained only with an amino acid mixture containing the same amino acids as those entering the general circulation after an oral intake of proteins with high biological value. Such an amino acid mixture for intravenous nutrition requires two components: the essential amino acids, and the non-essential amino acids. Many of the classical non-essential amino acids are necessary for optimal utilisation of the amino acid mixture. The proportions of all the individual amino acids are also of great importance from the nutritional point of view. An amino acid mixture, with a pattern optimal for growing infants, seems to be utilised better than other mixtures under all the conditions investigated.

The optimal utilisation of an amino acid mixture occurs when the energy need is covered. The ratio between energy and amino acids should be 150–200 kcal per gram amino acid nitrogen.

Amino acids and energy supplying nutrients should be given simultaneously in order to obtain an optimal nutritional effect. At the same time it is important to ensure an adequate supply of all other nutrients.

References

Abbott, WE and Albertsen, K (1963) *Nutr. Diet.*, *5*, 339
Allen, PC and Lee, HA (1969) In *A Clinical Guide to Intravenous Nutrition.*
Blackwell, Oxford
Allen, JG, Stemmer, E and Head, L (1956) *Ann. Surg.*, *144*, 349
Artz, CP (1959) *Ann. Surg.*, *149*, 841
Ashworth, A and Harrower, ADB (1967) *Brit. J. Nutr.*, *21*, 833
Bansi, HW (1963) In *Wissenschaftliche Veröffentlichungen der Deutschen
Gesellschaft für Ernährung, Band 11*. Dr Dietrich Steinkopff Verlag, Darmstadt.
Page 9
Bansi, HW, Jürgens, P, Müller, G and Rostin, M (1964) *Klin. Wschr.*, *42*, 232
Bässler, KH (1971) In *Balanced Nutrition and Therapy*. (Ed) K Lang, W Fehl and
G Berg. Georg Thieme Verlag, Stuttgart. Page 31
Belanger, R, Chandramohan, N, Misbin, R and Rivlin, RS (1972) *Metabolism*,
21, 855
Bergström, J, Fürst, P, Josephson, B and Norée, L-O (1970) *Life Sci.*, *9*, 787
Bergström, K, Blomstrand, R and Jacobson, S (1972) *Nutr. Metab.*, *14, Suppl.*,
118
Børresen, HC and Knutrud, O (1969) *Acta paediat. Scand.*, *58*, 420
Børresen, HC and Knutrud, O (1972) In *Parenteral Nutrition*. (Ed) AW Wilkinson.
Churchill Livingstone, Edinburgh and London. Page 176
Børresen, HC, Coran, AG and Knutrud, O (1970) In *Advances in Parenteral
Nutrition*. (Ed) G Berg. Georg Thieme Verlag, Stuttgart. Page 93
Broviac, JW (1974) *Clinical evaluation of Intralipid as a component in parenteral
nutrition: a controlled study.* Unpublished data
Bünte, H (1964) *Langenbeck's Arch. Klin. Chir.*, *308*, 187
Cahill, GF Jr (1972) In *Intravenous Hyperalimentation.* (Ed) G Cowan Jr and
W Scheetz. Lea & Febiger, Philadelphia. Page 52
Calloway, DH and Spector, H (1954) *Amer. J. clin. Nutr.*, *2*, 405
Calloway, DH and Margen, S (1967) *Fed. Proc.*, *26*, 629
Cannon, PB, Steffee, CH, Frazier, EJ, Rowley, DA and Stepto, RC (1947)
Fed. Proc., *6*, 390
Chan, JCM (1972) *Ped. Res.*, *6*, 7891
Chan, JCM, Malekzadeh, M and Hurley, J (1972a) *JAMA*, *220*, 1119
Chan, JCM, Asch, MJ, Lin, S and Hays, DM (1972b) *JAMA*, *220*, 1700
Christensen, HN, Wilber, PB, Coyne, BA and Fischer, JH (1955) *Surg. Forum*,
5, 434
Cox, WM Jr, Müller, AJ and Fickas, D (1942) *Proc. soc. exp. biol. Med.*, *51*, 303
Darke, SJ (1960) *Brit. J. Nutr.*, *14*, 115
Das, JB, Filler, RM, Rubin, VG and Eraklis, AJ (1970) *J. Ped. Surg.*, *5*, 127
Deckner, K, Brand, K and Kofrany, E (1970) *Klin. Wschr.*, *48*, 795
Deligné, P, Prochiantz, E, Bunodiere, M, Lauvergeat, J, Brault, D, Corcos, S,
Loygue, F and Maillard, G (1974) *Ann. Anésth. Franc.*, *15, Spécial 2*, 127
Dolif, D and Jürgens, P (1969) In *Advances in Parenteral Nutrition. Symposium
of the International Soc. of Parenteral Nutrition, Prague*. (Ed) G Berg.
G Thieme Verlag, Stuttgart
Doolan, PD, Harper, HA, Hutchen, ME and Alpen, EL (1965) *J. clin. Invest.*,
35, 888
Dudrick, SJ, Wilmore, DW, Vars, HM and Rhoads, JE (1968) *Surgery*, *64*, 134
Dudrick, SJ, Wilmore, DW, Vars, HM and Rhoads, JE (1969) *Ann.Surg.*, *169*, 974

Dudrick, SJ, Steiger, E, Wilmore, DW and Vars, HM (1970) *Lab.Anim.Care,*
20, 521
Dudrick, SJ, Steiger, E, Long, JM, Ruberg, RL, Allen, TR, Vars, HM and
Rhoads, JE (1972) In *Parenteral Nutrition.* (Ed) AW Wilkinson. Churchill
Livingstone, Edinburgh and London. Page 222
Ehle, SR and Jansen, GR (1965) *Food Techn., 19,* 1435
Elman, R (1937) *Proc.soc. exp. biol. Med., 37,* 610
Elman, R (1939) *Proc. soc. exp. biol. Med., 40,* 484
Elwyn, D (1970) In *Mammalian Protein Metabolism.* (Ed) HN Munro.
Academic Press, New York. Vol.4, page 523
FAO/WHO Expert Group (1965) *FAO Nutr. Meet. Rep. Ser. No.37*
Filler, RM, Eraklis, AJ, Rubin, VG and Das, JB (1969) *New Engl. J. Med., 281,*
589
Fishman, B, Whitman, RJ and Munro, HN (1969) *Proc. nat. acad. Sci., 64,* 677
Fleck, A, Shepherd, J and Munro, HN (1965) *Science, 150,* 628
Fomon, SJ (1967) *Infant Nutrition.* W Saunders, Philadelphia
Frost, DV (1959) In *Protein and Amino Acid Nutrition.* (Ed) AA Albanese.
Academic Press, New York and London. Page 225
Frost, DV and Sandy, HR (1949) *Fed. Proc., 8,* 383
Fürst, P, Josephson, B and Vinnars, E (1970) *Scand. J. clin. lab. Invest., 26,* 319
Garrow, JS (1969) *Reports on public health and medical subjects No.120.*
HMSO, London
Geiger, E (1951) *Fed. Proc., 10,* 670
Geyer, RP (1960) *Physiological Reviews, 40,* 150
Grotte, G (1971) In *Les Solutés de Substitution Rééquilibration métabolique.*
(Ed) GH Nahas and P Viars. Librairie Arnette, Paris. Page 509
Hallberg, D (1974) Lecture at the International Congress on Parenteral Nutrition,
Montpellier, September 1974
Hallberg, D, Schuberth, O and Wretlind, A (1966) *Nutr. Dieta, 8,* 245
Hallberg, D, Holm, I, Obel, A-L, Schuberth, O and Wretlind, A (1967)
Postgrad. Med., 42, A-71, A-87, A-99, A-149
Halmagyi, M and Kilbinger, G (1972) In *Parenteral Nutrition.* (Ed) AW Wilkinson.
Churchill Livingstone, Edinburgh and London. Page 283
Handler, P, Kamin, H and Harris, JS (1949) *J. biol. Chem., 179,* 283
Harper, AE (1958) *Annals NY Acad. Sci., 69,* 1025
Harper, AE (1968) *Amer. J. clin. Nutr., 21,* 358
Harper, AE (1970) In *Parenteral Nutrition.* (Ed) HC Meng and DH Laws.
Charles C Thomas, Springfield, Illinois. Page 181
Harper, AE, Najarian, JA and Silen, W (1956) *Proc. soc. exp. biol. Med., 92,* 558
Harper, AE and Rogers, OE (1965) *Proc. Nutr. Soc., 24,* 173
Hegsted, DM (1963) *Fed. Proc., 22,* 1424
Hegsted, DM (1964) In *Mammalian Protein Metabolism. Vol. II.* (Ed) HN Munro
and JB Allison. Academic Press, New York and London. Page 135
Heird, WC, Dell, RD, Driscoll, JM, Grebin, B and Winters, RW (1972a) *New*
Engl. J. Med., 287, 943
Heird, WC, Driscoll, JM, Schullinger, JN, Grebin, B and Winters, RW (1972b)
J. Ped., 80, 351
Hodges, JE, Fischer, BE and Nelson, EC (1963) *Amer. soc. brew. chem. Proc., 84*
Holm, I, Håkansson, I, Westling, K and Wretlind, A (1975a) *Opuscula Medica,*
Suppl.XXXIX, 154
Holm, I, Håkansson, I, Westling, K and Wretlind, A (1975b) Unpublished data

Holm, LE Jr and Snyderman, SE (1961) *JAMA, 175,* 100
Hussein, MA, Young, VB and Scrimshaw, NS (1968) *Fed. Proc., 27,* 485
Inoue, G, Fujita, Y and Niijama, E (1971) Data published by Munro (1972)
Jacobson, S (1972) *Nutr. Metab., 14, Suppl.,* 150
Jacobson, S and Wretlind, A (1970) In *Body Fluid Replacement in the Surgical Patient.* (Ed) CL Fox and GG Nahas. Grune & Stratton, New York. Page 334
Johnson, JA, Rooney, LW and Salem, A (1966) *Amer. chem. soc. Publ., 56,*153
Johnston, JD, Albritton, WL and Sun Shine, P (1972) *J. Ped., 81,* 154
Johnston, IDA and Spivey, J (1970) In *Advances in Parenteral Nutrition.* (Ed) G Berg. Georg Thieme Verlag, Stuttgart. Page 82
Johnston, IDA, Tweedle, D and Spivey, J (1972) In *Parenteral Nutrition.* (Ed) AW Wilkinson. Churchill Livingstone, Edinburgh and London. Page 189
Jordal, K (1965) *Internat. Zschr. Vitaminforsch, 35,* 26
Josephson, B, Fürst, P and Vinnars, E (1972) In *Parenteral Nutrition.* (Ed) AW Wilkinson. Churchill Livingstone, Edinburgh and London. Page 68
Jürgens, SP and Dolif, D (1968) *Klin. Wschr., 46,* 131
Jürgens, P and Dolif, D (1972) In *Parenteral Nutrition.* (Ed) AW Wilkinson. Churchill Livingstone, Edinburgh and London. Page 47
Kaplan, MW, Mares, A, Quintana, P, Strauss, J, Huxtable, RF, Brennan, P and Hays, DM (1969) *Arch. Surg., 99,* 567
Knutrud, O (1970) *Acta Anaesth. Scand., Suppl. 37,* 35
Kofranyi, E, Jekat, F, Brand, E, Hackenberg, K and Hess, B (1969) *Z. physiol. Chem., 350,* 1401
Lang, K (1972) In *Parenteral Nutrition.* (Ed) HC Meng and DH Law. Charles C Thomas, Springfield, Illinois. Page 160
Larsen, V and Brøckner, J (1965) *Acta chir. Scand., Suppl.343,* 191
Larsen, V and Brøckner, J (1969) *Scand. J. Gastroent., Suppl.4,* 41
Larson, PS and Chaikoff, IL (1937) *J. Nutr., 13,* 287
Lawson, LJ (1965) *Brit. J. Surg., 52,* 795
Levin, G (1973) *Näringsforskning, 17,* 17
Lidström, F (1954) *Acta chir. Scand., Suppl.186*
Lidström, F and Wretlind, A (1952) *Scand. lab. clin. Invest., 4,* 167
Liljedahl, S-O (1972) In *Parenteral Nutrition.* (Ed) AW Wilkinson. Churchill Livingstone, Edinburgh and London. Page 208
Malvey, P, Rousseau, C and Cardon, J (1961) *Presse Méd., 69,* 917
Mayer, G, Knuff, HC, Miller, B, Schmidt, H and Staib, I (1969) *Klin. Wschr., 47,* 1275
McNair, RD, O'Donnell, D and Quigley, W (1954) *Arch. Surg., 68,* 76
Miller, LL (1962) In *Amino Acid Pools.* (Ed) TT Holden. Elsevier, Amsterdam. Page 708
Moore, FD (1959) *Metabolic Care of the Surgical Patient.* W Saunders, Philadelphia and London
Munro, HN (1970) In *Balanced Nutrition and Therapy.* (Ed) K Lang, W Fekl and G Berg. Georg Thieme Verlag, Stuttgart. Page 1
Munro, HN (1972) In *Parenteral Nutrition.* (Ed) AW Wilkinson. Churchill Livingstone, Edinburgh and London. Page 34
Najarian, JS and Harper, HA (1956) *Proc. soc. exp. biol. Med., 92,* 560
El'Ode, JE, Dornseifer, TP, Keith, T and Powes, JJ (1966) *J. Food. Sci., 31,* 351
Panteliadis, C, Jürgens, P and Dolif, D (1975) *Infusionstherapie, 2,* 65
Peaston, MJT (1966) *Brit. Med. J., 2,* 388
Peaston, MJT (1967) *Postgrad. Med. J., 43,* 317

Recommended Dietary Allowances (1968) National Academy of Sciences, Washington, 7th Edition
Recommended Intakes of Nutrients for the United Kingdom: Department of Health and Social Security. Reports on public and medical subjects (1969). HMSO, London. No.120
Reissigl, H (1957) *Med. Klin.*, *52*, 1357
Rogers, QR and Leung, B (1973) *Federal Proc.*, *32*, 1709
Rooney, LW, Salem, A and Johnson, JA (1967) *Cereal Chem.*, *44*, 539
Roos, K-A (1973) *Näringsforskning*, *17*, 9
Rose, WC (1934-1935) *The Harvey Lectures*, *30*, 49
Rose, WC (1957) *Nutr. Abstr. Rev.*, *27*, 631
Rose, WC, Oesterling, MJ and Womack, M (1948) *J. Biol. Chem.*, *177*, 199
Schärli, A (1964) *Praxis*, *53*, 1215
Schärli, A (1965) *Int. Z. Vitaminforsch.*, *35*, 52
Schlappner, OLA, Shelley, WB, Ruberg, RL and Dudrick, SJ (1972) *JAMA*, *219*, 877
Shohl, AT and Blackfan, KD (1940) *J. Nutr.*, *20*, 305
Sirbu, ER, Margen, S and Calloway, DH (1967) *Amer. J. clin. Nutr.*, *20*, 1158
Stegink, G and Baker, GL (1971) *J. Ped.*, *78*, 595
Stegink, LD and den Besten, L (1972) *Science*, *178*, 514
Steinbereithner, K (1966) In *Modern Trends in Anaesthesia.* (Ed) TT Evans and TC Gray. Butterworth, London. Chapter 11
Sturman, JA, Gaull, G and Raiha, NCP (1970) *Sci.*, *169*, 74
Swenseid, ME, Feeley, RJ, Harris, CL and Tuttle, SG (1959) *J. Nutr.*, *68*, 203
Tuttle, SG, Bosset, SM, Griffith, WH, Mulcare, DB and Swenseid, ME (1968) *Amer. J. Clin.*, *16*, 225
Tweedle, DEF, Spivey, J and Johnston, IDA (1972) In *Intravenous Nutrition.* (Ed) AW Wilkinson. Churchill Livingstone, Edinburgh and London. Page 247
Watts, JH, Mann, AN, Bradley, L and Thompson, DJ (1964) *J. Gerontol.*, *19*, 370
Wilmore, DW, Groff, DB, Bishop, HC and Dudrick, SJ (1969) *J. Ped. Surg.*, *4*, 181
Womack, M and Rose, WC (1941) *J. biol. Chem.*, *141*, 375
Woodyatt, RT, Sansum, WD and Wilder, RM (1915) *JAMA*, *65*, 2067
Wretlind, A (1947) *Acta physiol. Scand.*, *13*, 45
Wretlind, A (1972) *Nutr. Metab. 14, Suppl.*, 1
Wurtman, RJ (1970) In *Mammalian Protein Metabolism.* (Ed) HN Munro. Academic Press, New York and London. Vol.4, page 445
Young, VR and Zamora, J (1958) *J. Nutr.*, *96*, 21
Young, VR, Hussein, EM, Murray, E and Scrimshaw, NS (1971) *J. Nutr.*, *101*, 54
Zimmerman, RA and Scott, HM (1965) *J. Nutr.*, *8*, 713

Changes in the Central Nervous System and their Role in the Metabolic Response to Injury

H B STONER

Experimental Pathology of Trauma Section, MRC Toxicology Unit, Medical Research Council Laboratories, Carshalton, England

Introduction

It is not possible to give a complete description of the part played by the central nervous system in the response to injury. Most information is available about changes in the neuroendocrine and thermoregulatory functions of the hypothalamus and in the behaviour of the monoaminergic neurons which arise from cells in the hind-brain, pass upwards and downwards in the central nervous system and seem to play some part in co-ordinating the response. The cerebral cortex and amygdala are concerned in the response, in the latter case, for instance, with the endocrine functions of the hypothalamus but very little is known of their precise functions. Practically all direct information on this subject has been derived from animal experiments.

Before attempting to describe the cerebral response to injury the effect of an injury on cerebral nutrition must be considered. Without adequate nutrition in the form of oxygen and substrates, particularly glucose, the function of the brain becomes disordered and soon ceases. As with all the effects of injury, local and general, the first task is to assess the role of hypoxia.

EFFECT OF INJURY ON CEREBRAL BLOOD FLOW

As might be expected with such an important organ as the brain great care is taken to preserve its blood supply. The cerebral blood flow is autoregulated so that in the ordinary way changes in blood pressure do not affect the flow rate. This autoregulation extends over a wider span of blood pressure than in other organs and it has frequently been shown that the mean arterial blood pressure can fall to about 40 mmHg before any decrease in cerebral blood flow occurs. Nevertheless, cerebral autoregulation can be interfered with in several ways. An important one is local damage to the brain (Reivich et al, 1971) since head injury often complicates injuries to other parts of the body. The amount of damage needed to do this seems quite large judging by the amount of trauma produced in experiments in which autoregulation has been successfully demonstrated (Fiechi et al, 1969; Koo & Cheng, 1974). Systemic hypoxia also interferes (Freeman & Ingvar, 1968) and autoregulation is said not to occur if the O_2 saturation of the arterial blood falls below 60% (Betz, 1972). Autoregulation can be demonstrated during anaesthesia but it is worth noting that most anaesthetics reduce the blood flow through the cerebral cortex towards the rate in the basal parts of the brain which remains unaltered (Goldman & Sapirstein, 1973; Goldman et al, 1973).

Taking this information into account some general conclusions can be drawn about the state of the cerebral blood flow in a number of commonly used shock models.

After injuries such as limb ischaemia where the blood pressure usually does not fall severely until the terminal stage one would not expect any change in cerebral blood flow during the 'ebb' phase. This was shown by direct measurement in the dog (Kovách & Fonyó, 1960). In the rat after a fatal 4 hr period of bilateral hind-limb ischaemia the blood pressure does not fall below 70–80 mmHg until near death and the concentrations of creatine phosphate and ATP, indirect measures of cerebral oxygenation, only decrease in the terminal stages (Stoner & Threlfall, 1954; Kovách & Fonyó, 1960).

In the artificial form of haemorrhagic shock produced by the standard Wiggers procedure in which the blood pressure is reduced by bleeding to low levels for long periods, e.g. 55 and 35 mmHg for consecutive 90 min periods in the dog, gross disturbances of cerebral blood flow occur. These changes are followed by decreases in many types of bio-electrical activity in the cortex and deeper parts of the brain, in reflex activity and in the concentrations of energy-rich phosphates (see Kovách & Fonyó, 1960; Peterson & Haugen, 1963,1965; Kovách, 1970; Kaasik et al, 1970a; Eklof et al, 1972). If the hypotension is sufficiently severe structural damage to the brain may follow (Brierley et al, 1969; Meldrum & Brierley, 1969). Under these conditions the fall in cerebral blood flow is probably the most important effect of the hypotension and the longer its consequences persist the poorer the prognosis (Simeone & Witoska, 1970; Fink et al, 1970). In this regard the changes in electrical activity are probably most important as the concentrations of energy-rich phosphates can revert to normal without proper recovery of function (Kaasik et al, 1970b; Duffy et al, 1972). These experiments, with the sudden onset of severe hypotension and reduction in cerebral blood flow, may serve as models for fatalities occurring in hypotensive anaesthesia, open-heart and dental surgery but not for the 'ebb' phase after more usual injuries in which the blood pressure is always above the critical level for the autoregulation of the cerebral blood flow.

Having established this difference between the Wiggers type of shock model and others based on limb ischaemia, burns, etc, I wish to limit the discussion to the changes in the central nervous system during the 'ebb' phase after the latter forms of experimental injury. (Noble-Collip drum injury can be eliminated as that injury causes direct brain damage [Otomo & Michaelis, 1960] with weakening of the blood-brain barrier.) The questions to be answered are: What effects does an injury have on the central nervous system which are not due to changes in blood flow? What changes occur before the hypoxia of the necrobiotic stage supervenes?

EFFECT OF INJURY ON SUBSTRATE UTILISATION BY BRAIN

Although the cerebral blood flow remains normal during the 'ebb' phase after many forms of injury it cannot be assumed that the utilisation of substrates by the brain continues at normal rates. The overall metabolism of the brain after injury has been reviewed by Kovách and Fonyó (1960) and Kovách (1970). They concluded that the utilisation of both oxygen and glucose was increased and that there was greater hexokinase activity. As pointed out above, the concentrations of energy-rich phosphates in the brain are unaltered at this stage but if creatine phosphate breaks down in response to electrical stimulation of the brain its re-synthesis is slower than normal in the injured rat. This, like the decreased incorporation of intracisternally administered ^{32}P into energy-rich phosphates (Kovách & Fonyó, 1965), may reflect the mitochondrial changes in the brain reported by several groups (Kovách & Fonyó, 1960; Panchenko, 1965; Somogyi et al, 1973) although it is difficult to relate mitochondrial function in vitro to that in vivo.

Much of the work on this topic is now old and some of it should be repeated using modern techniques. It would be particularly useful to determine the effect of injury on the utilisation of glucose and ketone bodies by the brain, using labelled substrates and analysing the data mathematically by methods such as those developed by Cremer and Heath (1974). From the incomplete evidence at present available and allowing for any changes in tissue temperature which may occur, the brain would appear to utilise blood-borne substrates in a fairly normal fashion during the 'ebb' phase.

THERMOREGULATION AFTER INJURY

In the small mammal, with its high surface-area/body weight ratio, thermoregulation is one of the most important functions of the central nervous system to be affected by injury. This effect dominates the metabolic changes of the 'ebb' phase.

It has been known for very many years that body temperature can fall after injury but it was Tabor and Rosenthal (1947) who stressed the importance of

181

this in small mammals and who showed that after limb ischaemia it was not due to failure of oxygen transport to the tissues. As postulated by them and later demonstrated by Stoner and Pullar (1963) with a gradient-layer calorimeter, it is due to decreased heat production. This is seen when the injured animal is at environmental temperatures below its thermoneutral zone. Under these conditions the rate of fall in core temperature is related directly to the severity of the injury and inversely to the ambient temperature (Stoner, 1961). Appreciation that the injured rat was unable to meet the requirements of its environment (Stoner, 1968) led to a detailed study of the matter.

Measurement of total O_2 consumption during the 'ebb' phase showed that the basal (minimal observed) O_2 consumption in the thermoneutral zone was unaltered and that at lower ambient temperatures O_2 consumption did not fall below this value. The critical temperature for heat production (Bligh & Johnson, 1973) was lowered according to the severity of the injury but when O_2 consumption did not respond to ambient temperature the slope of the regression line relating O_2 consumption and ambient temperature was the same as in uninjured rats (Stoner, 1969). As already emphasised, these changes were not due to failure of O_2 transport and, indeed, heat production can be pharmacologically stimulated in these injured rats, e.g. by increasing lipolysis with exogenous catecholamines (Stoner & Little, 1969). The changes only occurred in the thermoregulatory fraction of the total O_2 consumption indicating interference with central thermoregulation. In terms of the movable set-point theory (Hammel, 1968) the results suggested that injury lowered the set-point.

These observations were made on rats injured by limb ischaemia or scalding. The changes in O_2 consumption were found when fluid was lost from the circulation. Before fluid loss occurred the control of non-shivering thermogenesis appeared normal (Stoner & Marshall, 1971).

If the changes in thermoregulation were really due to a lower set-point then one would expect to find lower threshold temperatures (ambient and hypothalamic) for both the onset of shivering and the opening of the arteriovenous anastomoses in the rat's tail which control heat loss from that organ. These temperatures have been determined in rats injured by limb ischaemia (Table I). The first conclusions from the results are that some interference with thermoregulation occurs during the period of limb ischaemia and that the changes cannot be explained by an alteration in set-point since the thresholds move apart instead of in the same direction. While the tourniquets were in place lower temperatures were needed to stimulate shivering and higher ones to open the A-V anastomoses. When the tourniquets were removed these differences were exaggerated.

Although this disturbance in thermoregulation would present a severe disability to a rat in many environments, an injured rat at 20°C should have no difficulty for it would not need to shiver or open A-V anastomoses, and yet the body temperature falls. A fall in body temperature under these conditions implies inhibition of non-shivering thermogenesis (NST). In the rat this form of heat

TABLE I. Features of Thermoregulation in Control Rats and Rats Injured by 4 hr Bilateral Hind-limb Ischaemia

Stage	Oxygen consumption	Threshold (°C)			
		Shivering		Tail Heat Loss	
	$(1[STP]/kg/hr^{-1})$ $(T_a = 20°C)$	T_a	T_{hypo} $(T_a = 20°C)$	T_{hypo} $(T_a = 20°C)$	T_c $(T_a = 20°C)$
		mean ± SEM			
Controls	1.77±0.05 (11)	20.0±1.0 (11)	34.8–36.4$^\mathcal{f}$ (11)	39.8±0.16 (9)	39.2±0.4 (15)
During limb ischaemia	2.09±0.06* (11)	14.0±1.6† (13)	~31	40.5±0.22# (9)	39.1±0.1 (5)
'Ebb' phase after limb ischaemia	1.23±0.07* (6)	11.3±1.7* (10)	no response	no response	–

No of rats shown in parentheses; $\mathcal{f}$ = range
Difference from controls significant * P $<$ 0.001, † P $<$ 0.01, # P $<$ 0.02
Data from Little and Stoner (1968); Stoner (1969,1971,1972); Stoner and Little (1969); Stoner and Marshall (1971)

production is the continuous variant in thermoregulation being especially important when the ambient temperature is below the critical temperature but above the threshold for the onset of shivering. The control of NST during limb ischaemia was unaffected (Stoner & Marshall, 1971) but afterwards when fluid loss occurred, the ambient temperature at which heat transfer from brown adipose tissue commenced was significantly lower than in controls (Stoner, 1974).

A popular way of considering thermoregulation is through the use of neuronal net models. A particularly useful family of models which accept most of the phenomena of mammalian thermoregulation, has been developed by Bligh (1973). An adaptation of one of these models for the rat, where NST is the continuous variant, is shown in Figure 1. In this model cold stimuli activate, first, the effector pathway to NST and then if the stimulus is large enough to overcome a threshold mechanism at A, the effector pathway to shivering, while at the same time inhibiting the heat loss pathways. In the same way hot stimuli inhibit heat production and activate heat loss pathways, overcoming a threshold mechanism at B. The changes in the injured rat can be fitted to this model as follows. During limb ischaemia inhibition at A and B is increased so that colder and hotter stimuli are needed to evoke thermoregulatory responses and the temperature gap between the thresholds is widened. Later, when the tourniquets are removed, inhibition at

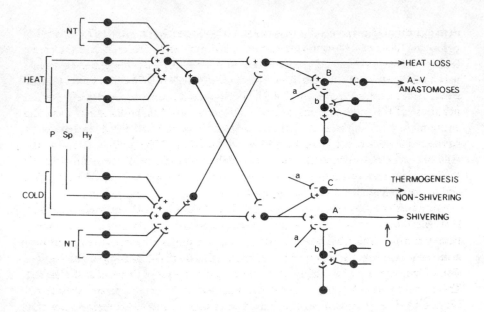

Figure 1. Neuronal model for thermoregulation by the rat hypothalamus after Bligh (1973). Hy = hypothalamic thermoreceptors; Sp = spinal thermoreceptors; P = peripheral thermoreceptors; NT = non-thermal afferents. For explanation of A, B, C and D see text

these points is reinforced and there is also inhibition at C, depressing NST. The precise nature and sites of origin of the non-thermal afferent impulses which lead to these changes are not known. Since the inhibition at C occurs when fluid is lost from the circulation the afferent impulses in this case may arise in volume receptors.

There is a further way in which injury can affect thermoregulation. Shivering is dependent on an input to the brain from the baroreceptors and if this is reduced shivering becomes attenuated (Mott, 1963). We have confirmed Mott's findings and this effect could obviously play a part if hypotension accompanied the injury. The site of this interaction in the brain is not known but is believed to be on the efferent pathway (Figure 1, D). This phenomenon is not concerned in the inhibition of shivering during limb ischaemia as the blood pressure is raised at that time.

Given that the thermoregulatory mechanism depends in real life on some such neuronal net as that shown in Figure 1 and that the changes produced by injury represent interference with that mechanism by non-thermal afferent nerve impulses, which neurotransmitter is concerned? Bligh (1973) has proposed that the transmitter for the 'cross-over neurones' is noradrenaline (NA). It has also been shown (Stone & Mendlinger, 1974), and we have confirmed, that NA injected into the cerebral ventricular system will inhibit shivering in the rat. Consequently, of the possible transmitters NA seemed to be the one to examine first.

6-hydroxydopamine is taken up by catecholaminergic nerve terminals and

184

destroys them (Kostrzewa & Jacobowitz, 1974; Sachs & Jonsson, 1975). As this compound does not cross the blood-brain barrier it can be injected into the cerebral ventricular system and used as a tool to destroy the catecholaminergic terminals near the walls of the ventricles while leaving the NA cell bodies intact (Ungerstedt, 1968; Uretsky & Iversen, 1969). Serotoninergic neurons are not affected, nor those of the tubero-infundibular dopaminergic system. On the other hand the entire neurons of the nigrostriatal and mesolimbic dopaminergic systems are damaged (Ungerstedt, 1973). As used by us, 6-OHDA (250 μg into a lateral ventricle one week before test) caused severe depletion of NA in all the main areas of the hypothalamus containing noradrenergic terminals, especially the POAH region and *n. dorsomedialis* (Stoner & Marshall, 1975a).

Although rats treated in this way have disabilities (appetite and weight loss) at first, thermoregulation, after recovery from the initial hypothermia, seems superficially normal. Shivering began at the same environmental ambient temperature as in untreated rats. However, this treatment with 6-OHDA prevented the depression of the threshold for the onset of shivering after injury (Unpublished Results). This implies that NA is the transmitter concerned in the effect, presumably at A (Figure 1). The synapses concerned must be caudal to the POAH region since the direct injection of 6-OHDA into this part of the brain had no effect on the response to injury. It was not possible to decide whether NA was also involved in the effect of injury on the heat loss side.

CENTRAL MONOAMINERGIC NEURONS-ASCENDING FIBRES

There are several systems of monoaminergic neurons in the brain (Dahlstrom & Fuxe, 1964; Fuxe, 1965; Loizou, 1969; Ungerstedt, 1971; Maeda & Shimizu, 1972). The main ones from our point of view are the NA and serotonin (5HT) fibres which arise from groups of cells in the hind-brain. The NA fibres arise mostly from the cells of the *locus coeruleus* in the anterior part of the floor of the 4th ventricle and from other smaller nuclei in the hind-brain. The cells of origin of the 5HT fibres are mostly in the region of the median raphé. Fibres of both types ascend and descend in the brain and spinal cord. Those going to the hypothalamus ascend mostly in the medial forebrain bundle from which they are widely distributed to its nuclei and regions. Terminals containing NA are particularly dense around the cells of the magnocellular nuclei, the *n. dorsomedialis* and the POAH region. Serotoninergic terminals are similarly distributed but are more difficult to examine by fluorescence histochemistry and other techniques and hence have been less closely studied than the NA fibres in the response to injury. Of the various dopaminergic fibre systems only the tubero-infundibular system are positively known to be concerned in the response to injury. Adrenergic neurons have been reported in the hypothalamus but their function is not known.

A severe injury such as bilateral hind-limb ischaemia in the rat activates the NA system, stimulating first the fibres which go to the magnocellular nuclei and later

185

those which supply the POAH region and the *n. dorsomedialis* (Stoner & Elson, 1971; Stoner et al, 1973; Stoner & Marshall, 1975b). These conclusions, based on changes in the concentration and turnover of NA and in its fluorescence histochemistry, are supported by increases in the hypothalamic concentration of the major metabolite of NA secreted by the terminals, 3-methoxy-4-hydroxy-phenylethylene glycol sulphate (MOPEG-SO$_4$) [Stoner & Hunt, Unpublished Results].

The function of these NA fibres in the response to injury is not clearly understood. Removal of these NA terminals by injecting 6-OHDA into a lateral cerebral ventricle increased the mortality rate and shortened the survival time after limb ischaemia in the rat (Stoner & Marshall, 1975a). Some of the neurons will no doubt be concerned in producing the changes in thermoregulation, as described above, but this would only account for a few of them. In general NA is thought to be an inhibitory transmitter in this region of the brain. In many ways this makes it even more difficult to visualise its function since at this time the activity of the neurotransducer cells of the hypothalamus is increased (v.i.).

Serotoninergic neurons are also activated by injury. This conclusion is based on biochemical measurements which have mostly shown changes in 5HT concentration or turnover in the region of the cells of origin in the hind-brain after mild stress (Barchas & Freedman, 1963; Thierry et al, 1968). Foot-shock has been shown to increase the 5-hydroxyindole acetic acid (5HIAA) concentration in the hypothalamus (Bliss et al, 1968) and a rise in the concentration of this 5HT metabolite is usually taken to indicate increased neural activity. After a more severe injury such as limb ischaemia no changes in 5HT or 5HIAA concentrations were seen in the hypothalamus but the 5HIAA concentration in the hind-brain rose during limb ischaemia and the 5HT concentration was elevated during the 48 hr after a non-fatal period of ischaemia (Stoner & Elson, 1971). The physiological importance of these changes is not known although many of these neurons are involved in the same types of activity as the NA neurons, e.g. thermoregulation.

CENTRAL MONOAMINERGIC NEURONS-DESCENDING FIBRES

Less is known about the descending NA fibres. Some supply the *n. tractus solitarius* and dorsal nucleus of the vagus. These fibres did not show any changes after injury when examined by fluorescence histochemistry (Stoner & Marshall, 1975b). However, the turnover of NA in the hind-brain increased during limb-ischaemia (Stoner et al, 1973) and there was a progressive rise in the MOPEG-SO$_4$ concentration in the hind-brain, particularly in its caudal part (Stoner & Hunt, Unpublished). An increase in neuronal activity at this time could be anticipated since this part of the hind-brain contains the cardiovascular centres which would be expected to be affected by injury. There is physiological evidence for this. Tilting can be used to test the reactivity of the cardiovascular centres. Little

(1975) has found that the rise in blood pressure in response to a head-up tilt in the rat is reduced during limb ischaemia and even more so after the tourniquets have been removed. Similar changes were seen after scalding. These changes may be due to the inhibitory effect of the descending NA fibres on the cardiovascular centres (e.g. de Jong et al, 1975; Struyker Boudier et al, 1975).

The role in the response to injury of the NA fibres distributed down the spinal cord is not known. Similarly, little can be said about the function of the descending 5HT fibres. For instance, it is not known if they play any part in the transient hyperexcitability followed by progressive deterioration in the reflex activity of the spinal cord described by Peterson and Haugen (1963, 1965).

CENTRAL CHOLINERGIC NEURONS

The central cholinergic neurons are in some ways more difficult to study than the NA and 5HT neurons. The areas of the brain concerned in homoeostasis are supplied with cholinergic fibres from two main ascending pathways (Shute & Lewis, 1966). The dorsal fibres come from the dorsolateral part of the mesencephalic reticular formation and the ventral fibres from the region of the *substantia nigra* and posterior part of the diencephalon. From what is known of the functions of these fibres it is clear that they are concerned in homoeostasis, in temperature control and the regulation of the neurons which produce hypothalamic releasing hormones such as corticotrophine-releasing hormone. Consequently these fibres must be concerned in the response to injury but there is little direct information about their behaviour under these conditions. In view of the increased activity in both the anterior and posterior lobes of the pituitary it is assumed that the activity of these ascending cholinergic fibres is also increased after injury and that they are concerned in relaying the afferent information to the effector parts of the brain.

Cholinergic neurons are present in all parts of the brain and Kovách and Fonyó (1960) described a large rise in the acetylcholine content of the whole cerebrum in the terminal stages of traumatic shock. The mechanism of this is not known but part of it could be secondary to the fall in body temperature of the injured rat leading to decreased utilisation of acetylcholine.

HYPOTHALAMIC NEUROTRANSDUCER CELLS

Hypothalamic neurons which also secrete hormones have been described as neurotransducer cells. They can be divided into two groups depending on whether the hormones are related to the posterior or anterior lobes of the pituitary.

Posterior Pituitary Hormones

The neurons which synthesise antidiuretic hormone (ADH) and oxcytocin and secrete them in the posterior lobe of the pituitary have their cell bodies in the magnocellular supraoptic and paraventricular nuclei. Noxious stimuli, haemorrhage, limb ischaemia and surgical operations all lead to a rapid increase in secretion by these cells. Both nuclei secrete both hormones although the proportions for the individual nuclei may differ in different species. Both hormones are secreted in response to injury but different stimuli lead to the secretion of different proportions of ADH and oxytocin (Dyball, 1968).

The stimuli to the cells in these nuclei come from osmo-receptors and, particularly in the case of haemorrhage, from volume receptors in the thorax via the vagi. Other types of afferent fibres must also be involved in injuries such as limb ischaemia for stimulation occurs while the tourniquets are in place (Dexter et al, 1953). The cells in the magnocellular nuclei are thought to be stimulated by cholinergic fibres and inhibited by noradrenergic ones (Pickford, 1939; Moss et al, 1972; Ganong, 1974). This matter is not, however, completely settled and there are reports of these neurons being stimulated by NA (Kühn, 1974; Garay and Leibowitz, 1974; Milton & Paterson, 1974). Hence, it is difficult to define the role of the secretion of NA in these nuclei after injury. Is it, for instance, concerned in regulating the proportion of the two hormones secreted in the posterior lobe?

The value of secreting a pressor and antidiuretic hormone after injury is obvious. The posterior lobe hormones also stimulate glycogenolysis in the liver to produce hyperglycaemia (Clark, 1928; Imrie, 1929) and Hems and Whitton (1973) have recently suggested that this action contributes to the hyperglycaemia after injury and is also beneficial in causing transference of the water stored in conjunction with glycogen from the liver to the plasma.

Anterior Hypophysis

As a result of recent work in many laboratories it is now clear that the anterior lobe of the pituitary is firmly under the control of a system of neurons scattered through the anterior part of the hypothalamus. These neurons secrete the releasing and, in some cases, release-inhibiting hormones which are carried in the vessels of the pituitary portal system to the anterior lobe (see Schally et al, 1973; Besser & Mortimer, 1974). Stimulation of these cells leads to the well-known liberation of ACTH from the pituitary after injury. In man injury is also accompanied by an increase in secretion of growth hormone (Glick et al, 1965; Ross et al, 1966; Salter et al, 1972) whereas in the rat injury decreases the secretion of growth hormone (Krulich et al, 1974). Prolactin secretion is controlled by a release-inhibiting hormone. Secretion of this factor is inhibited after injury with an increase in the secretion of prolactin in both rat and man (Krulich et al, 1974).

Rather less is known about the neurotransmitters which affect these transducer cells than in the case of the cells in the magnocellular nuclei (Ganong, 1974). For corticotrophin-releasing hormone it appears that acetylcholine stimulates and NA inhibits secretion (Hillhouse et al, 1975). In other cases NA is thought to stimulate secretion. Dopamine and 5HT are also postulated as neurotransmitters in these reactions (Ganong, 1974; Lu & Meites, 1973; Berger et al, 1974). The whole matter lacks finality and its investigation is obviously more difficult than in the case of the posterior pituitary hormones because of the scattered distribution of the cells which secrete the hormones. Nevertheless it requires detailed study, particularly as the liberation of ACTH, growth hormone and prolactin can be altered by commonly used drugs such as morphine and barbiturate (George et al, 1974; Ajika et al, 1972).

The hypothalamic releasing hormones and their activities form a rapidly expanding field of research. Most of it concerns their responses to physiological changes within the body and to mild stress. More work is needed on their responses to serious injuries which endanger life. The afferent pathways by which the incoming impulses reach the cells have been described (Stoner, this volume). It has been suggested (McCann et al, 1973) that the afferent pathways are similar for all the hormones and that the differential patterns of release are brought about by specific intrahypothalamic mechanisms.

HYPOTHALAMIC DEFENCE AREA

Before we can consider the effects of all these changes in the brain on the metabolism of the injured animal another cerebral mechanism must be mentioned. There is an area in the posterior part of the hypothalamus which is known as the 'defence area' and which is under cortical control. When this part of the hypothalamus is stimulated there is mass excitation of the sympathetic system to increase blood pressure and cardiac output and direct blood from the skin, kidneys and gastrointestinal tract to the muscles where the blood vessels are dilated by cholinergic fibres (Abrahams et al, 1964). This reaction is brought into play by the cerebral cortex in response to danger and is intended to put the animal in a suitable state of alert. Consequently, in many cases, this reaction will have taken place before the injury is inflicted. In some species an alternative response to danger is 'playing dead' with a fall in blood pressure and widespread vasodilatation. This can be reproduced by stimulating an area in the anterior part of the hypothalamus. These responses and the parts of the brain concerned have been recently reviewed by Folkow and Neil (1971).

METABOLIC EFFECTS OF CENTRAL NERVOUS SYSTEM OUTFLOW

The information reaching the brain of the injured animal via afferent nervous impulses and the blood is converted, in the interactions described above, into a neuro-endocrine outflow with a wide range of metabolic effects.

Sympathetic-adrenal Medullary System

The autonomic outflow which begins before injury in the defence reaction

(Natelson et al, 1973) and continues afterwards leads to the liberation of adrenaline from the adrenal medulla and of noradrenaline at sympathetic nerve endings in fat, liver and other tissues. This results in the mobilisation of the stores of triglyceride and glycogen, probably in that order. The triglyceride in the fat depots is broken down to non-esterified fatty acids which will be transported through the body bound to plasma albumin if there is adequate circulation through the fat depots (Stoner, 1962; Stoner & Matthews, 1967; Kovách et al, 1970). These fatty acids will either be utilised as such or converted to ketone bodies or triglycerides in the liver (Heath & Stoner, 1968; Barton, 1971). The glycogen is converted directly, or indirectly through the Cori Cycle to glucose which accumulates in the extracellular space (Stoner, 1958).

Other Neuroendocrine Responses

Other neuroendocrine responses to injury involve hormones producing rapid effects. Injury stimulates the cells of the magnocellular nuclei to secrete ADH and oxytocin from the posterior lobe of the pituitary. The ADH produced in this way could, as discussed above, contribute to the stimulation of glycogenolysis and, hence, to the hyperglycaemia.

The other rapidly acting hormones are those of the pancreas. Change in the concentration of plasma glucose is the prime stimulus for changes in the secretion rates of insulin and glucagon. However, the secretion of both hormones is also under nervous control. Glucagon secretion can be stimulated by both cholinergic (vagal) and noradrenergic (sympathetic) nerves which form the termination of pathways coming down from the hypothalamus (Frohman & Bernardis, 1971). It is thought that the sympathetic innervation is involved in the glucagon response to injury (Bloom et al, 1974). It must, however, be remembered that glucagon secretion can also be stimulated by circulating adrenaline and by some amino acids, such as arginine, which could increase in the plasma after injury. The most important stimulus for insulin secretion by the β-cells is probably the plasma glucose concentration but these cells are also under central control through their double innervation (Porte et al, 1973; Woods & Porte, 1974). The parasympathetic fibres stimulate and the sympathetic fibres and circulating adrenaline inhibit insulin secretion. After an injury the circulating insulin concentrations may be appropriate for the hyperglycaemia or they may be depressed if the injury has caused a powerful stimulus to the sympathetic adrenal medullary system (see Stoner & Heath, 1973 for references). This latter effect, coupled with the insulin resistance which accompanies injury, could impede the utilisation of plasma glucose.

The anterior pituitary hormones secreted at the behest of the hypothalamic releasing hormones have slower and more prolonged actions, particularly if they act through a second endocrine gland. The precise roles of the corticosteroids, growth hormone and prolactin which can increase in the circulation after injury are not known. Participation by the adrenal steroids is essential but it is not clear whether anything is gained by having more than the concentrations necessary for their permissive actions. These hormones have been linked with growth hormone in attempts to explain the insulin resistance after injury. However, the species differences in the growth hormone response to injury — increased secretion in man, decreased in rat — could raise doubts about its importance.

These actions of the central nervous system mobilise the energy stores of the body into readily utilisable forms, glucose, non-esterified fatty acids and ketone bodies. Despite interactions in their subsequent metabolism this would seem, teleologically, useful, at least at a time when 'fight or flight' are possible. However, the continuing neuroendocrine response after an actual injury introduces other dimensions to the response. An element of conservation appears, e.g. in insulin resistance. Some of these hormonal alterations represent changes in metabolic control at or near the cell surface. The central nervous system also affects metabolism through its control of body temperature. In the small mammal this is mainly done by controlling the rate of oxidative metabolism.

At first sight, the two aspects of the neuroendocrine response during the 'ebb' phase appear to be in opposition and the possible significance of this will be considered later (Stoner, this volume).

References

Abrahams, VS, Hilton, SM and Zbrozyna, AW (1964) *J. Physiol. (Lond), 171*, 189
Ajika, K, Krulich, L and McCann, SM (1972) *Proc. Soc. exp. biol. Med. NY, 141*, 203
Barchas, JD and Freedman, DX (1963) *Biochem. Pharmac., 12*, 1232
Barton, RN (1971) *Clin. Sci., 40*, 463
Berger, PA, Barchas, JD and Vernikos-Danellis, J (1974) *Nature (Lond.), 248*, 424
Besser, GM and Mortimer, CH (1974) *J. clin. Path., 27*, 173
Betz, E (1972) *Physiol. Rev., 52*, 595
Bligh, J (1973) *Temperature Regulation in Mammals and Other Vertebrates.* North-Holland, Amsterdam
Bligh, J and Johnson, KG (1973) *J. appl. Physiol., 35*, 941
Bliss, EL, Ailion, J and Zwanziger, J (1968) *J. Pharmacol., 164*, 122
Bloom, SR, Vaughan, NJA and Russell, RCG (1974) *Lancet, ii*, 546
Brierley, JB, Brown, AW, Excell, BJ and Meldrum, BS (1969) *Brain. Res., 13*, 68
Clark, GA (1928) *J. Physiol. (Lond.), 64*, 324
Cremer, JE and Heath, DF (1974) *Biochem. J., 142*, 527
Dählstrom, A and Fuxe, K (1964) *Acta physiol. Scand., 62, Suppl. 232*, 5
Dexter, DD, Stoner, HB and Green, HN (1953) *Brit. J. exp. Path., 34*, 625
Duffy, TE, Nelson, SR and Lowry, OH (1972) *J. Neurochem., 19*, 959
Dyball, REJ (1968) *Brit. J. Pharmacol., 33*, 319
Eklof, B, MacMillan, V and Siesjö, BK (1972) *Acta physiol. Scand., 86*, 515
Fieschi, C, Bozzao, L, Agnoli, A, Nardini, M and Bartolini, A (1969) *Exp. brain Res., 7*, 111

Fink, RA, Burham, WA, Owen, TL, Dixon, AC and Goldstein, JD (1970) *Neurology, 20,* 408

Folkow, B and Neil, E (1971) *Circulation.* Oxford University Press, London. Page 342

Freeman, J and Ingvar, DH (1968) *Ex. brain. Res., 5,* 61

Frohman, LA and Bernardis, LL (1971) *Amer. J. Physiol., 221,* 1596

Fuxe, K (1965) *Acta physiol. Scand., 64, Suppl. 247,* 37

Ganong, WF (1974) *Life Sciences, 15,* 1401

Garay, KF and Leibowitx, SF (1974) *Federation Proc., 33,* 563

George, JM, Reier, CE, Lanesa, RR and Rower, JM (1974) *J. clin. endocrinol. Metab., 38,* 736

Glick, SM, Roth, J, Yalow, RS and Berson, SA (1965) *Recent Progr. horm. Res., 21,* 255

Goldman, H and Sapirstein, LA (1973) *Amer. J. Physiol., 224,* 122

Goldman, H, Sapirstein, LA, Murphy, S and Moore, J (1973) *Proc. Soc. exp. biol. Med. NY, 144,* 983

Hammel, HT (1968) *Ann. rev. Physiol., 30,* 641

Heath, DF and Stoner, HB (1968) *Brit. J. exp. Path., 49,* 160

Hems, DA and Whitton, PD (1973) *Biochem. J., 136,* 705

Hillhouse, EW, Burden, J and Jones, MT (1975) *Neuroendocrinology, 17,* 1

Imrie, CG (1929) *J. Physiol. (Lond.), 67,* 264

Jong, W de, Nijkamp, FP and Bohus, B (1975) *Arch. int. Pharmacodyn., 213,* 272

Kaasik, AE, Nilsson, L and Siesjö, B (1970a) *Acta physiol. Scand., 78,* 433

Kaasik, AE, Nilsson, L and Siesjö, B (1970b) *Acta physiol. Scand., 78,* 448

Koo, A and Cheng, KK (1974) *Microvascular Res., 8,* 151

Kostrjewa, RM and Jacobowitz, DM (1974) *Pharm. Rev., 26,* 200

Kovách, AGB (1970) *J. clin. Path., 23, Suppl. (Roy. Coll. Path.), 4,* 202

Kovách, AGB and Fonyó, A (1960) In *The Biochemical Response to Injury.* (Ed) HB Stoner and CJ Threlfall. Blackwell, Oxford. Page 129

Kovách, AGB and Fonyó, A (1965) *Acta physiol. Acad. Sci. Hung., 27,* 27

Kovách, AGB, Rosell, S, Sándor, P, Koltay, E, Kovách, E and Tomka, N (1970) *Circ. Res., 26,* 733

Krulich, L, Hefco, E, Illner, P and Read, CB (1974) *Neuroendocrinology, 16,* 293

Kuhn, ER (1974) *Neuroendocrinology, 16,* 255

Little, RA (1975) *J. Physiol. (Lond.)* (In press)

Little, RA and Stoner, HB (1968) *Quart. J. exp. Physiol., 53,* 76

Loizou, LA (1969) *Brain Res., 15,* 563

Lu, KH and Meites, J (1973) *Endocrinology, 93,* 152

Maeda, T and Shimizu, N (1972) *Brain Res., 36,* 19

McCann, SM, Ajika, K, Fawcett, CP, Hefco, E, Illner, P, Negro-Vilar, A, Orias, R, Watson, JT and Krulich, L (1973) In *Hormones, Metabolism and Stress.* (Ed) S Németh. Slovak Academy of Sciences, Bartislava. Page 67

McCutcheon, EP, Frazier, DT and Boyarsky, LL (1971) *Proc. Soc. exp. biol. Med., 136,* 1063

Meldrum, BS and Brierley, JB (1969) *Brain Res., 13,* 101

Milton, AS and Paterson, AT (1974) *J. Physiol. (Lond.), 241,* 607

Moss, RL, Urban, I and Cross, BA (1972) *Amer. J. Physiol., 223,* 310

Mott, J (1963) *J. Physiol. (Lond.), 166,* 563

Natelson, BH, Smith, GP, Stokes, PE and Root, AW (1973) *Amer. J. Physiol., 224,* 1454

Otomo, E and Michaelis, M (1960) *Proc. Soc. exp. biol. Med. NY, 104,* 259
Pásztor, A, Sarkadi, Á, Tomka, I and Okrutay, K (1972) *Acta physiol. Acad. sci. Hung., 42,* 411
Panchenko, LF (1966) *Federation Proc., 25,* T482
Peterson, CG and Haugen, FP (1963) *Amer. J. Surg., 106,* 233
Peterson, CG and Haugen, FP (1965) *Ann. Surg., 161,* 485
Pickford, M (1939) *J. Physiol. (Lond.), 95,* 226
Porte, D, Girardier, L, Seydoux, J, Kanazawa, Y and Posternak, J (1973) *J. clin. Invest., 52,* 210
Reivich, M, Marshall, WJS and Kassell, N (1971) In *Cerebral Vascular Diseases.* (Ed) J Moossy and R Janeway. Grune & Stratton, New York. Page 63
Ross, H, Johnston, IDA, Welborn, TA and Wright, AD (1966) *Lancet, ii,* 563
Sachs, G and Jonsson, G (1975) *Biochem. Pharmacol., 24,* 1
Salter, CP, Fluck, DC and Stimmler, L (1972) *Lancet, ii,* 853
Schally, AV, Arimura, A and Kastin, AJ (1973) *Science, 179,* 341
Shute, CCD and Lewis, PR (1966) *Brit. med. Bull., 22,* 221
Simeone, FA and Witoszka, M (1970) *Amer. J. Surg., 119,* 427
Somogyi, J, Cremer, JE and Ikrényi, K (1972) *Adv. exp. med. Biol., 33,* 345
Stone, EA and Mendlinger, S (1974) *Res. comm. chem. path. Pharmac., 7,* 549
Stoner, HB (1958) *Brit. J. exp. Path., 39,* 635
Stoner, HB (1961) *Scientific Basis of Medicine (Ann. Rev.).* Athlone Press, London. Page 172
Stoner, HB (1962) *Brit. J. exp. Path., 43,* 556
Stoner, HB (1968) *Ann. NY Acad. Sci., 150,* 722
Stoner, HB (1969) *Brit. J. exp. Path., 50,* 125
Stoner, HB (1971) *J. Physiol. (Lond.), 214,* 599
Stoner, HB (1972) *J. appl. Physiol., 33,* 665
Stoner, HB (1974) *J. Physiol. (Lond.), 238,* 657
Stoner, HB and Elson, PM (1971) *J. Neurochem., 18,* 1837
Stoner, HB, Elson, PM and Koltay, E (1973) *J. Neurochem., 21,* 223
Stoner, HB and Heath, DF (1973) *Brit. J. Anaesth., 45,* 244
Stoner, HB and Little, RA (1969) *Brit. J. exp. Path., 50,* 107
Stoner, HB and Marshall, HW (1971) *Brit. J. exp. Path., 52,* 650
Stoner, HB and Marshall, HW (1975a) *Brit. J. exp. Path., 56,* 157
Stoner, HB and Marshall, HW (1975b) *Brain Res.* (In press)
Stoner, HB and Matthews, J (1967) *Brit. J. exp. Path., 48,* 58
Stoner, HB and Pullar, JD (1963) *Brit. J. exp. Path., 44,* 586
Stoner, HB and Threlfall, CJ (1954) *Biochem. J., 58,* 115
Struyker Boudier, H, Smeets, G, Brouwer, G and Van Rossum, JM (1975) *Arch. int. Pharmacodyn., 213,* 285
Tabor, H and Rosenthal, SM (1947) *Amer. J. Physiol., 149,* 449
Thierry, AM, Fekete, M and Glowinski, J (1968) *Europ. J. Pharmac., 4,* 384
Ungerstedt, U (1968) *Eur. J. Pharmacol., 5,* 107
Ungerstedt, U (1971) *Acta physiol. Scand., 82, Suppl. 367,* 1
Ungerstedt, U (1973) *Neurosci. Res., 5,* 73
Uretsky, NJ and Iversen, LL (1969) *Nature, Lond., 221,* 557
Woods, SC and Porte, D (1974) *Physiol. Rev., 54,* 596

An Integrated Neuro-endocrine Response to Injury

H B STONER

Experimental Pathology of Trauma Section, MRC Toxicology Unit, Medical Research Council Laboratories, Carshalton, England

SUBSTRATE MOBILISATION

In the injured animal there is a metabolic conflict between increased production of easily used substrates and the inhibition of their metabolism. The prime result of increased sympathetic and adrenal medullary activity at the beginning of the response to an injury, or even before it occurs, is a superabundance of circulating substrates in readily usable forms, non-esterified fatty acids, glucose and ketone bodies. In an uninjured animal such an increase in the plasma concentrations of these substrates would accelerate their rates of disposal. In the case of the plasma glucose the utilisation rate increases as the square of its concentration (Heath & Corney, 1973). For non-esterified fatty acids and ketone bodies the rate of uptake from the plasma is directly related to their concentrations in the plasma (Fine & Williams, 1960; Cunningham, 1973; Barton, 1973). Consequently, if these excess substrates were taken up by the cells and metabolised, unless the metabolic pattern was altered, all the ketone bodies and most of the other compounds, except for those which could be stored as glycogen, would be rapidly oxidised and so, in a sense, lost. Admittedly, some of the energy exposed would be trapped and used as adenosine triphosphate (ATP) but once the ATP is hydrolysed the energy associated with its special bonds is used and cannot be recalled. As part of a defence reaction, conditioning the body for sudden effort, the risk of losing these energy stores might be well worth running. In these circumstances the advantages of having supplies of ATP, both actual and potential, readily available could be very great, the difference between life and death.

If the mobilisation of energy stores could be restricted to the 'fight or flight' type of situation in which they are needed, all would be well. An injury

194

provokes the same response whether it is inflicted during this state of preparedness or whether it occurs accidentally. The afferent pathways might be different in the two cases but the effector pathways and the end result would be the same. Then with the possibility of being incapacitated and unable to hunt for food and water, the inability to conserve these important substrates might be very serious especially for carbohydrate, the stores of which are smaller than those of fat.

METABOLIC RESTRAINTS

After an injury a series of metabolic restraints are imposed which have the effect of conserving available substrates. Insulin is necessary for the uptake of glucose by cells. If the injury is very severe the secretion of insulin which would normally occur in response to the hyperglycaemia is inhibited by circulating adrenaline and the sympathetic nervous system (Porte et al, 1966, Stoner & Heath, 1973). Even with less severe injuries in which the plasma insulin concentration rises appropriately for the plasma glucose concentration, insulin resistance occurs (Frayn, 1975).

In these conditions the rate of removal of glucose from the plasma no longer varies as the square of its concentration but is practically independent of it (Heath & Corney, 1973). These methods of conservation are quite effective for glucose, which is either extracellular at the time of the injury or is secreted by the liver shortly afterwards. Glucose which is broken down in the cells, passing through glycolysis to the tricarboxylic acid cycle, is uninfluenced by an effective lack of insulin at the cell surface and is thus lost.

Conservation of fat is more difficult and fortunately there is more of it. If the injury is severe the fat depots will be poorly perfused and the newly-formed non-esterified fatty acids will not be removed by the plasma (Stoner & Matthews, 1967; Kovách et al, 1970). Provided there is sufficient insulin the high glucose concentrations may favour re-esterification in the fat cells but neither of these changes can be looked upon as more than chance methods of conservation. Once the albumin-bound non-esterified fatty acids escape into the circulating plasma they will be extracted by the tissues in accordance with their concentrations. Injury does not interfere with this process (Heath & Stoner, 1968). Injury does, however, inhibit the direct oxidation of non-esterified fatty acids. In the liver some may be directed towards triglyceride but the proportion converted to ketone bodies is increased (Barton, 1971).

Ketone bodies secreted into the general circulation by the liver are taken up by the tissues according to their concentration in the plasma (Barton, 1973) and oxidised. There is really no way of storing these useful compounds. For many compounds there is a side pool on their metabolic pathway into which they can be shunted and so delay their final destruction. Examples of this are glycogen, lactate and the Cori cycle and liver triglyceride. No such pool exists

195

for the ketone bodies and, except for the slight delay for their interconversion, they must be oxidised. Barton (1973) has shown that after 4 hr bilateral hind-limb ischaemia in the post-absorptive rat the average blood concentrations of ketone bodies were raised, the mean total rate of disposal was increased and the mean contribution of ketone bodies to the whole body O_2 consumption rose from 7 to 15 per cent.

CONTROL OF METABOLIC RATE

Although the stores of fat, and hence of ketone bodies, are relatively large the continued utilisation of these substrates in the absence of readily available glucose would, in the long term, lead to considerable losses (Moore, 1971). Once triglycerides have been hydrolysed and reach the plasma the possibilities for controlling their metabolism are few. The only effective measure would be to lower the metabolic rate of the body and keep the whole mechanism running at a lower level of energy expenditure. This could be achieved by allowing the metabolic rate to fall towards the basal level. The basal metabolic rate is strictly defined as the rate of metabolic free energy production calculated from measurements of heat production or oxygen consumption in an organism in a rested, awake, fasting and thermoneutral state (Bligh & Johnson, 1973). In this paper basal rate refers to the 'minimum observed' rate of oxygen consumption in a thermoneutral environment. Normally when the environmental temperature falls below the thermoneutral zone the oxygen consumption rises to meet the demand for heat. It is this increase which would have to be prevented or reduced in the injured animal. Using the normal control mechanisms of the body the best that could be done would be to keep metabolism near the basal level. A fall in oxygen consumption below the basal level indicates either failure of oxygen transport or damage to the intracellular oxidative mechanisms or both, and in the case of the injured animal means that it has passed from the 'ebb' phase to the final, necrobiotic stage.

It would seem that the overall reduction in oxidation needed to conserve the body's substrates might be achieved if alterations could be made to the thermo-regulatory mechanisms.

ROLE OF THERMOREGULATION

The central control of body temperature could be altered in one of two ways. Thermoregulation is probably best described as a system for the proportional control of body temperature by means of a movable set-point (Hammel, 1968). Lowering the set-point would have the desired result. The body would then tend to a lower core temperature, the critical temperature for the onset of non-shivering thermogenesis would be lower as would the threshold temperatures for the onset of shivering. At any environmental temperature below the normal thermoneutral zone oxygen consumption and heat production would be less than in an uninjured animal. The alternative method would be by inhibiting

196

(or increasing existing inhibition of) the effector pathways which excite non-shivering thermogenesis, shivering and thermoregulatory heat loss. From the point of view of heat production the effect of this could be the same as lowering the set-point. One difference from that method lies on the heat loss side. When the set-point is moved the thresholds for shivering and thermoregulatory heat loss move in the same direction. Hence, lowering the set-point reduces the threshold temperatures at which the arterio-venous anastomoses of the heat loss mechanism in the rat's tail open. In the second method inhibition can be applied to both heat production and heat loss mechanisms. Another difference between the two methods lies in the parts of the brain concerned. The 'home' of the set-point is in the pre-optic anterior hypothalamic region whereas interference with the effector pathways seems to take place in more caudal parts of the hypothalamus.

Of these two possibilities the body seems to have adopted the second. There is no evidence that injury lowers the set-point but there is a wealth of evidence showing increased inhibition of the effector pathways after injury. In the previous lecture I showed that during limb ischaemia in the rat the threshold temperatures for the onset of shivering were lowered and those for the onset of thermoregulatory heat loss were raised, increasing the separation between these thresholds, and that when the tourniquets were removed and fluid loss occurred non-shivering thermogenesis was also inhibited.

No real reason can be given for this choice. Perhaps choice is not involved. It may be that this is the only way a change of this type can be produced by non-thermal afferent impulses. The effects appear to depend on noradrenergic nerve fibres which must arise from the noradrenergic nuclei of the hind-brain. These nuclei are concerned in the responses to trauma and associated with the other centres involved. They are, therefore, probably in a position to send up an inhibitory message to the thermoregulatory centres which reflects the severity of the injury.

Although I have set out above the reasons why it could seem a good idea for the injured animal to conserve its substrates by reducing oxidation in this way, there is an element of risk involved and penalties may be incurred. All methods of thermoregulation are inhibited so that it is more difficult for an injured rat to lose excess heat if this should arise. This is not a very likely eventuality but it could happen and would certainly increase the chance of death. A more likely event would be a fall in environmental temperature which would impose too big a strain on the inhibited heat production mechanisms. The core temperature could then fall too far and if it fell below 30° C the injured animal would have great difficulty in recovering unaided (Hemingway, 1963). Shivering also requires an adequate input from the baroreceptors and will become attenuated if the blood pressure fell severely (Mott, 1963).

Without adequate non-shivering thermogenesis, and with greater difficulty in activating either heat loss or shivering, the animal is very much more affected by environmental temperature after injury. It is, therefore, not too surprising that there is an optimum environmental temperature for survival (Tabor & Rosenthal, 1947; Green & Stoner, 1950; Haist, 1960; Stoner, 1969a). The optimum temperature is always below the thermoneutral zone. In the injured rat it is about 20°C. The optimum temperature is raised if the injured animal is given fluid replacement therapy. For instance, in the mouse injured by limb ischaemia fluid therapy raises the optimum environmental temperature for survival from 19° to 25°C. Since the oxygen consumption of the injured rat would only maintain a normal core temperature in a thermoneutral environment, at the optimum environmental temperature the core temperature will fall but not so far that unaided recovery is impossible.

STABILISATION OF THE 'EBB' PHASE

The object of this defence seems to be to stabilise the situation during the 'ebb' phase. The longer this phase can be maintained and the more substrates that can be conserved the better placed the animal will be for recovery and the 'flow' phase. In the same way the greater the stores of carbohydrate at the time of injury the better the chances of survival (Threlfall & Stoner, 1954). Evidence that this sort of change is occurring is provided by the changes in oxygen consumption (Stoner, 1969b). In a normal rat oxygen consumption starts to increase above the basal rate when the environmental temperature falls below 28°C. In the 'ebb' phase after injury the increase does not commence until a lower environmental temperature has been reached; 20°C in the rat after 4 hr bilateral hind-limb ischaemia. The size of this change varies with the severity of the injury but once oxygen consumption starts to increase the gain of the response is the same as in the controls. Similarly, in injured rats in a 20°C environment the irreversible disposal rate of glucose is less than in controls in that environment and approximates to the rate in normal rats at 30°C (Heath & Corney, 1973). Should this defence fail the hypoxia of the necrobiotic stage would accelerate the uptake and breakdown of glucose and lead to the accumulation of lactate.

In this way it is possible to view all these reactions associated with the 'ebb' phase as defensive. One set of centrally determined responses is designed to mobilise the energy stores and stimulate the metabolism to meet the requirements of a 'fight or flight' situation (Cannon, 1929) and this is followed, if the occasion demands, by another set of responses designed to inhibit metabolism and conserve substrate. If the initial 'danger' situation is successfully resolved only the first set of responses may be seen. The second group of responses is characteristic of the first part of the response to actual injury and as Hunter (1794) wrote: "There is a circumstance attending accidental injury which does not belong to disease, namely, that the injury done, has in all cases a tendency to produce both the disposition and means of cure".

198

Species Variation

This theory which I have developed in an attempt to encompass the early changes in the body following injury, particularly in regard to energy metabolism, is based on observations of the response in small mammals particularly the rat. In these species with a large surface area/weight ratio heat production is very important if the body temperature is to be maintained constant and non-shivering thermogenesis is the continuous variable in their thermoregulation. It should be no surprise, therefore, that thermoregulation is intimately concerned in any scheme to limit energy expenditure and conserve substrate. Since the thermoregulation mechanisms largely decide the level of oxidation and hence the rate of metabolism in all environments other than a thermoneutral one, the changes in these mechanisms after injury would be expected to determine the metabolism of the 'ebb' phase. How far can these ideas be extrapolated to a larger animal such as man?

Extrapolation to Man

In the larger mammals non-shivering thermogenesis is less important, at least in adults (Heldmaier, 1971). The continuous variable in thermoregulation is now some form of controllable heat loss. It must be admitted from the outset that very little is known about the effect of injury on thermoregulation in man. Much more is known about the metabolic effects after injury but, again, more about events in the 'flow' phase than in the 'ebb' phase.

The metabolic changes in man shortly after an injury are very similar to those in the rat. The glycogen stores are mobilised in the same way to produce hyperglycaemia and the removal of the glucose from the plasma is impeded by an effective lack of insulin (see Stoner & Heath, 1973 for references). Triglyceride stores are converted to non-esterified fatty acids at an excessive rate (Carlson, 1970) and the concentration of ketone bodies in the blood is also increased under some conditions (Smith et al, 1975). The effect of injury on total O_2 consumption is less well defined (Gump et al, 1970). In many patients with injuries other than burns it seems to be little altered during the acute 'ebb' phase. This may be because it has often been measured in a thermoneutral environment or one close to it.

There has been no direct investigation of the effect of injury on thermoregulation in man and there is little indirect information available. A fall in body temperature during the terminal stages after severe injuries has been known for a long time (see Wiggers, 1950). In the early stages there is some evidence, from the small increases in body temperature which are occasionally seen, that heat loss mechanisms are inhibited (Wright & Devine, 1944; Hardy & Raudin, 1952; Green, Stoner, Whiteley and Eglin, unpublished results). Temperature falls in severely burned patients (Harrison et al, 1964) imply that their heat production

199

mechanisms are unable to meet the increased demand.

CONCLUSION

These fragments of evidence suggest that injured man is using similar methods to the rat for his defence against injury. Differences in size, in the importance of non-shivering thermogenesis, etc. mean that different aspects of the response will have greater survival value in different species. We know a good deal now about the rat and how it defends itself against injury. The theory which has been outlined here only refers to events during injury and the ebb phase of the response. This is the part of the response we know least about in man. If we can establish the correctness of the theory it would be a great help when we come to determine the relative importance of the human responses. This information must be available if the responses are to be assisted by therapy, e.g. by the use of optimum environmental temperatures, insulin, corticosteriods, etc. At present these are used on an empirical basis which may not be satisfactory.

References

Barton, RN (1971) *Clin. Sci., 40,* 463
Barton, RN (1973) *Biochem. J., 136,* 531
Bligh, J and Johnson, KG (1973) *J. appl. Physiol. 35,* 941
Cannon, WB (1929) *Bodily Changes in Pain, Hunger, Fear and Rage* Appleton, New York
Carlson, LA (1970) *In Energy Metabolism in Trauma* (Ed) R Porter and J Knight. Churchill, London. Page 155
Cunningham, VJ (1973) *Biochem. J., 136,* 545
Fine, MB and Williams, RH (1960) *Amer. J. Physiol., 199,* 403
Frayn, KN (1975) *Europ. J. clin. Invest.* (In press)
Green, HN and Stoner, HB (1950) *Biological Actions of the Adenine Nucleotides.* Lewis, London
Gump, FE, Kinney, JM and Price, JB (1970) *J. surg. Res., 10,* 613
Haist, RE (1960) In *The Biochemical Response to Injury.* (Ed) HB Stoner and CJ Threlfall. Blackwell, Oxford. Page 313
Hammel, HT (1968) *Ann. rev. Physiol., 30,* 641
Hardy, JD and Raudin, IS (1952) *Ann. Surg., 136,* 345
Harrison, HN, Moncrief, JA, Duckett, JW and Mason, AD (1964) *Surgery, 56,* 203
Heath, DF and Corney, PL (1973) *Biochem. J., 136,* 519
Heath, DF and Stoner, HB (1968) *Brit. J. exp. Path., 49,* 160
Heldmaier, G (1971) *Z. vergl. Physiol., 73,* 222
Hemingway, A (1963) *Physiol. Rev., 43,* 397
Hunter, J (1794) *A Treatise on the Blood, Inflammation and Gunshot Wounds.* Nicol, London
Kovách, AGB, Rosell, S, Sándor, P, Koltay, E, Kovách, E and Tomka, N (1970). *Circ. Res., 26,* 733

Krebs, HA (1954) *Bull. Johns Hopkins Hosp., 95,* 45

Moore, FD (1971) In *Manual of Preoperative and Postoperative Care, 2nd Edn..* (Ed) JM Kinney, RH Egdahl and GD Zuidema. Saunders, Philadelphia. Page 19

Mott, J (1963) *J. Physiol., 166,* 563

Porte, D, Graber, AL, Kuzuya, T and Williams, RH (1966) *J. clin. Invest., 45,* 228

Smith, R, Fuller, DJ, Wedge, JH, Williamson, DH and Alberti, KGGM (1975) *Lancet, i,* 1

Stoner, HB (1969a) *Postgrad. med. J., 45,* 555

Stoner, HB (1969b) *Brit. J. exp. Path., 50,* 125

Stoner, HB and Heath, DF (1973) *Brit. J. Anaesth., 45,* 244

Stoner, HB and Matthews, J (1967) *Brit. J. exp. Path., 48,* 58

Tabor, H and Rosenthal, SM (1947) *Amer. J. Physiol., 149,* 449

Threlfall, CJ and Stoner, HB (1954) *Quart. J. exp. Physiol., 39,* 1

Wiggers, C (1950) *Physiology of Shock.* Commonwealth Fund, New York

Wright, RD and Devine, J (1944) *Med. J. Aust., 1,* 21

Causative Factors and Afferent Stimuli Involved in the Metabolic Response to Injury

H B STONER

Experimental Pathology of Trauma Section, MRC Toxicology Unit, Medical Research Council Laboratories, Carshalton, England

Introduction

To appreciate the factors which determine the metabolic response to injury one must first understand how that response is divided into different stages. These stages have been defined and described by Cuthbertson (1942, 1970). The first part of the response to injury is the 'ebb' phase which is characterised for the most part by a general depression of the body's activities. What follows depends on the severity of the injury. With non-fatal injuries the 'ebb' phase is followed by the 'flow' phase and the metabolic changes associated with recovery. When the injury is so severe that it leads to death the changes of the 'ebb' phase are prolonged into a phase which we have called necrobiosis. This phase contains those metabolic changes which characterise the final downward spiral to death. Since these stages in the response can be distinguished from one another it is reasonable to suppose that they have different causes or that if the causes are not completely different at least their relative importance in the three phases is different.

THE EBB PHASE

The 'ebb' phase is set in motion by injury. A large number of conditions qualify as injuries, haemorrhage, burns, fractures, soft tissue damage by crush, ischaemia, sepsis, diarrhoea. As the responses set in motion by these injuries are very similar we should seek to express the almost infinite variety in general terms.

It is commonly agreed that the important components of these injuries are:

1. Fluid loss.
2. Afferent sensory impulses
3. Toxic factors.

It has been clear for many years that the causative factors lie within these groups. In the past too much time has been wasted arguing for one factor as *the* cause to the exclusion of the others. The fact that these arguments could continue for a century with experiment and counter-experiment of apparently equal validity means that no one cause is responsible on all occasions. A more profitable approach is surely to try to determine the relative importance of the various factors in different types of injury. In this connection it is important to decide which are the factors which initiate changes in the body after an injury and which are those which prolong the response or alter its outcome. For instance, what factors in an injury lead the patient towards necrobiosis rather than towards recovery and the 'flow' phase?

There are three main factors:

Fluid Loss

Fluid loss is now widely accepted as the major initiating cause of the response in most cases. The lost fluid can be whole blood, as when vessels are divided, something more or less closely related to plasma, as in the exudate from a burn, and in the oedema of tissues damaged by crushing, ischaemia or infection or consist of water and electrolytes with very little protein as in the 'rice-water' stools of cholera.

Clinically the most important type of fluid loss is haemorrhage. This is true for both military and civil casualties. Despite the work of Grant and Reeve (1951) in World War II the large amount of blood which could be lost was not fully appreciated until the Korean War (Prentice et al, 1954).

The volume of fluid loss needed to produce death has been well discussed by Millican (1960; 1965) and today there is no need to reiterate old arguments about methods of measurement or whether loss of plasma, and particularly of its proteins, is more serious than loss of whole blood. Initially, the loss of circulating volume is more important than the nature of the fluid lost. Without treatment a loss of fluid from the circulation equivalent to 3–5% body weight is usually fatal. A loss of this size is equally dangerous whether it be as frank haemorrhage or as exudate into a post-ischaemic limb (Little, 1972, a,b) or an infected peritoneal cavity (Stoner et al, 1967).

In several cases the mechanism of the fluid loss is fairly well understood. In bleeding to the exterior from severed vessels the mechanism is obvious but one must not forget that large amounts of blood can be shed into the tissues from the damaged vessels around a closed fracture. Similarly, the cavities of the thorax and abdomen can hold large volumes of blood. Significant degrees of haemorrhage usually arise from direct trauma to vessels. Medical conditions causing extravasation of red cells seldom give rise to sufficient losses to cause

203

concern on that account.

The fluid lost in burns and soft tissue injuries is due to increased vascular permeability which has been closely studied under the heading of 'inflammation'. The changes are complex. The increase in permeability occurs in two stages. The first, which can be short-lived, is restricted to the post-capillary venules and in many cases is thought to involve a mediator such as histamine, serotonin or bradykinin. The second stage is usually more important and prolonged and affects capillaries as well. There are, however, many features of the permeability changes in damaged tissues which remain unexplained.

Limb ischaemia, for instance, is followed by extensive exudation into the limbs of a fluid little different from plasma yet anoxia per se is a poor stimulus to increased permeability (Henry, et al, 1947; Nairn, 1951) and it is difficult to find evidence of vascular damage in the limbs by the carbon labelling technique (Strock & Majno, 1969; Little, 1972a).

Fluid loss can be very important in bacterial infections and bacterial exotoxins can produce striking changes in vascular permeability (Miles & Wilhelm, 1960; Stoner, 1972). *Cl. welchii* α-toxin produces a well-marked biphasic response on intraperitoneal injection which can be prevented by passive immunisation (Stoner et al, 1967). In this case the effects of the organism cannot be entirely accounted for by the α-toxin for in passively immunised guinea-pigs the intraperitoneal injection of a very large number of *Cl. welchii* will cause a marked and widespread increase in venular permeability with loss of sufficient fluid from the circulation to cause death (Stoner et al, 1967). The whole question of the role of α-toxin in gas gangrene has been discussed by MacLennan (1962) and Bullen (1970). In most infections the exudate has a protein concentration akin to plasma. In cholera, on the other hand, enormous amounts of a more or less isotonic fluid free of protein are lost through an intact intestinal mucosa.

The rate of fluid loss is an essential factor in assessing its importance. The more slowly the loss occurs the longer the time available to the body to meet the challenge. In experimental studies fluid loss is usually rapid. This is particularly the case with the well-known Wiggers' protocol for haemorrhagic shock in the dog and Bassin et al, (1971) have shown how the responses produced by this protocol differ from those seen in most accident patients suffering from haemorrhage. More realistic models for haemorrhage have been devised by these authors and by Schmidt and Schmeir (1968).

In considering the rate of loss one must also consider the rate at which the blood volume is being restored from the fluid reserves within the body. Replacement of lost red cells, except by those stored in the spleen, is slow but replacement of fluid can be rapid and insofar as this restores the circulating fluid volume it reduces the size of the primary injury. It must be emphasised that increased vascular permeability is confined to the damaged tissues and that in other regions of the body the vessel walls retain their normal characteristics. Outward passage of fluid in the damaged tissues is met by the inward passage of fluid from the undamaged tissues. The faster the latter process occurs the better. The rapidity with which flying birds and new-born rabbits can compensate in this way plays a large part in their greater resistance to fluid loss (Djojosugito et al, 1968; Kovách et al, 1969; Kovách & Balint, 1969; Little, 1974).

The importance of fluid loss as a causative factor is shown by the beneficial effect of fluid replacement (Rosenthal, 1960). Whole blood is the best replacement after haemorrhage but for other experimental injuries 0.9% saline is often adequate. In rats subjected to 4 h bilateral hind-limb ischaemia in a $20°C$ environment the mortality rate is usually 75–80% and this can be reduced to zero by the intraperitoneal injection at the time of removal of the tourniquets of a volume of 0.9% saline equivalent to 12–15% body weight (Stoner, 1966). After this form of injury massive saline therapy will even save rats in the terminal stage if the saline is given by both intravenous and intraperitoneal routes (Koletsky and Klein, 1955). Work on the role of electrolytes in therapy has emphasised the increased requirement for sodium after injury (Rosenthal and Millican, 1954).

Afferent nervous impulses

Although few people today would go along with Crile, who at the end of the last century proposed that afferent nerve impulses were the main cause of shock, there can be no doubt that nociceptive afferent impulses are generated by almost any injury which could cause shock, that these impulses will not be without effect on the responses of the body to that injury and that in recent years too little attention has been paid to them.

O'Shaughnessy and Slome (1934) and Slome and O'Shaughnessy (1938) were the last to champion afferent nerve impulses as the major cause of shock and while subsequent workers have not adopted their extreme position they have frequently shown by nerve section, local anaesthesia, spinal anaesthesia and spinal cord sections that such impulses are involved (Bell, et al, 1937; Blalock & Cressman, 1939; Lorber, et al 1940; Eversole, et al 1944; Overman & Wang, 1947). It is however, impossible to assess the relative importance of the nervous factors despite the many experiments performed.

Although in this connection we may be thinking of severe pain stimuli these are often not a feature of serious injuries (Beecher, 1945) and we must not forget the widespread changes which can follow milder stimulation. What is commonly called 'stress' comes under this heading and the afferent impulses generated by such things as restraint, immobilisation and other environmental disturbances can provoke major hormonal changes, particularly in adrenocortical secretion. This aspect has perhaps been confused by the word 'stress' for it is never very clear whether the word applies to the stimulus or the response. It would always be better to define the actual stimulus involved, although this may be difficult.

Although pain stimuli may be concerned in such changes as the rise in blood pressure during limb ischaemia in man (Stoner & Green, 1945) other pressor and accelerator reflexes arise from muscle (Alam & Smirk, 1937, 1938a,b). Similarly, afferent impulses from receptors inside and outside the central nervous system which are stimulated by the pressure, volume, composition and temperature of the blood will all contribute to the final picture.

The pathways taken by these afferent stimuli, apart from those from cardio-vascular and pulmonary receptors, are not well defined. Nociceptive afferent impulses from the damaged tissue ascend in the dorsal spino-thalamic tracts (Swingle, et al 1944). In some of this type of work ACTH secretion has been used as an indicator. Nociceptive stimuli causing ACTH release pass upwards to the pons on the controlateral side of the cord to the injury and thence, probably via the medial fore-brain bundle, to the hypothalamus (Gibbs, 1969a, Greer, et al 1970; Feldman, et al 1971). This may not be the only pathway by which stimuli reach the neurotransducer cells which secrete hypothalamic releasing hormones (Gibbs, 1969b) and the exact method of stimulating these cells may vary with the type of injury (Greer et al, 1970).

It would be wrong to think of the hypothalamus and hindbrain as the only targets for the afferent impulses arising in injury. The hippocampus and amygdala are also concerned in the endocrine responses and must receive afferent information. The thalamus and sensory cortex must also be informed. Furthermore, the actual occurrence of the injury may have been anticipated by the triggering of the hypothalamic defence area by impulses from higher centres brought into play by suitable afferent stimuli. Indeed, all parts of the brain are probably affected in one way or another. It must also be remembered that nervous reflexes with the afferent path arising in the damaged area and the efferent path in the sympathetic outflow can extend the amount of tissue damage. Barnes and Trueta (1942) showed in rabbits that the application of a tourniquet to one limb caused vascular spasm in the opposite limb and, in similar experiments on rats, Bielschowsky and Stoner (unpublished results) found a decrease in the adenosine triphosphate concentration in the muscle of the contralateral leg which could be prevented by denervation of either leg. Changes of this sort can occur in injured man as shown by the case reported by Green, et al (1951).

Toxic Factors

Many substances may be considered under this heading and some undoubtedly play a part in causing the response to injury. Rather than give long lists of the compounds which have been examined from this point of view over the years I would prefer to try to classify them and to determine whether they could be initiating or continuing factors. It has often been thought that the existence and importance of toxic factors could be shown by cross-circulation experiments and many such have been done (e.g. Bell et al, 1937; Rapport, et al, 1945;

Green, et al, 1947; Little et al, 1948). However, the results have been variable and never sufficiently definite to be accepted as conclusive evidence in either direction.

Toxic factors may be classified first into the exogenous and the endogenous.

Exogenous toxic factors are those which do not occur normally in the body. In most cases they are microbial products.

The effects of *Cl. welchii* α-toxin have already been mentioned. This exogenous toxin usually arises during the course of a wound infection. However, in some species (dog and goat but not man or rat) the spores of this organism are harboured in tissues such as muscle where they may be activated by a local injury which will cause tissue hypoxia. Hence, in dogs the effusion in a post-ischaemic limb can contain α-toxin (Aub, et al, 1944, 1945; Lindsey, et al, 1959) which will contribute to the clinical picture.

Bacterial exotoxins are not the only microbial products involved in the production of shock. Endotoxins have been thought to be concerned in two ways. In 'septic shock' where there is invasion of the blood stream with Gram negative organisms, fever, circulatory collapse with hypotension, respiratory distress and acute changes in mental state it is reasonable to attribute the syndrome to the liberation of bacterial endotoxin which could, in this case, be classed as an initiating factor. Guenter, et al, (1969) have shown that *E. coli* and its endotoxin produce the same biological effects.

During the past fifteen years endotoxin shock has been intensively studied particularly in the dog although there are important species variations and the responses of the monkey most closely resemble those of man (Vaughn, et al, 1968). It is also unfortunate that in most experiments the endotoxin has been given as a single intravenous injection and not as a prolonged infusion which might mimic the natural disease more closely.

Fine and his colleagues (Fine, et al, 1960; Fine, 1961; Fine, et al, 1968; Palmerio & Fine, 1969; Cuevas & Fine, 1971, 1972) have proposed that endotoxin derived from the normal bacterial flora of the gut plays a part in haemorrhagic and other forms of traumatic shock. In these conditions it is not an initiating factor but one which has been claimed to account for irreversibility and death. This question has been reviewed in some detail (Stoner, 1972). Attempts to substantiate the theory, including recent studies in which endotoxin has been assayed by the *Limulus* lysate technique (e.g. Herman, et al, 1974), have not been successful when the gut mucosa has been undamaged. In situations where the injuries are accompanied by a break in the continuity of the intestinal mucosa the endotoxin which is certainly present in the lumen, can penetrate the body and play a part.

Endogenous factors may be subdivided into particulate and non-particulate factors.

(a) Several types of circulating particle can appear after an injury and play a part in the response to it, particularly in the later stages. Of these particles the best known, although not necessarily the most dangerous, are fat emboli. These are frequently more a pathological than a clinical finding and their origin, mode of action, etc. is fully discussed by Sevitt (1962), Szabo (1970), Watson (1970) and Prys-Roberts, et al (1970).

Other particles are derived from the blood. The clot promoting activity of extracts of damaged tissues is greater than that of normal tissue (Quastel & Racker, 1941; Stoner & Green, 1947) and in vivo small clots — 'sludge' — are found in the blood leaving a damaged area (Knisely, et al, 1945; Knisely, et al, 1947; Bigelow, et al, 1949; Brooks, et al, 1950). In the necrobiotic stage more general changes in consistency of the blood can occur with aggregation of red cells (Fahraeus, 1960) and disseminated intravascular coagulation (Hardaway, 1970). The latter is a late phenomenon when death is close and is shown by the rapid development of a consumptive coagulopathy.

None of these particles can be considered as initiating factors in the response to injury since they are produced after it has begun. Nevertheless, they could certainly play a part in directing the course of the response. Pulmonary embolisation from any cause could prejudice recovery, anatomically interfering with pulmonary function, laying the foundation for delayed lung complications and hindering oxygen transport. Pulmonary emboli also generate afferent vagal stimuli which can be deleterious in these conditions (Green and Stoner, 1950a).

(b) Non-particulate toxic factors range from electrolytes to large protein molecules. It would take too long even to list all the substances which have been suggested for this role. None has attained the distinction of being considered as a general toxic factor after injury. Some may play a significant part under special conditions or contribute to the general decline of the necrobiotic stage. A few comments will be made about some of them.

Electrolytes

Potassium keeps its place as a possible toxic factor but only in the terminal stages. Injured animals are more sensitive than normal to the toxic action of K^+ (Tabor & Rosenthal, 1945) and there is some evidence that it might account for the sudden death after limb ischaemia in animals at thermoneutral invironmental temperatures (Van der Meer, et al, 1966).

Low-molecular weight substances

Many proposed toxic factors fall into this category. Many of them might fill out a small corner of the full picture of the response but it is very doubtful if any could be the sole cause. Once a compound is put up as a possibility it is exceedingly difficult to eliminate it.

For example, adenosine triphosphate (ATP), the soluble component of Dyckerhoff's myotoxin (Dyckerhoff & Schörcher, 1939; Dyckerhoff, et al, 1939) seemed a possibility at one time (Green, 1943; Bielschowsky & Green,

1943; Green & Stoner, 1950b) and finally we thought we had eliminated it on the grounds that ATP did not leave injured muscle before it was broken down and deaminated to the non-toxic inosinic acid or inosine (Threlfall & Stoner, 1957). However, now that more sensitive analytical methods are available several groups have claimed to demonstrate adenine nucleotides in the blood draining exercising or post-ischaemic muscles (e.g. Forrester & Lind, 1969; Forrester, 1972) and this group of compounds is now being proposed for a role in the autoregulation of tissue blood flow and reactive hyperaemia. Such a role would be most likely in those tissues such as brain and heart where dephosphory-lation precedes deamination in the breakdown of ATP. However, the methods used in some of these experiments have been questioned (Bockman, et al, 1975). The amounts of nucleotide involved are very small and it is doubtful if they would have any general effect, particularly as the breakdown products of ATP are much less toxic than the parent compound. In general far too little attention is paid to the quantitative aspects of putative toxic factors. It is most essential that enough of the material should be available to produce the effects claimed.

Many compounds in this group are normal metabolites which have become displaced by the injury. Since they are usually acidic their accumulation in the plasma is reflected in the fall in its alkali reserve and finally pH. In some cases more specific effects may be seen. Amino acids accumulate in the plasma after limb ischaemia in the rat (Hoar & Haist, 1944; Stoner & Green, 1948). Competition by these amino acids for the carrier for the uptake of tryptophan by cells may partly explain the decrease in the rate of irreversible disposal of tryptophan after limb ischaemia (Stoner, et al, 1975).

Large molecular weight substances

The appearance of intracellular macromolecules in the plasma after injury should usually be taken as evidence of cellular damage either at the site of the injury or in distant organs. There are many examples. Montagnani and Simeone (1953) showed that myoglobin rapidly appeared in the blood and lymph after limb ischaemia, as did glutamate-oxaloacetate transaminase (Albaum & Milch, 1957). Lewis (1967, 1969) has shown that after thermal injury cytoplasmic enzymes appear in the lymph from the damaged area before mitochondrial ones. Acid hydrolases increase in activity in the blood after haemorrhage due, it is thought, to increased permeability of lysomes in liver and ileum (Courtice, et al, 1974). Most of this work has been done on enzymes since they are more easily measured in the blood and lymph than other intracellular macromolecules.

Activation of the triggered enzyme systems (Macfarlane, 1969) by trauma could prove more important than the leakage of intracellular enzymes into the plasma. This group of five complicated multistage enzyme systems, the blood clotting system, the fibrinolytic mechanism, the renin-angiotensin system, the kinin system and complement, is clearly implicated in the response to injury although the precise role of the many components is ill-understood.

Lefer and his colleagues (Lefer & Glenn, 1972) have claimed that when there is splanchnic hypoperfusion from any cause there is activation of the lysomal enzymes in the pancreas leading to the formation of a small peptide with myocardial depressant properties which enters the general circulation via the thoracic duct. This theory has not yet been adequately confirmed by independent groups (Harden & Garrott, 1973). It has been known for a long time that thoracic duct lymph is toxic after injury to the hind-limb (Blalock, 1943; Katzenstein, et al, 1943) but as these authors used dogs the toxicity might have been due to *Cl. welchii* α-toxin.

CONCLUSION

The order in which these putative toxic factors has been discussed might be considered unusual but is deliberate. They have been arranged in order of certainty. If an infecting organism produces an exotoxin there is no doubt that it will play some part in the response even if not a major one. Similarly, it seems most probably that an endotoxin plays a part in the general disturbance of a Gram negative septicaemia. The significance of the particulate factors is rather less certain although they may be important if numerous or large and impede flow through important areas of the circulation. Where they do have a role, these particulate factors must be classed as continuing factors which prolong the response by interfering with tissue perfusion and thus precipitating the onset of necrobiosis. Although many non-particulate factors have been suggested it is difficult to single out one as a factor of real importance. It is doubtful if any of them could initiate the response. Most arise when the response has been going for some time. Some, like K^+, could be important in special circumstances. Others, such as myoglobin and cellular enzymes, are probably more indicators of tissue damage than toxic factors.

So much for listing and classifying those features of an injury which could play a part in causing the response to it. The next important question is how do these factors set in motion all the different metabolic responses to injury and how are they related to the three stages of the response?

The loss of fluid from the circulation and the afferent nociceptive stimuli, being closely linked with the production of the injury, are associated with the 'ebb' phase. The severity of the injury is probably best measured by the volume of fluid lost. There is a rough correlation between this and the size of the response. The main metabolic changes during this stage reflect the reflex activation of various neuroendocrine systems although the responses are complicated by other events occurring at that time such as the effect of the injury on thermoregulation.

Continuing fluid loss in excess of the amounts which can be compensated for the autoregulation of organ blood flow coupled with embolic and other toxic phenomena, will lead to poor tissue perfusion and so to the necrobiotic stage. The characteristic of that stage is failure of O_2 transport however produced and the changes in blood and tissues reflect the increasing lack of O_2.

THE FLOW PHASE

It is rather more difficult to link the 'flow' phase with specific features of the injury. Since it follows an injury the same factors could be involved. Comparisons in man of the effects of surgical operations of differing severity indicate that the primary injury must exceed some threshold (simple herniorrhaphy) before this response can be detected (Kinney et al, 1970). Above this a close quantitative relationship between the size of the response and the injury is not very obvious. Fracture of long bones provides a powerful and seemingly disproportionate stimulus. The most usual measure of the 'flow' phase is the nitrogen balance. It has been shown that the negative balance which can persist for a long time during the recovery period cannot be explained by the immobilisation of the patient (Cuthbertson, 1929) or the breakdown of extravasated blood (Campbell & Cuthbertson, 1970). One of the difficulties is explaining the duration of the response. This becomes simpler in the special case of burns where the continuing loss of fluid from the burn and the need to produce heat equivalent to that used for the evaporation of fluid from the burned surface provide continuing stimulation.

Some of the topics in the last three paragraphs will be considered in more detail in my other lectures. In this one I have assumed a smooth progression from injury to recovery or death. Clinically this is not always the case. After recovery has begun the patient may suffer a relapse due to a variety of complications. This will inevitably affect the response by superimposing on the 'flow' phase elements of the 'ebb' or necrobiotic phases. For this reason one should beware of generalisations and it should not be assumed that because a group of patients were studied on, say, the fourth day after their accident, they were all equally in the 'flow' phase. Each patient must be considered on his merits paying due attention to any complications such as further haemorrhage, continuing drainage, etc. This matter is important because such patients often form the subject of study and the basis of publications.

References

Alam, M and Smirk, FH (1937). *J. Physiol., 89,* 372
Alam, M and Smirk, FH (1938a). *J. Physiol., 92,* 167
Alam, M and Smirk, FH (1938b). *Clin. Sci. 3,* 253
Albaum, HG and Milch, LJ (1957). *Amer. J. Physiol. 190,* 533
Aub, JC, Brues, AM, Dubos, R, Kety, SS, Nathanson, IT, Pope, A and
    Zameenik, PC (1944). *War Medicine, 5, 71*

Aub, JC, Brues, AM, Ketty, SS, Nathanson, IT, Nutt, AC, Pope, A and
  Zamecnik, PC (1945). *J. Clin. Invest. 24*, 845
Barnes, JM and Trueta, J (1942). *Brit. J. Surg. 30*, 74
Bassin, R, Vladeck, BC, Kim, SI and Shoemaker, WC (1971). *Surgery 69*, 722
Beecher, HK (1945). *Ann. Surg. 123*, 96
Bell, JR, Clark, AM and Cuthbertson, DP (1937). *J. Physiol. 92*, 361
Bielschowsky, M and Green, HN (1943). *Lancet ii*, 153
Bigelow, WG, Heimbecker, RO and Harrison, RC (1949). *Arch. Surg. 59*, 667
Blalock, A (1943). *Bull. Johns Hopkins Hosp. 72*, 54
Blalock, A and Cressman, RD (1939). *Surg. Gynec. Obstet. 68*, 278
Bockman, EL, Berne, RM and Rubio, R (1975). *Pflügers Arch. 355*, 229
Brooks, F, Dragstedt, LR, Warner, L and Knisely, MH (1950). *Arch. Surg. 61*,387
Bullen, JJ. In *Microbial Toxins.* (Ed) SJ Ajl, S Kadis and TC Montie. Academic
  Press, New York. Vol.1, page 233
Campbell, R and Cuthbertson, DP (1970). *Quart. J. exp. Physiol. 55*, 338
Courtice, FC, Adams, EP, Shannon, AD and Bishop, DM (1974). *Quart. J. exp.
  Physiol. 59*, 31
Cuevas, P and Fine, J (1971). *Surg. Gynec. Obstet. 133*, 81
Cuevas, P and Fine, J (1972). *Surg. Gynec. Obstet. 134*, 953
Cuthbertson, DP (1929). *Biochem. J. 23*, 1328
Cuthbertson, DP (1942). *Lancet i*, 433
Cuthbertson, DP (1970). In *Energy Metabolism in Trauma.* (Ed) R Porter and
  J Knight. Churchill, London. Page 98
Djojsugito, AM, Folkow, B and Kovách, AGB (1968). *Acta physiol. scand.
  74*, 114
Dyckerhoff, H and Schörcher, F (1939). *Biochem. Z. 300*, 183
Dyckerhoff, H, Schörcher, F and Torres, J (1939). *Biochem. Z. 300*, 193
Eversole, WJ, Kleinberg, W, Overman, RR, Remington, JW and Swingle, WW
  (1944). *Amer. J. Physiol. 140*, 490
Fåhraeus, R (1960). In *The Biochemical Response to Injury.* (Ed) HB Stoner
  and CJ Threlfall. Blackwell, Oxford. Page 161
Feldman, S, Conforti, N and Chowers, I (1971). *J. Endocr. 51*, 745
Fine, J (1961). *Federation Proc. 20*, 166
Fine, J, Frank, ED, Ravin, HA, Rutenberg, SH and Schweinburg, FB (1960).
  In *The Biochemical Response to Injury.* (Ed) HB Stoner and CJ Threlfall.
  Blackwell, Oxford. Page 377
Fine, J, Palmerio, C and Rutenberg, S (1968). *Arch. Surg. 96*, 163
Forrester, T (1972). *J. Physiol. 224*, 611
Forrester, T and Lind, AR (1969). *J. Physiol. 204*, 347
Gibbs, FP (1969a). *Amer. J. Physiol. 217*, 78
Gibbs, FP (1969b). *Amer. J. Physiol. 217*, 84
Grant, RT and Reeve, EB (1951). *Spec. Rep. Ser. Med. Res. Coun. (Lond) 277*
Green, HD, Bergeron, GA, Little, JM and Hawkins, JE (1947). *Amer. J.
  Physiol. 149*, 112
Green, HN (1943). *Lancet ii*, 147
Green, HN and Stoner, HB (1950a). *Biological Actions of the Adenine
  Nucleotides.* Lewis, London
Green, HN and Stoner, HB (1950b). *Brit. med. J. i*, 805
Green, HN, Stoner, HB, Whiteley, HJ and Eglin, D (1951). *Brit. J. Surg. 39*,80
Greer, MA, Allen, CF, Gibbs, FP and Gullickson, C (1970). *Endocrinology,
  86*, 1404

Guenter, CA, Fiorica, V and Hinshaw, LB (1969). *J. appl. Physiol. 26*, 780
Kinney, JM, Long, CL and Duke, JH (1970). In *Energy Metabolism in Trauma* (Ed) R Porter and J Knight. Churchill, London. Page 103.
Hardaway, RM (1970). *J. Clin. Path. 23. (Roy. Coll. Path.) 4*, 110
Harden, TK and Garrett, RL (1973). *Proc. Soc. exp. biol. med. 144*, 56
Henry, J, Goodman, J and Meehan, J (1947). *J. clin. Invest. 26*, 1119
Herman, CM, Kraft, AB, Smith, KR, Artnak, EJ, Chisholm, FC, Dickson, LG, McKee, AE, Homer, LD and Levin, J (1974). *Ann. Surg. 179*, 910
Hoar, WS and Haist, RE (1944). *J. biol. Chem. 154*, 331
Katzenstein, R, Mylon, E and Winternitz, MC (1943). *Amer. J. Physiol. 139*, 307
Kinney, JM, Long, CL and Duke, JH (1970). In *Energy Metabolism in Trauma* (Ed) R Porter and J Knight. Churchill, London. Page 103
Knisely, MH, Bloch, EH, Eliot, TS and Warner, L (1947). *Science, 106*, 431
Knisely, MH, Eliot, TS and Bloch, EH (1945). *Arch. Surg. 51*, 220
Koletsky, S and Klein, DE (1955). *Amer. J. Physiol. 182*, 439
Kovách, AGB and Bálint, T (1969). *Acta physiol. hung. 35*, 231
Kovách, AGB, Szász, E and Pilmayer, N (1969). *Acta physiol. hung. 35*, 109.
Lefer, AM and Glenn, TM (1973). *Adv. Exp. Med. Biol. 33*, 367
Lewis, GP (1967). *J. Physiol. 191*, 591
Lewis, GP (1969). *J. Physiol. 205*, 619
Lindsey, I, Wise, HM, Knecht, AT and Noyes, HL (1959). *Surgery, 45*, 602
Little, JM, Green, IID and Hawkins, JE (1948). *Amer. J. Physiol. 151*, 554
Little, RA (1972a). *Br. J. exp. Path. 53*, 180
Little, RA (1972b). *Br. J. exp. Path. 53*, 341
Little, RA (1974). *J. Physiol. 238*, 207
Lorber, V, Kabat, H and Welte, EJ (1940). *Surg. Gynec. Obstet. 71*, 469
Macfarlane, RG (1969). *Proc. Roy. Soc. B 173*, 259
MacLennan, JD (1962). *Bacteriol. Rev. 26*, 177
Miles, AA and Wilhelm, DL (1960). In *The Biochemical Response to Injury*. (Ed) HB Stoner and CJ Threlfall. Blackwell, Oxford. Page 51
Millican, RC (1960). In *The Biochemical Response to Injury*. (Ed) HB Stoner and CJ Threlfall. Blackwell, Oxford. Page 269
Millican, RC (1965). In *Shock and Hypotension*. (Ed) LC Mills and JH Moyer. Grune & Stratton, New York. Page 351
Montagnani, CA and Simeone, FA (1953). *Surgery 34*, 169
Nairn, RC (1951). *J. Path. Bact. 63*, 213
O'Shaughnessy, L and Slome, D (1934). *Brit. J. Surg. 22*, 589
Overman, RR and Wang, SC (1947). *Amer. J. Physiol. 148*, 289
Palmerio, C and Fine, J (1969). *Arch. Surg. 98*, 679
Prentice, TC, Olney, JM, Artz, CP and Howard, JM (1954). *Surg. Gynec. Obstet. 99*, 542
Prys-Roberts, C, Greenbaum, R, Nunn, JF and Kelman, GR (1970). *J. clin. Path. 23, Suppl (Roy. Coll. Path.) 4*, 143
Quastel, JH and Racker, E (1941). *Br. J. exp. Path., 22*, 15
Rapport, D, Guild, R and Canzanelli, A (1945). *Amer. J. Path. 143*, 440
Rosenthal, SM (1960). In *The Biochemical Response to Injury*. (Ed) HB Stoner and CJ Threlfall. Blackwell, Oxford. Page 397
Rosenthal, SM and Millican, RC (1954). *Pharmacol. Rev. 6*, 489
Schmidt, HD and Schmier, J (1968). *Pflüger's Arch. 298*, 336
Sevitt, S (1962). *Fat Embolism*. Butterworths, London
Slome, D and O'Shaughnessy, L (1938). *Brit. J. Surg. 25*, 900

213

Strock, PE and Majno, G (1969). *Surg. Gynec. Obstet. 129*, 309

Stoner, HB (1966). In *Research in Burns*. (Ed) AB Wallace and AW Wilkinson. Livingstone, Edinburgh. Page 159

Stoner, HB (1972). *Symposia Soc. Gen. Microbiol. 22*, 113

Stoner, HB, Bullen, JJ, Cushnie, GH and Batty, I (1967). *Br. J. exp. Path. 48*, 309

Stoner, HB, Cunningham, VJ, Elson, PM and Hunt, A (1975). *Biochem. J. 146*, 659

Stoner, HB and Green, HN (1945). *Clin. Sci. 5*, 159

Stoner, HB and Green, HB (1947). *Br. J. exp. Path. 28*, 127

Stoner, HB and Green, HN (1948). *Br. J. exp. Path. 29*, 121

Swingle, WW, Kleinberg, W, Remington, JW, Eversole, WJ and Overman, RR (1944). *Amer. J. Physiol. 141*, 54

Szabo, G (1970). *J. clin. Path. 23, Suppl. (Roy. Coll. Path.) 4*, 123

Tabor, H and Rosenthal, SM (1945). *Publ. Hlth. Reps. Wash 60*, 373

Threlfall, CJ and Stoner, HB (1957). *Br. J. exp. Path. 38*, 339

Van der Meer, C, Valkenburg, PW, Ariëns, AT and Van Benthem, RMJ (1966). *Amer. J. Physiol. 210*, 513

Vaughn, DL, Gunter, CA and Stookey, JL (1968). *Surg. Gynec. Obstet. 126*, 1309

Watson, AJ (1970). *J. clin. Path. 23 Suppl (Roy. Coll. Path.) 4*, 132

Effect of Injury on Protein Requirements

J C WATERLOW and P M SENDER

London School of Hygiene and Tropical Medicine, London, England

Introduction

In discussing the protein requirements of normal people the assumption is always made that the needs for energy and other nutrients are fully met, but this may not be true in surgical patients after injury in whom the energy expenditure may be greatly increased during the 'flow' phase. However the patient is being fed, it may be difficult to get enough energy into him and under these circumstances protein and amino acids cannot be efficiently utilised, however adequate the amount or well designed the mixture.

We can consider requirements under two heads: the requirement for maintenance and that for growth, tissue formation or repair. Each of these can again be divided into two parts, the requirement for total N and that for essential amino acids.

MAINTENANCE REQUIREMENT – TOTAL N

Nitrogen is needed for maintenance to balance the obligatory losses of N in urine, faeces and through the skin on a protein free diet. In a normal adult in a temperate climate the obligatory losses on a protein free diet amount to 50–60 mg N/kg/day (Table I). FAO/WHO (1973) decided not to use these direct values to estimate the maintenance requirement, but instead determined what they called the 'safe level' of protein intake from the minimum amount of good quality protein (egg, milk) needed to maintain N balance. This amount is about 30% greater than the sum of the obligatory losses, perhaps because even at this low level of protein intake utilisation of N is not 100% sufficient, a matter which needs to be further investigated.

215

TABLE I. Obligatory N Losses in Adult Men on a Protein-free Diet

	mg N/kg/day
Urine	37
Faeces	12
Skin	3
Miscellaneous	2
	—
	54 = 2.0 mg N/basal kcal

(From FAO/WHO 1973)

The minimum N intake needed to secure balance was estimated from studies which cover a total of about 200 individuals of both sexes. The coefficient of variation was found to be about 15%. The 'safe level' is defined as the mean requirement to maintain N balance + 30% (+ 2SD). This should cover the requirement over 97% of the range of individual variation. The safe level at selected ages is shown in Table II.

TABLE II. Safe Level of Intake of Good Quality Protein — egg or milk — (after addition of 30% to cover individual variability)

Age	Safe level g protein/kg/day
< 3 months	2.40
3—6 months	1.85
6—9 months	1.62
9-11 months	1.44
1 year	1.27
2— 5 years	1.19—1.01
5—10 years	1.01—0.82
15 M	0.67
15 F	0.59
Adult M	0.57
Adult F	0.52

If we apply a correction for quality, on the conservative assumption that the protein value of a mixed diet is 70% of that of egg or milk, then the requirement of the adult man is 0.8 g mixed protein per kg per day, or 60 g for a 75 kg man. This is about two-thirds of what people actually eat in Western countries.

Many people have argued that these safe levels are unacceptably low, since almost all diets in which the staple is a cereal (other than maize), would, on these criteria, provide an adequate protein supply. However the best established requirements are those from balance studies in neonates on breast milk and older infants on various forms of cow's milk. Experience in countries whose protein malnutrition is common shows that these values are realistic, and if they are accepted the values for adults should be based on the same principles.

ESSENTIAL AMINO ACID REQUIREMENT FOR MAINTENANCE

In good quality proteins such as those of meat, milk and eggs the essential amino acids make up about 50% by weight of the protein. Studies by several groups in the USA have shown that such a mixture is unnecessarily rich for maintenance in adults. It can be diluted with substantial amounts of non-essential N, e.g. glycine or ammonium salts, without loss of nutritive value until the proportion of essential amino acids falls to about 25%. Rose's balance studies on the requirement for each individual essential amino acid led to an even lower proportion of essential amino acids to total N. The pattern of essential amino acid requirements for maintenance, based largely on Rose's figures, is shown in Table III. The total is only 15% by weight of the overall protein requirement.

TABLE III. Essential Amino Acid Requirements of Adults (Sexes Combined)

Based on total protein requirement of 0.55 g/kg/day

	mg/g protein
Isoleucine	18
Leucine	25
Lysine	22
Methionine + cystine	24
Phenylalanine + tyrosine	25
Threonine	13
Tryptophan	6.5
Valine	18
Total	151.5

(From FAO/WHO 1973)

The reason only such small amounts of essential amino acids are needed is simply that maintenance means the replacement of amino acids lost by endogenous oxidation. On a low protein intake just sufficient for maintenance, adaptive changes occur which result in a reduced oxidation of amino acids. Krebs (1972) has pointed out that the K_m of the amino acid oxidising enzymes is such that their activity will fall when the substrate concentration is low. In addition, there is no doubt that adaptive changes occur in the amounts of these enzymes. One of the best studied examples is threonine dehydratase in the liver; the

217

activity of this enzyme may vary 100-fold under different nutritional conditions (Pitot & Peraino, 1964). The three branched-chain amino acids, valine, leucine and isoleucine, are metabolised mainly by muscle. It used to be thought that adaptive changes do not occur in muscle enzymes. However, recent work has shown that the activity of the keto-acid dehydrogenase which catalyses the first step in oxidation is reduced in rats on a low protein diet (Reeds, 1974; Sketcher et al, 1974). At the same time the activity of the amino acid activating enzymes is increased (Stephen, 1968). The effect of these adaptive enzyme changes is that essential amino acids, instead of being oxidised, are reutilised for protein synthesis. Tracer studies show that on low protein diets about 95% of the amino acid flux is recycled. Under these circumstances the limiting factor in maintenance diets is likely to be total N rather than essential amino acids.

TOTAL NITROGEN REQUIREMENT FOR GROWTH AND REPAIR

A good example of rapid tissue growth is provided by the infant recovering from malnutrition and protein depletion (Ashworth et al, 1968; Ashworth, 1969). If given enough food such an infant may gain 20 g/kg/day, which is about 20 times the normal rate of growth. If the tissue deposited contains 25 mg N/g, this baby is laying down 500 mg N/kg/day and the growth requirement is about five times the maintenance requirement. These infants seem to be able to utilise food N very efficiently; provided that the protein quality is adequate there is no need to give a large excess of N. In practice the main problem is not the provision of adequate protein but of adequate energy (see below).

The situation may be very different with injury and repair because there may be a factor which is not present in the babies — a block in protein synthesis, so that food N is not efficiently utilised. If an adult has had a cumulative negative N balance of −300 g in 20 days, to restore this loss of protein at the same rate, i.e. 15 g N/day, or 200 mg N/kg/day, it will be necessary to give an intake of at least three times the maintenance requirement. The magnitude of the loss which may have to be made good in an adult is not always appreciated. However, the real problem, it seems to us, is whether, when the 'catabolic' phase is over, the adult can speed up his rate of protein synthesis in the same way as the recovering child. Another facet of this problem is whether, if utilisation is inefficient, N retention can be improved by increasing the intake. More information is needed on these points.

Essential Amino Acid Requirement for Growth and Repair

Since for growth and repair there has to be a net deposition of essential amino acids, these have to be supplied from the food and cannot be made available by recycling. The pattern in which the essential amino acids are needed is obviously determined by the pattern of amino acids in the protein deposited. This is likely

218

TABLE IV. Essential Amino Acid Composition of Mixed Muscle Protein

	mg/g protein
Isoleucine	45
Leucine	82
Lysine	91
Methionine + cystine	39
Phenylalanine + tyrosine	77
Threonine	46
Tryptophan	12
Valine	48
	440

(From EJ Bigwood 'Protein and amino acid functions' 1972)

to be mainly muscle. The amino acid composition of mixed muscle protein is shown in Table IV. The eight essential amino acids account for nearly 50% by weight of the protein. Thus the pattern of requirement for growth and repair is much richer in essential amino acids than that for maintenance, and in any particular situation the actual requirement will depend on the relative sizes of the growth and maintenance components. The only way to deal with this is by being over-generous, by specifying a pattern which will cover most levels of growth and repair. FAO/WHO (1973) were faced with the same problem when specifying an ideal amino acid pattern as a basis for calculations of protein quality. It would obviously be impractical to have two patterns, one for maintenance and one for growth. Therefore, to be on the safe side, they specified a pattern based on the amino acid requirements of pre-school children and containing 36% essential amino acids. This probably underestimates protein quality for adults, but it is a fault on the right side.

The 'repair' mixture should therefore have an amino acid composition similar to that of milk, egg or meat. It should be provided in amounts adequate to cover maintenance and tissue deposition, say 2 g protein/kg/day, i.e. about three times the maintenance requirement.

ENERGY REQUIREMENT FOR MAINTENANCE AND GROWTH

Payne and Waterlow (1971) have proposed as a generalisation that the maintenance requirement of energy may be taken as the basal metabolic rate (BMR) x 1.5. This is based on animal studies in which growth is measured at different levels of energy intake. The intake which provides zero growth is the maintenance requirement. On this basis the energy requirement for maintenance in an adult man is about 37 kcal/kg/day; in the infant it is about 80 kcal/kg/day (Payne & Waterlow, 1971).

219

Most of our information about the energy requirement for growth has been obtained from work on children recovering from malnutrition, but the principles apply equally well to adults laying down new tissue during recuperation from injury. As has been said, the child recovering from malnutrition grows extremely fast. During this rapid growth phase it has been found that, provided there is an adequate supply of protein, the rate of weight gain is related linearly to the energy intake. A recent detailed study in Jamaica gave a value of 4.8 kcal/g for the gross energy cost of weight gain. This gross cost includes two elements: the energy stored as protein and fat, and the energy cost of synthesis or deposition. The composition of the tissue gained is not known exactly, but indirect evidence suggests that it contained about 35% fat and 12% protein. If the new tissue contained less fat and more protein, the energy cost of deposition would be less. For tissue such as muscle, containing only protein and no fat, the energy cost would be about 2 kcal per g tissue, or 10 kcal per g protein laid down. In the example we are considering, of a patient recovering from injury, in whom we are trying to promote a positive N balance of 15 g N per day, equivalent to 94 g protein per day, the extra energy needed for this deposition of protein would be nearly 1000 kcal per day. This is a very large increment, and for many patients it is likely to be the energy intake rather than the protein intake which limits the rate of recuperation.

PROTEIN TURNOVER AFTER INJURY

We have suggested that the 'catabolic' loss of nitrogen after injury might be caused by a block in protein synthesis rather than an increase in the rate of breakdown of protein. The suggestion has led to some misunderstanding (Brennan et al, 1975) which may derive from failure to be clear about terminology. We use the terms *breakdown* or *degradation* of protein to denote the process by which the polypeptide chain is hydrolysed to its constituent amino acids. The word *catabolism* is best reserved for the oxidation of amino acids, leading to excretion of their nitrogen as urea. It is now generally accepted that protein synthesis (S) and breakdown (B) are going on continuously. In the normal subject in the steady state there is a balance between S and B, just as there is a balance between nitrogen intake (I) and excretion (E). These two balances are related.

The simplest conception of protein metabolism consist of two pools, an amino acid or 'metabolic' pool and a protein pool. The flux, denoted by Q, is the rate at which amino N is entering or leaving the metabolic pool. If we suppose that the amount of amino N in the metabolic pool is constant, the rates of entry and exit will be equal, so that:

$$Q = S + E = B + I \tag{1}$$

This equation is based on the assumption that pathways of amino acid metabolism, other than synthesis to protein or excretion, are quantitatively unimportant. It follows from equation (1) that $S - B = I - E$. This shows how the two balances mentioned above are related. Any difference between synthesis and breakdown of protein must be reflected by a change in the conventional N balance (intake minus output).

A change from N equilibrium to negative N balance could be produced in two ways — by a decrease in S or an increase in B or by a combination of both processes. Since amino acids cannot be stored as such, if there is a block in synthesis the unused amino acids will be oxidised (catabolised) and their nitrogen excreted. Thus a decrease in synthesis will be accompanied by *an increase in amino acid catabolism without any necessity for an increase in protein breakdown*. Perhaps failure to distinguish between catabolism and breakdown is one reason for resistance to the idea that the catabolic loss of nitrogen in injury may not be due to increased protein breakdown.

MEASUREMENT OF RATES OF PROTEIN SYNTHESIS AND BREAKDOWN

Measurement of these rates depends on determining the flux, Q, through the amino acid pool. It is evident from equation (1) that once Q is known, measurements of I and E enable us to calculate B and S.

We have measured Q in two ways:

(a)   An amino acid labelled with ^{14}C is given by constant intravenous infusion. James et al (1974) discuss the pros and cons of different ^{14}C amino acids. As an example, we may consider $1\text{-}^{14}C$-leucine. After some hours the specific radioactivity (SR) of leucine in the plasma reaches a constant plateau. At plateau isotope must be entering and leaving the plasma at the same rate.

If q^* = rate of infusion of isotope (dpm.h^{-1})
      C_p = plateau SR in plasma (dpm.mmole^{-1})
      Q_L = flux of infused amino acid (leucine) (mmole/h^{-1})

then $q^* = Q_L C_p$, and $Q_L = q^*/C_p$ (2)

This gives us the flux of the particular labelled amino acid which is infused, in this case leucine. We normally also collect expired air, and measure the rate of output of $^{14}CO_2$. This gives us the proportion of the leucine flux which is oxidised and excreted, denoted E_L. Finally, we have to convert this into the rate of total protein synthesis. To do this, it is necessary to know the average leucine content of total body protein, which from measurements on the rat we take to be about 8% (Block & Weiss, 1956). Then the rate of total protein synthesis,

$$S = \frac{100}{8}(Q_L - E_L) \times 24 \times \frac{131}{1000} \ \text{g.d.}^{-1}$$

where 131 is the molecular weight of leucine.

(b) ^{14}C cannot be given to children or to adults in the child-bearing age. Therefore a method was devised for determining N flux by measurement

221

of the rate of excretion of ^{15}N in urinary urea during continuous infusion of ^{15}N glycine (Picou & Taylor-Roberts, 1969). ^{15}N abundance in urinary urea reaches a plateau after about 10 h in children and 24—30 h in adults (Crane, Picou, Smith & Waterlow, to be published).
There are two basic assumptions:

(i)   that the metabolism of glycine reflects that of total amino-N, so that the proportion of ^{15}N glycine excreted is urea in the same as the proportion of total amino-N excreted as urea.

(ii)   that the synthesis of urea and the synthesis of protein occur from the same metabolic pool, and only from that pool.

On the basis of these assumptions, one can write:

$$\frac{q^*}{Q_N} = \frac{e_u^*}{E_u} \tag{3}$$

where q*, as before = rate of infusion of isotope
$\qquad\qquad\quad Q_N$ = total N flux
$\qquad\qquad\quad e_u^*$ = rate of excretion of ^{15}N in urea
$\qquad\qquad\quad E_u$ = rate of excretion of urea N
Since Q_N = $E_{TN} + S_N$
where E_{TN} = rate of total N excretion
$\qquad\quad S_N$ = rate of total N synthesis to protein

Substituting from equation 3:

$$S_N = q^* \cdot \frac{E_u}{e_u^*} - E_{TN} \tag{4}$$

All these quantities on the righthand side can be measured, and so S_N is determined.

Admittedly it is difficult to prove the validity of the basic assumptions on which this equation depends. However, in a recent study in which ^{15}N glycine and ^{14}C leucine were infused together in the same patients, the two tracers gave results which were in satisfactory agreement (Golden & Waterlow, to be published).

Results

We know of only two studies of the effect of injury on protein turnover. Both were concerned with the effect of elective operations. O'Keefe et al (1974) infused $1\text{-}^{14}C$-leucine in five patients before and after abdominal operations. The results are shown in Table V. They suggest that after operation there was a small decrease in synthesis rate, with no increase in breakdown. A difficulty in interpreting this finding is that before operation the patients were receiving a normal diet, whereas afterwards they were given only water and electrolytes. Therefore

222

TABLE V. Effect of Abdominal Operations on Rates of Protein Synthesis and Breakdown Measured by Continuous Infusion of 1-[^{14}C]-leucine

Subject	Sex	Synthesis, g/kg/day		Breakdown, g/kg/day	
		Pre-op	Post-op	Pre-op	Post-op
H	F	4.10	–	3.92	–
F	M	3.58	2.83	4.06	3.54
B	M	4.65	4.45	5.87	5.68
K	F	2.25	1.98	1.23	2.47
G	F	–	3.32	–	3.92
M	M	3.62	3.57	3.37	4.50
Mean		3.64	3.23	3.69	4.02

Mean urinary N excretion, g/mg; pre-op 6.8; post-op 8.8

(Data from O'Keefe, 1974)

it is possible that the negative N balance after operation and the decrease in protein synthesis were a result not of injury but of the withdrawal of dietary protein.

This particular problem does not arise in the second study, which in fact was carried out seven years ago (Crane, Picou, Smith & Waterlow, to be published). ^{15}N glycine was given to 11 patients before and after elective orthopaedic operations. In preliminary experiments it was found that if the isotope was administered in repeated oral doses every 4 h, a plateau of ^{15}N abundance was achieved in urinary urea, which was no less constant than that obtained with intravenous infusion. Since the intermittent dose was clearly more convenient than infusion, all the patients were tested in this way. As there was no interference with the gastrointestinal tract, the patients were able to each as much, or nearly as much, after the operation as they did before.

The results are summarised in Table VI. There was a small negative N balance

TABLE VI. Protein Turnover in 11 Patients Before and After Elective Orthopaedic Operations.   Mean ± SD

	Pre-operative	Post-operative
N balance, g/day	-1.2 ± 1.40	-5.1 ± 3.74
Synthesis, g protein/kg/day	2.77 ± 0.64	2.51 ± 0.51
Breakdown, g protein/kg/day	2.90 ± 0.65	3.00 ± 0.72

Data of Crane, Picou, Smith and Waterlow, to be published

after operation. On average, there was a decrease in the rate of protein synthesis, which was not large enough to be statistically significant. There was no change in the rate of breakdown.

Discussion

Obviously a critical appraisal of these results should begin with an examination of the methods used for measuring protein turnover, since they are not yet well established. A detailed analysis of the methods is in preparation (Waterlow, Garlick and Millward, Elsevier Press). Apart from our early work with ^{14}C lysine (Waterlow, 1967), and the two investigations reported here, there are four other studies in which total protein turnover has been measured by constant infusion or repeated dosage of labelled amino acids in normal adults. The results are summarised in Table VII. The ^{14}C amino acids tend to give rather higher results than ^{15}N, except in the study of Golden and Waterlow. The reasons for this are

TABLE VII. Rates of Total Protein Synthesis in Adults

Author	Subjects No	Age	Amino acid	Synthesis rate g/kg/day
O'Keefe (1974)	52	75	1-[^{14}C] leucine	3.64 ± 0.89
Sender et al (to be published)	30	65	U-[^{14}C] tyrosine	4.68 ± 0.77
Golden and Waterlow (to be published)	66	91	1-[^{14}C] leucine	2.67 ± 0.71
Crane et al (to be published)	20	65	^{15}N glycine	2.77 ± 0.64
Young et al (1975)	20	23	^{15}N glycine	3.0 ± 0.2
Young et al (1975)	69	91	^{15}N glycine	1.9 ± 0.2

Mean ± SD

not clear. The problems associated with each variant of the method are discussed in the individual papers. It is satisfactory, however, that the average rate of protein turnover found in the orthopaedic patients agree well with those obtained in healthy young men by Young et al (1975).

We are far from having demonstrated unequivocally that injury causes a block in protein synthesis. The main criticism of both the studies reported here is that the trauma was not very severe, so that the negative N balance was small. We are at present trying to remedy this by measurements of protein turnover in more seriously injured patients.

There is one other investigation which points in the same direction, although it did not involve trauma. Twenty years ago workers in Denmark developed a method of measuring rates of total protein synthesis and breakdown by multi-exponential analysis of the excretion of ^{15}N in the urine after a single dose of ^{15}N glycine (Olesen et al, 1954).

The results were analysed in terms of a model containing two protein pools, one turning over fast and the other slowly. In normal subjects the combined synthesis rate in the two pools was very similar to that found by us and by Young et al (1975). The Danish workers immobilised three subjects by encasing them in plaster to the neck, and repeated the turnover measurement (Schonheyder et al, 1954). Immobilisation produced a negative N balance ranging from 6.6-11.2 g per day. In two of the subjects for whom the data were analysed in full, there was a substantial decrease in the calculated rate of protein synthesis in the slowly turning over pool, with no change in the overall rate of breakdown.

The method is inconvenient, because measurements have to be continued for 5-10 days. We also believe that the attempt to distinguish two protein pools put more on the data than they can bear (Waterlow, Garlick and Millward, in preparation). Nevertheless, we have no criticism of the conclusions of this pioneer experiment. It may be permissible to analyse the results in a simpler way. If it is assumed that 48 h after the dose of ^{15}N glycine, all the isotope which is not going to be incorporated in protein has been excreted in the urine, and if it is also assumed that over this period recycling of isotope from protein is insignificant, then one can write:

$$\frac{e^*_{max}}{d^*} = E/(E + S)$$

where $\frac{e^*_{max}}{d^*}$ is the cumulative excretion of ^{15}N

E is the rate of N excretion (g per day)
S is the rate of N synthesis (g per day).

Since $\frac{e^*_{max}}{d^*}$ and E are measured, S can be determined.

The results of this calculation are shown in Table VIII. They show that in all three subjects immobilisation caused a substantial fall in the rate of synthesis with no change in the rate of breakdown.

As far as we know, measurements of protein turnover have not been made in injured animals, but there is indirect evidence from animal experiments which

225

TABLE VIII. Rates of Total Protein Synthesis in Subjects before and after
Immobilisation in a Plaster Cast. (Recalculated from Schonheyder et al, 1954)

Subject		N excretion	N balance	Cumulative excretion of ^{15}N in 48 h	Synthesis	Break-down
		g/day	g/day	% of dose	gN/day	gN/day
HV	normal	11.5	0	26	32.7	32.7
	immobilised	22.7	-11.2	56	17.8	29.0
EB	normal (1)	10.9	0	22	38.6	38.6
	normal (2)	10.4	+0.5	27	28.1	28.6
	immobilised	18.0	-6.6	43	23.9	30.5
ES	normal	11.55	-0.35	27	31.2	31.55
	immobilised	19.2	-8.0	48	20.8	28.8

Note: In the original paper data are given for N intake and total N excretion
(urine + faeces).
Urinary N excretion calculated on assumption that faecal N = 10% of intake

might lead us to expect a block in protein synthesis. Cuthbertson's experiments
suggest strongly that the greater part of the excess N which is lost after injury is
derived from muscle. For many years we have been particularly interested in
protein turnover in muscle. This tissue seems to be much more labile than has

TABLE IX. The Effect of a Protein-free Diet on the Rate of Protein Synthesis
in Rat Gastrocnemius muscle

Days on diet	Body weight	Muscle weight	Fractional rate of protein synthesis
	g	g	% per day
0	108	0.82	18.7
1	102	0.84	9.7
2	98	0.82	8.7
3	96.5	0.84	8.2
9	85.5	0.79	5.1
21	76.5	0.71	4.3

Each value is the mean of 5—6 rats

been thought. The fractional synthesis rate of mixed muscle protein in the weanling rat is 25-30% per day, falling to about 12% per day at 2 months and 5% per day at a year (Millward, 1975; Millward et al, 1975a). Table IX shows that nutritional stress produces a rapid and profound decrease in the rate of synthesis of muscle protein (Garlick et al, 1975). As Millward has shown (Millward et al, 1973; Millward, 1975), this decrease is accompanied by a reduction in RNA content and a fall in the activity or 'efficiency' of RNA (mg protein synthesised per mg RNA). The breakdown rate can be estimated as the difference between the rate of protein synthesis and the net loss or gain of protein over a suitable interval. Although deprivation of dietary protein causes a net loss of muscle weight and of muscle protein, no increase in breakdown rate has been found. Starvation in the rat produces an immediate fall in the rate of muscle protein synthesis, but it is only after two days that the breakdown rate begins to rise. Injection of a glucocorticoid (triamcinolone) in the rat caused a loss of muscle protein and RNA, with a small fall in synthesis rate, but again there was no indication of an increase in breakdown (Millward et al, 1975b).

Of course, nutritional deprivation is not the same as injury, nor would we claim that there are no conditions which increase the rate of muscle protein breakdown. These experiments, however, do support the idea that muscle protein synthesis is extremely labile, and that variations in it are the most important determinants of changes in muscle protein mass. This is in sharp contrast to the situation in liver, where changes are probably effected mainly by alterations in the rate of protein breakdown (Waterlow & Garlick, 1975).

Acknowledgments

We should like to acknowledge our gratitude to Professor Charles G Clark, Department of Surgery, University College Hospital, for his interest and for the facilities he has given; and to Dr WPT James for his guidance and help. We are grateful to Dr SJD O'Keefe for allowing us to use material from his unpublished report for the degree of MSc.

References

Ashworth, A (1969) *Brit. J. Nutr., 23,* 835
Ashworth, A, Bell, R, James, WPT and Waterlow, JC (1968) *Lancet, ii,* 600
Bigwood, EJ (Ed) (1972) *Protein and Amino Acid Requirements, Chapter 5.* Pergamon Press, Oxford
Block, RJ and Weiss, KW (1956) *Amino Acid Handbook.* Charles C Thomas, Springfield, Illinois
Brennan, M, Tweedle, D and Moore, FD (1975) *Lancet, i,* 38
FAO/WHO (1973) *Energy and Protein Requirements. Tech. Rep. Ser. No. 522.* WHO, Geneva
Garlick, PJ, Millward, DJ, James, WPT and Waterlow, JC (1975) *Biochim.*

biophys. Acta, 414, 71

James, WPT, Sender, PM, Garlick, PJ and Waterlow, JC (1974) In *Dynamic Studies with Radioisotopes in Medicine 1974, Volume I.* International Atomic Energy Agency, Vienna. Page 461

Krebs, HA (1972) In *Advances in Enzyme Regulation, Volume 10.* (Ed) G Weber. Pergamon Press, New York. Page 387

Millward, DJ (1975) In *Alcohol and Abnormal Protein Biosynthesis: Biochemical and Clinical.* (Ed) MA Rothschild, M Oratz and SS Schreiber. Pergamon Press, New York. Page 203

Millward, DJ, Garlick, PJ, James, WPT, Nnanyelugo, DO and Ryatt, JS (1973) *Nature, Lond., 241,* 204

Millward, DJ, Garlick, PJ, Stewart, RJC, Nnanyelugo, DO and Waterlow, JC (1975a) *Biochem. J., 150,* 235

Millward, DJ, Nnanyelugo, DO, Bates, P and Heard, CRC (1975b) *Proc. nutr. Soc., 35,* 48A

O'Keefe, SJD (1974) Project report for MSc, University of London

O'Keefe, SJD, Sender, PM and James, WPT (1974) *Lancet, ii,* 1035

Olesen, K, Heilskov, NCS and Schonheyder, F (1954) *Biochim. biophys. Acta, 15,* 95

Payne, PR and Waterlow, JC (1971) *Lancet, ii,* 210

Picou, D and Taylor-Roberts, T (1969) *Clin. Sci., 36,* 382

Pitot, HC and Peraino, C (1964) *J. biol. Chem., 240,* 3039

Reeds, PJ (1974) *Brit. J. Nutr., 31,* 259

Schonheyder, F, Heilskov, NSC and Olesen, K (1954) *Scand. J. clin. Lab. Invest., 6,* 178

Sketcher, RD, Fern, EB and James, WPT (1974) *Brit. J. Ntr., 31,* 333

Stephen, JML (1968) *Brit. J. Nutr., 22,* 153

Waterlow, JC (1967) *Clin. Sci., 33,* 507

Waterlow, JC and Garlick, PJ (1975) In *Alcohol and Abnormal Protein Biosynthesis: Biochemical and Clinical.* (Ed) MA Rothschild, M Oratz and SS Schreiber. Pergamon Press, New York. Page 67

Young, VR, Steffee, WP, Pencharz, PB, Winterer, JC and Scrimshaw, NS (1975) *Nature, Lond., 253,* 192

Injury and Plasma Proteins

A FLECK

Department of Biochemistry, Western Infirmary, Glasgow, Scotland

Introduction

The changes in the plasma proteins after injury have been the subject of study for many years. Cuthbertson and Tompsett in 1935 described the fall in albumin concentration and increase in the globulin fraction which occurred after injury. As new techniques have developed they have been applied to studies of the effects of the metabolic changes induced by injury on plasma proteins.

CHANGES IN CONCENTRATION OF PLASMA PROTEINS AFTER INJURY

The changes in the main plasma protein fractions and changes in plasma proteins are summarised in Tables I and II.

Electrophoretic Pattern

The changes in albumin, α_1, α_2, β and γ globulins observed on electrophoresis of serum from injured patients are summarised in Table I, and have been discussed in detail by Owen (1967) and Werner and Cohnen (1969).

All investigators agree that after trauma, albumin concentration decreases reaching a minimum around the third to sixth day and gradually returning towards normal concentration which, depending on the severity of the injury, may be attained after seventeen days (Ballantyne & Fleck, 1973a) but after more severe injuries such as burning, may take a month or more to regain the normal concentration (Prendergast et al, 1952). It is also generally agreed that the α_1 and α_2 globulin fractions increase. This increase is probably accounted for by

229

TABLE I. Changes in Plasma Proteins after Injury. 1. Electrophoresis Pattern

Increased	Decreased
α_1 globulins	Albumin
α_2 globulins	
	β globulins*
γ globulins, only if infection present	γ globulins (transient and slight)
	*See text — increased after burns

TABLE II. Changes in Plasma Proteins after Injury. 2. Acute Phase Reactants

	Increased	Decreased	Rapid	Response Intermediate	Slow
		Albumin		Min. d5	
α_1 globulins	α_1 antitrypsin		Max.d3		
	α_1 acid glycoprotein		Max.d3		
		α_1 lipoprotein	Min.d3		
α_2 globulins	ceruloplasmin				Max.d3-9
	haptoglobin		Max.d3		
β globulins		transferrin		Min.d3-6	
		β lipoprotein			Min.d3-9
γ_1 region	C-reactive protein		Max.d1-2		
	Fibrinogen		increase d1-12+		

the observation that most of the components of the α_1 and α_2 globulins increase in concentration after injury (Table II).

The behaviour of β globulins after injury seems not to be so consistent, e.g. Werner and Cohnen (1969) report a decrease whereas Owen (1967) suggests that β globulin generally remains unchanged and our findings (Fleck et al, 1970) are consistent with this. Owen (1967) does however comment that the concentration of the major component of the β globulin fraction — transferrin — usually decreases rapidly after injury.

Specific Proteins — Acute Phase Reactants

The acute phase reactants have been described by Koj (1970) as the plasma proteins which show an increase in concentration in the acute phase of inflammation. The pattern of changes in the acute phase reactants and some other plasma proteins after laparotomy, herniorrhaphy and thyroidectomy is summarised in Table II (Crockson et al, 1969; Werner, 1969; Werner & Cohnen, 1969).

Because there are few extensive simultaneous studies of the changes in a large number of serum proteins after injury (Crockson et al, 1966; Werner & Cohnen, 1969), it is impossible to compare accurately the extent of the changes in each protein. Another reason for the difficulty in comparing the extent of changes is that many important studies have been carried out after accidental injury so that there is no pre-injury 'base line' for comparison in these patients. However, attempts have been made to obtain rough comparisons of the extent of the changes in the various plasma proteins after injury. It must be noted that the degree of the change is strongly influenced by the magnitude of the injury.

Albumin

The timing of the fall in albumin concentration after injury has been summarised above. After serious burning injury, the plasma albumin concentration may fall to very low levels (less than 20g/l) [Prendergast et al, 1952] and infusions of blood or plasma may be required for many weeks in order to maintain the concentration around 25g/l. After moderate injury, however, the fall in albumin concentration is of the order of 25-30% (Ballantyne & Fleck, 1973a).

Fibrinogen

Quantitatively the response of fibrinogen is the next in importance to albumin and there is widespread agreement that fibrinogen concentration increases, occasionally very considerably, after injury (Cuthbertson & Tompsett, 1935; Crockson et al, 1966; Davies et al, 1970; Koj, 1970; Owen, 1967). Increases up to twice the upper limit of the normal range, maintained for nine days after operations on the femur in elderly patients have been reported (Davies et al, 1970). The average increase was of the order of 60-70% in these patients.

In contrast, in younger patients, the same authors report that the increase, although present, was of lesser magnitude.

C-reactive Protein (CRP)

This protein, the role of which is not clear, is scarcely detectable in the serum of 'normal' individuals. It seems to appear consistently after injury or inflammation and it has been suggested (Crockson et al, 1966) is the best single screening test of an 'acute phase reaction'. On electrophoresis it migrates in the γ_1 region.

α_1 Globulins

Taking this electrophoretic group together, α_1 antitrypsin and α_1 acid glycoprotein both increase fairly rapidly by usually at least 50% (Ballantyne & Fleck, 1973a; Crockson et al, 1966). The α_1 lipoprotein decreases by about 50% (Werner & Cohnen, 1969). Together this probably accounts for the early increase in total α_1 globulins after injury.

α_2 Globulins

Ceruloplasmin and haptoglobin are the examples quoted from this group. Both show moderately rapid increases of the order of 50-100% (Crockson et al, 1966; Werner & Cohnen, 1969).

β Globulins

Transferrin and β lipoprotein consistently show a decrease in concentration after injury. In both cases the decrease seems to be of the order of 25-50% (Werner & Cohnen, 1969).

γ Globulins

The immunoglobulins IgG, IgA, IgM seem not to change significantly after injury (Ballantyne & Fleck, 1973a), unless there is a source of infection as in burns where the increases may be considerable (Prendergast et al, 1952).

CHANGES IN PLASMA PROTEIN METABOLISM AFTER INJURY

Catabolism

The catabolism of albumin, fibrinogen and gamma G globulin (IgG) have been studied after injury, using ^{125}I or ^{131}I-labelled protein. The calculation of catabolic rate has been mainly by the U/P method. The more recent studies of albumin catabolism after moderate injury by Ballantyne and Fleck (1973b) are in agreement with those of Mouridsen (1967) in the failure to find a significant increase in the absolute catabolic rate of albumin after injury. The fractional catabolic rate (which is the fraction of the total intravascular albumin catabolised per day) however, was increased (Ballantyne & Fleck, 1973b) for a period of several days.

In contrast, Davies et al have consistently reported increased catabolism of albumin (1962, 1969), fibrinogen (1970) and IgG (1969) after severe burning injury. The increased catabolism of albumin and IgG in the series of burned patients studied by them was proportional to the increase in resting metabolic rate.

The distribution of albumin in the body, expressed as extravascular : intravascular ratio (EV/IV) is markedly increased after injury (Ballantyne & Fleck, 1973b) with the greatest changes being found after burning (Davies et al, 1969).

Synthesis

An attempt has been made to calculate rates of synthesis of albumin and IgG in burned patients in studies using ^{131}I labelled proteins by making allowances for the changes in the circulating albumin and IgG pools (Davies et al, 1969). Calculated in this way the synthesis rate of albumin after severe burning injury increased in the first few days, then decreased through normal about five days, then became subnormal for at least twenty days. In the same study the calculated synthetic rate of IgG similarly rose rapidly after the injury, then fell slightly but remained elevated for more than twenty days.

A similar study carried out on fibrinogen also showed an increased rate of synthesis after injury (Davies et al, 1970).

Direct measurement of synthesis rates of plasma proteins by the ^{14}C carbonate method following injury have rarely been carried out, probably mainly because of the technical complexities of the method. In experimental rabbits Ballantyne et al (1973a) found that albumin synthesis was significantly decreased on the third day after femoral fracture and they concluded that the decrease in plasma albumin concentration after injury could be accounted for by the decrease in its synthesis.

In contrast Koj and McFarlane (1968) found that the administration of endotoxin to experimental rabbits led to increased synthesis of both albumin and fibrinogen 48 hours after the injection of endotoxin, albumin synthesis was increased by about 60%, whereas fibrinogen synthesis was increased by 400%. This increase is twice as large as the figure obtained from the indirect calculations of Davies et al (1970), who found, in human subjects after orthopaedic operations, that the early increase in fibrinogen synthesis was of the order of 200%.

CONTROL OF PLASMA PROTEIN METABOLISM

Nutrition

It is generally accepted that albumin synthesis in the liver is rapidly reduced in protein deprivation (Rothschild et al, 1970; Hoffenberg, 1970; Jeejeebhoy et al, 1973).

In contrast it seems that the catabolic rate does not decrease immediately after the onset of protein deprivation but only after the concentration of plasma albumin has decreased significantly.

When protein repletion is begun the synthesis rate of albumin responds with a very rapid increase which thereafter gradually declines (Hoffenberg, 1970). The catabolic rate increases very gradually as the plasma albumin concentration rises. In nutritionally depleted human subjects with reduced plasma albumin concentration, the absolute catabolic rate of albumin is significantly reduced (Hoffenberg et al, 1966; Ballantyne & Fleck, 1973b). In contrast with albumin, fibrinogen synthesis is not initially sensitive to protein deprivation (Jeejeebhoy, 1973).

Disease

Because of the considerable losses of albumin in nephrosis, both catabolism and synthesis of albumin have been studied in experimental animals and patients with this condition. Both the intravascular and extravascular pools are greatly reduced in nephrosis as is the extravascular : intravascular (EV/IV) ratio of albumin (Ballantyne, 1971). The absolute catabolic rate of albumin may be reduced, the fractional rate is elevated and the synthesis rate is also increased (Ballantyne, 1971; Hoffenberg, 1970).

In active rheumatoid arthritis, the fractional catabolic rate of albumin is increased in proportion to the activity of the disease in an affected joint (Ballantyne et al, 1971).

Discussion

That an increase in the extravascular : intravascular (EV/IV) ratio of albumin occurs after injury is generally agreed. The explanation may lie in post-injury sodium retention, reduced lymphatic return and wound or burn oedema leading to an expansion of the extravascular space. In malnutrition and other disease the tendency, in contrast, is for a reduction in the EV/IV ratio which may be regarded as tending to retain maximal IV concentration (e.g. of albumin) at the expense of the extravascular pool. After mild to moderate injury the changes in albumin concentration are compatible with the observed decrease in synthesis but with the normal absolute catabolic rate maintained. This would lead to the increased fractional catabolic rate reported by Ballantyne and Fleck (1973b). The extension of this argument cannot however apply in the severely burned patient in whom the absolute catabolic rate and synthesis rate are initially increased. The later fall in the synthesis rate may be due to inadequate supply of amino acids to the liver (i.e. 'protein malnutrition') because of the difficulty in meeting the enormously increased energy and protein demands of these patients.

The prolonged increase in catabolic rate in the presence of reduced total pool and low intravascular albumin in severely burned patients is in notable contrast with the reduced catabolism in the primary malnourished individual. The explanation may be in the endocrine changes which accompany severe injury (Fleck,

234

1976). Increases in adrenocortical hormone output lead to increased albumin catabolism (Rothschild et al, 1958). These hormones may also by increasing the supply of amino acids to the liver from muscle (Munro, 1970), effect an increase in albumin synthesis (Jeejeebhoy et al, 1973). It might be expected, however, that the increased gluconeogenesis promoted by the increases in secretion of cate-cholamines and glucagon early in the injury response (Fleck, 1976) might reduce the free amino acids in the liver sufficiently to reduce protein synthesis.

It is apparent that the metabolic interactions are complex and that the changes in plasma proteins after injury cannot be explained by blood loss (see Baar & Topley, 1956), only by altered metabolism. Different patterns of synthesis and catabolism have been found for each plasma protein studied (Jeejeebhoy et al, 1973).

Studies on liver polysomes confirm that no clear single gross trend in liver protein synthesis is likely to be found after injury. Polysome patterns in rat liver after injury and RNA synthesis studies are compatible with a general increase in protein synthesis up to 12h, followed by a decrease to 18h; which in turn is followed by a lesser increase at 24h after the injury (Khan et al, 1974).

The details of the mechanism of control of synthesis and catabolism of plasma proteins remains to be elucidated, especially of the changes which occur after injury.

References

Baar, S and Topley, E (1956) *Acta med. Scand., 153,* 319
Ballantyne, FC (1971) *Studies on Albumin Metabolism in Injury and Disease.* PhD Thesis, University of Glasgow
Ballantyne, FC and Fleck, A (1973a) *Clin. Chim. Acta, 44,* 341
Ballantyne, FC and Fleck, A (1973b) *Clin. Chim. Acta, 46,* 139
Ballantyne, FC, Fleck, A and Carson Dick, W (1971) *Ann. rheum. Dis., 30,* 265
Crockson, RA, Payne, CJ, Ratcliff, AP and Soothill, JF (1966) *Clin. chim. Acta, 14,* 435
Cuthbertson, DP and Tompsett, SL (1935) *Brit. J. exp. Path., 16,* 471
Davies, JWL, Liljedahl, S-O and Birke, G (1969) *Injury, 1,* 43
Davies, JWL, Liljedahl, S-O and Reizenstein, P (1970) *Injury, 1,* 178
Davies, JWL, Ricketts, CR and Bull, JP (1962) *Clin. Sci., 23,* 411
Fleck, A (1976) 'The Early Metabolic Response to Injury', in *Shock.* (Ed) IMcA Ledingham. Elsevier Scientific Publishers, Amsterdam (in press)
Fleck, A, Ballantyne, FC, Green, J, Tilstone, WJ and Cuthbertson, DP (1970) In *Proc. 8th Internat. Congr. Nutrition, Prague 1969.* Excerpta Medica, International Congress 213, Amsterdam
Hoffenberg, R (1970) 'Control of Albumin Degradation in vivo and in the Perfused Liver' in *Plasma Protein Metabolism Regulation of Synthesis, Distribution and Degradation.* (Ed) MA Rothschild and T Waldmann. Academic Press, London
Hoffenberg, R, Black, E and Brock, JF (1966) *J. clin. Invest., 45,* 143
Jeejeebhoy, KN, Bruce-Robertson, A, Ho, J and Sodtke, U (1973) 'The Comparative Effects of Nutritional and Hormonal Factors on the Synthesis

of Albumin, Fibrinogen and Transferrin', in *Protein Turnover, Ciba Foundation Symposium 9 (new series).* (Chairman) AS McFarlane. Associated Scientific Publishers, Amsterdam

Khan, SN, Tilstone, WJ, Fleck, A and Broom, I (1974) *Proc. nutr. Soc., 33,* 93A

Koj, A (1970) 'Synthesis and Turnover of Acute-Phase Reactants', in *Energy Metabolism in Trauma, Ciba Foundation Symposium.* (Ed) R Porter and J Knight. J & A Churchill, London

Koj, A and McFarlane, AS (1968) *Biochem. J., 108,* 137

Mouridsen, HT (1967) *Clin. Sci., 33,* 345

Munro, HN (1970) 'Free Amino Acid Pools and their Role in Regulation', in *Mammalian Protein Metabolism, Volume 4, Chapter 34.* (Ed) HN Munro. Academic Press, New York

Owen, JA (1967) 'Effect of Injury on Plasma Proteins', in *Advances in Clinical Chemistry, Volume 9.* (Ed) H Sobatka and CP Stewart. Academic Press, London. Page 9

Prendergast, JJ, Fenichel, RL and Daly, BM (1952) *Arch. Surg., 64,* 733

Rothschild, MA, Oratz, M and Schreiber, SS (1970) 'Albumin Metabolism', in *Plasma Protein Metabolism Regulation of Synthesis, Distribution and Degradation.* (Ed) MA Rothschild and T Waldmann. Academic Press, London

Rothschild, MA, Schreiber, SS, Oratz, M and McGee, HL (1958) *J. clin. Invest., 37,* 1229

Werner, M (1969) *Clin. Chim. Acta, 25,* 299

Werner, M and Cohnen, G (1969) *Clin. Sci., 36,* 173

Surgical Hypermetabolism and Nitrogen Metabolism

J M KINNEY

Department of Surgery, Columbia University College of Physicians and Surgeons, New York, USA

Introduction

Cuthbertson followed his initial observations on the metabolic response to injury by dividing the response into the early or 'ebb' phase of depressed vitality lasting for a day or so, and followed by resurgence of vitality which he termed the 'flow' phase and which seemed to bear a certain resemblance to inflammation (Cuthbertson, 1942) [Figure 1]. The flow phase can be divided into a catabolic phase, lasting days to weeks, and the later anabolic phase, lasting weeks to months. The surgeon, all too often, considers the time scale of the metabolic response to injury according to the time needed for healing of the operative wound to adequate tensile strength. This process has usually reached a satisfactory functional end point within the first 10 to 14 days. In contrast the catabolic course of the patient with the resolving abcess, the healing intestinal fistula or the major burn being resurfaced is a process which extends over many weeks. But regardless of whether the catabolic phase lasts 10 days or 60 days the process of anabolic recovery will still lie ahead of the patient. The last thing to return in surgical convalesence is the ability to work a full day without fatigue. This recovery is not complete until there is restoration of both muscle mass and muscle function, with part, if not all, of the adipose tissue loss being restored.

The catabolic response to injury and infection is characterised not only by weight loss and weakness, but resting hypermetabolism, increased nitrogen excretion, carbohydrate intolerance and increased mobilisation of fat. Du Bois et al (1924) commented on the parallel increase in resting energy expenditure and nitrogen excretion. Cuthbertson (1932) reported a similar parallel behaviour between the increased oxygen consumption and increased nitrogen excretion following long-bone fracture. Subsequent studies have confirmed this parallel

RESPONSE TO INJURY OR SEPSIS IN MAN

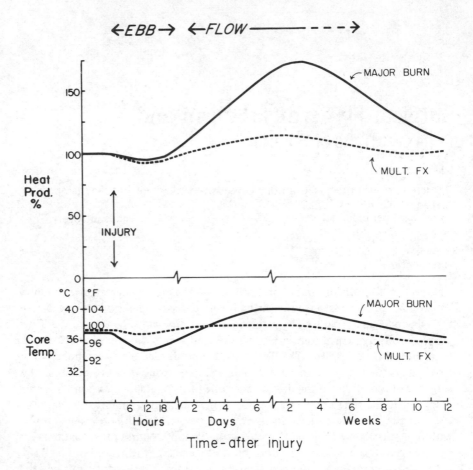

Figure 1. A schematic representation of the changes in human heat production and core temperature when divided by the 'ebb' and 'flow' phase of Cuthbertson

behaviour when both are decreased, as in starvation, or a variety of surgical conditions which exhibit parallel rises in resting energy expenditure and nitrogen excretion. Surgical patients with a severe catabolic response represent an ill-defined combination of the metabolic changes of starvation, of physical injury and the additional changes which result from fever and major infection. Therefore, this discussion will use the factors of energy metabolism and nitrogen excretion as the central subject for a discussion of the evolving metabolic picture in surgical catabolism.

238

The caloric expenditure under basal conditions per square meter of body surface area reaches a peak during the first five years of life of approximately 60 to around 40 kcal/m^2/hr (Talbot, 1921). The metabolic rate then decreases from the ages of 5 to 20 years. This steady decline is interrupted by increased metabolism at puberty which occurs slightly earlier for the female than the male. From the ages of 20 to 85, there is a slow but steady decrease from approximately 40 to 34 kcal per square metre per hour. There is a general relationship between nitrogen excretion and the resting energy expenditure which in turn is a function of the body cell mass (Brody, 1945). A value of 2 mg of urinary nitrogen per basal kcal has been accepted as applying to mammals in general. For adult man, however, the average endogenous urinary nitrogen excretion has been determined experimentally to be only 1.3 to 1.4 mg of nitrogen per basal kcal (Food and Nutrition Board, National Academy of Sciences, 1974). If one accepts 1.35 mg of nitrogen per basal kcal as an average figure for the endogenous nitrogen excretion of 2.5 g per day, to this figure must be added approximately 0.9 g per day for faecal nitrogen loss and 300 mg per day lost from sweat, skin desquamation, and so forth. Summing up these values, the minimum nitrogen loss of a 70 kg man, consuming no protein, is estimated to be 3.7 g per day, or a protein loss of 23 g per day (0.33 g per kg of body weight), which must be replaced under normal conditions.

The average American diet is said to have approximately 15% of the calories supplied as protein. It seems obvious that the average American intake of protein is considerably in excess of the minimum endogenous protein loss calculated in the report of Recommended Dietary Allowances by the National Academy of Sciences (1974). Future studies are needed to define why there is a correlation between resting energy expenditure and nitrogen excretion, to examine which tissues are involved and whether this is mainly related to urea synthesis or is a general correlation involving many pathways of nitrogen metabolism. Perhaps the energetics are somehow linked to a few, selected amino acids as proposed by Lusk (1931) in explaining the specific dynamic action of foodstuffs. Present information does not explain why these two factors tend to decrease and increase together.

METABOLIC RESPONSE TO STARVATION

Starvation in man can be considered in successive phases, each of which must guarantee a supply of appropriate fuel for the brain. The classic study of total starvation in normal, adult man was performed by Benedict in 1912 (Benedict, 1915) [Figure 2]. During 31 days of total starvation, his subject's weight fell from 60.6 to 47 kg, 22%. The heat production of Benedict's subject fell steadily over the first 18 days from 1760 to 1260 kcal per day. The nitrogen excretion

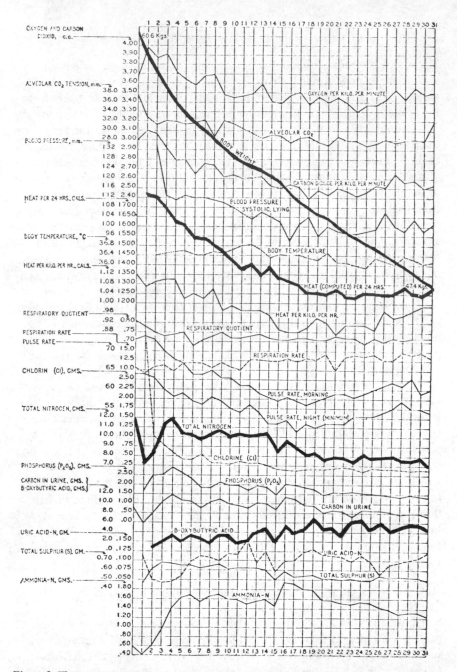

Figure 2. The master graph of data from the study of 31 days of total starvation in normal adult man. This is reproduced from Benedict (1915) with heavy lines drawn to emphasise body weight, daily heat production, total nitrogen excretion and urinary excretion of β-hydroxybuteric acid

240

was erratic for the first three days, and thereafter decreased from 12 to 8 g per day in parallel with the decreasing energy metabolism. Neither variable changed from the 18th to the 31st day of starvation. It has been generally assumed that nitrogen excretion and energy metabolism are also reduced in approximately parallel fashion during chronic partial starvation. It is of interest that the depleted patient who demonstrates a decreased, or absent clinical response to injury or infection, also shows a limited, or absent, increase in both energy expenditure and nitrogen excretion.

The available carbohydrate reserves for the brain are limited to the 70 g of liver glycogen, which are depleted in the first one to two days of starvation. Maintenance of glucose homeostasis depends upon an increase in glucose production (gluconeogenesis) and limitation of extracerebral glucose oxidation. The main signal initiating this adaptive response appears to be a small decrease of 10 to 15 mg in circulating glucose levels. This results in decreased insulin (Cahill et al, 1966) and increased glucagon blood levels (Marliss et al, 1970). Lipolysis is stimulated to provide energy for muscle and liver. The liver shifts to ketone production which is used for fuel by muscle, along with fatty acids (Owen & Reichard, 1971).

New glucose production arises from lactate, glycerol and amino acids. The lactate is assumed to be glucose-derived and the glycerol is a limited source arising from triglyceride breakdown. Thus, amino acids represent the major source of new glucose, and muscle protein represents the predominant source of amino acids

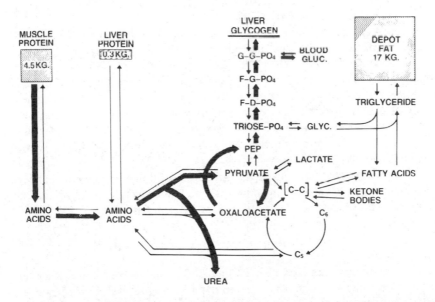

Figure 3. A schematic diagram has been constructed to represent general metabolic pathways connecting the protein of muscle and liver with liver glycogen, adipose tissue and the TCA cycle. Heavy lines have been drawn to emphasise certain pathways of gluconeogenesis

when extra gluconeogenesis is required (Figure 3). Clinical studies have shown that the output of amino acids from muscle is dominated by alanine and glutamine. The splanchnic uptake is greatest for these two amino acids, the gut being the site of glutamine utilisation, while ananine is taken up solely by the liver (Felig & Wahren, 1974).

Alanine accounts for only 7% of the amino acids in muscle protein, but for 30 to 40% of the amino acid output from muscle. Felig et al (1969) suggested a glucose-alanine cycle between muscle and liver. Approximately two-thirds of the alanine coming from muscle is derived from glucose, with some evidence that the branched chain amino acids are preferentially catabolised in muscle and provide the major source of nitrogen for synthesis of alanine from glucose-derived pyruvate in muscle (Odessey et al, 1974; Felig & Wahren, in press).

The alanine output from muscle is progressively increased during the first 3 days of starvation, while the extraction of alanine by the liver is also increased (Saudek & Felig, 1974). As fasting continues, the urinary nitrogen loss, particularly urea, drops to 3 or 4 g per day within 4 to 6 weeks of starvation. During this time, hepatic glucose release is reduced to a range of 40 to 50 g per day. The kidney contributes an additional 40 g of glucose per day. At the same time, the brain, which normally consumes 100 to 125 g of glucose per day, begins to depend on ketones for approximately half of its total fuel requirements (Owen et al, 1967). It may be that the brain begins to utilise ketone bodies at the point when muscle utilisation has been exceeded causing blood ketone levels to become sufficiently elevated (Garber et al, 1974).

After prolonged starvation, the low output of glucose from the liver is not due to altered hepatic mechanisms, but rather to a decrease in the level of gluconeogenic substrates being brought to the liver. Recent studies by Sherwin et al (1975) suggest that substrates, particularly ketones may provide the signal for protein-sparing in muscle tissue. Therefore, ketones appear to have a dual role in the late stage of starvation, serving as a 'substrate' as well as a 'signal'. Insulin may be important in a permissive role to allow the protein-sparing effect of hyperketonaemia, since protein breakdown is accelerated in the hyperketonaemia of severe diabetic acidosis.

In summary, the twin goals of starvation metabolism are the maintenance of glucose homeostasis and protein conservation, while meeting the obligatory needs for energy in the form which can be utilised by each tissue.

INFLUENCE OF FEVER AND INFECTION

The correlation between resting hypermetabolism and increased nitrogen excretion was originally thought to be due to the presence of fever. European investigators had referred to the 'traumatic fever' of injury, even before the increased nitrogen excretion had been identified as part of the metabolic response. In the early part of this century, the influence of fever on nitrogen metabolism received increasing attention. The body temperature of a normal subject was raised by a hot bath and it was observed that nitrogen excretion was not increased despite the elevation of body temperature by several degrees (Graham & Pulton, 1912). Various reports in the literature state that the hypermetabolism with exercise is not correlated with an increased nitrogen excretion. It appears that as long as the caloric intake is adequate to meet the extra demands of physical activity, body protein will not be broken down (Campbell & Webster, 1921).

The relationship of resting metabolism to body temperature in various forms

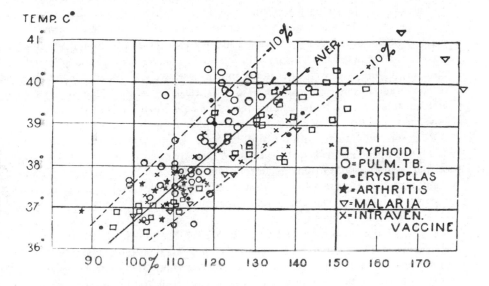

Figure 4. The relation of basal metabolism to body temperature is shown for six different fevers. The continuous line shows the average and the dotted lines are drawn to represent metabolism 10 per cent above and 10 per cent below the average. (Reproduced by permission from EF Du Bois 'Basal Metabolism in Health and Disease', 2nd Edition. Lea & Febiger, Philadelphia. Page 390)

of fever is shown in Figure 4. The average increase in metabolism with fever has led to the widespread acceptance that every degree Fahrenheit rise in body temperature can be expected to produce a 7.2% increase in metabolic rate (13% increase for every degree Centigrade). It is obvious from Figure 4 that there is a relatively wide deviation from the average. It seems clear that the surgical patient with major infection such as peritonitis is behaving much more like the patient with typhoid fever than one with pulmonary tuberculosis, even though each condition is usually associated with 2 to 3 degrees F rise in body temperature.

The overall uniformity of the results of studies of fever and metabolic rate in clinical infection suggested to Du Bois (1924) that this might be the result of a general law regarding the velocity of chemical reactions. The Van't Hoff Law states: "With a rise in temperature of 10 degrees centigrade, the velocity of chemical reaction will increase between 2 and 3 times". Nearly all of the clinical fever experiments fell within these limits. In other words, the response of a fever patient closely resembles the behaviour of chemical reactions which might be studied in the test tube at varying temperatures.

The relationship of body temperature to resting energy expenditure was studied in a group of surgical patients (Kinney & Roe, 1962; Roe & Kinney, 1965). During the post-operative course the patients tended to follow the '7% rule' of Du Bois as an average, but there was a significant number of patients who deviated above and below that level, similar to the clinical infection studies from which the original average value was obtained. It was of interest that fracture patients who suffered significant weight loss without secondary complications showed the predicted relationship between body temperature and energy metabolism during the early days after injury, but progressively less energy metabolism response (and less nitrogen excretion) as weight loss progressed. One wonders whether this response to depletion produced a similar metabolic setting to the presumed depletion of the Bellevue Hospital patients with pulmonary tuberculosis. The surgical patients with the most extreme elevations of energy metabolism and nitrogen excretion above the predicted increase due to their extent of fever, were the patients with extensive peritonitis and major third degree burns. Future studies are needed to separate the influence of fever on visceral organs such as the liver from its influence on muscle and adipose tissue.

Reiss (1959), studying infections in rats, Madden (1950), studying turpentine abscesses in dogs, Levenson and associates (1957), studying burns in rats, and Blocker et al (1955), studying human burns, were all able to demonstrate that amino acid incorporation into certain proteins was normal or increased at the height of the reaction to injury or infection. Therefore, the increased urinary nitrogen excretion under these circumstances could not be due to a simple decrease in anabolism. Both anabolism and catabolism might be accelerated, with catabolism predominating, to account for the net loss of nitrogen. But all tissues do not participate equally in this response. The amino acid incorporation in these studies dealt only with dog plasma protein, the proteins of rat liver, gastrointestinal tract, plasma, and human plasma protein. In burned rats, the protein turnover of organs such as the liver markedly increased, but the content changed very little, whereas the protein content of the carcass fell, despite a lower turnover rate, and accounted for most of the extra urinary loss. The protein content of liver and kidneys of starved rats with infection did not decrease, but both fell in starved control animals. This is consistent with the different effects of glucocorticoids on protein metabolism, which depends upon the particular tissue or organ being studied.

Beisel and co-workers (1967) conducted extensive metabolic studies in experimental infection in man. Their studies revealed that circulating amino acids began to drop for 1 or 2 days before the febrile period began. An endogenous mediator substance is elaborated from polymorphonuclear leukocytes in the presence of

244

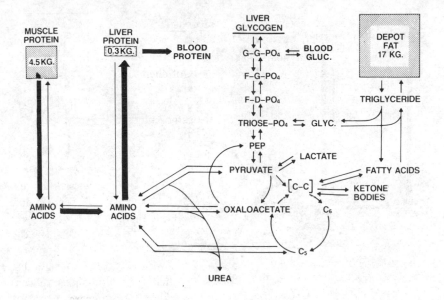

Figure 5. A schematic diagram of general metabolic pathways is used to emphasise in heavy lines, the pathways which are catabolic for muscle but anabolic for liver in the presence of acute infection

various infective agents. (Wannemacher et al, 1972). This material has been demonstrated during infections of both animals and man. Chemical characterisation is not complete but has proceeded far enough to show that this substance is not endotoxin derived from gram negative bacteria (Pekarek et al, 1974). It is of particular interest that the assay for the material is based on the demonstration of more rapid uptake of amino acids and zinc from the circulating blood stream into liver cells; this amino acid uptake is not for gluconeogenesis but rather for the synthesis of acute phase proteins as part of the metabolic response to infection (Figure 5). It is noteworthy that the liver is responsible not only for the majority of new glucose formation during catabolic states but also for the acute phase protein synthesis since all the acute phase proteins are glycoproteins. Stimulation of this process represents muscle protein breakdown which is in addition to the amount of breakdown which would be predicted by extra urea excretion and this is consistent with the fact that the most rapid and extreme muscle wasting is observed in the well muscled young male with injuries and secondary infection (Figure 6).

THE INFLUENCE OF INJURY

Cuthbertson has described the flow phase as having a resemblance to inflammation, which appears to be important before anabolic processes can complete

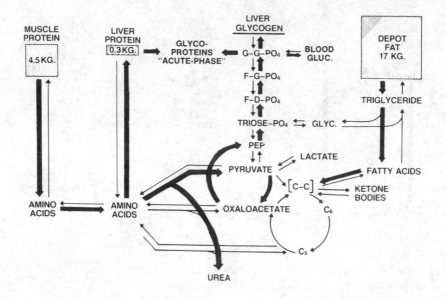

Figure 6. The schematic diagram of general metabolic pathways is shown to emphasise the stimulus to both gluconeogenesis, acute phase protein synthesis and increase far mobilisation in septic, catabolic states

convalescence. One might consider this inflammatory-like response as necessary to remove the products of tissue injury and rebuild normal tissue. The concept seems plausible in the presence of extensive infection such as peritonitis or as a result of both infection and circulating toxic products presumed to be present in the patient with a major burn. Before measurements of energy expenditure were available there were estimates of large increases in energy expenditure following injury, with the corollary that body protein was degraded in a desperate attempt to find additional tissue fuel. The fact that fatty acids are readily mobilised from adipose tissue to supply 2-carbon fragments for general fuel needs must be combined with the fact that these fatty acids cannot provide for the synthesis of carbohydrate intermediates such as pyruvate, glucose or glycogen. The synthesis of carbohydrate intermediates and new glucose formation must depend largely upon the breakdown of body protein, particularly muscle protein. Measurements of the protein and calorie contribution to the tissue loss of surgical catabolism reveal that protein, which is normally 10 to 12% of the weight loss in the early weeks of partial and total starvation, may decrease slightly after tissue depletion with partial starvation, but seldom is increased to account for more than 14% of weight loss during extreme catabolic states. Contribution of calories from protein to the resting metabolic expenditure is commonly between 12 and 22% of the RME (Duke et al, 1970). In other words, fat continues to provide from 80 to 90% of the calories even in severe surgical catabolism. This information supports the

246

concept that the increased nitrogen loss in surgical catabolic states has to do with demands for specialised syntheses which utilise the amino acids from muscle protein, and not merely the provision of 2-carbon fragments to meet general demands for tissue fuel.

Resting hypermetabolism after long-bone fracture in the rat has been linked by Cairnie et al (1957) to the breakdown of tissue protein. These workers propose that the same pathways which are involved in the extra heat production following protein ingestion, known as specific dynamic action, are also involved with body protein breakdown causing surgical hypermetabolism as a kind of 'endogenous specific dynamic action'. This idea was consistent with the work of Myers (1954) showing the prompt increase in oxygen uptake of the splanchnic bed, when hypertonic amino acids solutions were infused. It seemed possible that metabolic events associated with either urea synthesis or the hepatic handling of the deaminated amino acid residue were associated with this increase in heat production. In this case, the entire increase should be demonstrable across the splanchnic bed. Studies by Gump et al (1970), utilising catheterisation of the hepatic vein in febrile surgical patients with abdominal infections, have demonstrated that only approximately half of the increase in cardiac output and oxygen consumption above predicted normal values could be accounted for across the splanchnic bed. Therefore, surgical hypermetabolism, at least when involved with infection, appears to involve increased utilisation of non-protein fuel in tissues other than the liver.

The increment in nitrogen excretion and heat production following experimental fracture has been shown to be abolished when rats have been fed a protein free diet which is adequate in energy, while an increased response is observed in animals which have been fed a 30% protein diet (Munro & Chalmers, 1945). Caldwell (1970) studied the influence of environmental temperature on the metabolism of rats following burns. He found that rats kept at 30°C after injury had less metabolic response and that this experimental group showed fewer fatalities and more rapid recovery than did the experimental group housed at 20°C. Cuthbertson and Tilstone (1967) demonstrated an acceleration in healing of skin wounds in rats at 30°C. Campbell and Cuthbertson (1967) also showed in the rat that the increased energy metabolism and nitrogen excretion after long-bone fracture was essentially prevented by keeping animals at 30°C rather than at 20°C. Subsequent studies by this group on the nitrogen excretion after fractures in man indicate a definite reduction in nitrogen excretion when patients were cared for at the higher temperature. These results are in general agreement with the behaviour of burn patients in elevated ambient temperatures. The decrease in metabolic response after elevation of the ambient temperature seems harder to explain after long-bone fracture than in the burned patient. Tilstone and Cuthbertson (1970) feel that the most likely explanation is that the animal or man at 30°C is just below the temperature at which heat stress will begin in the non-acclimatised subject and will thus avoid any non-obligatory increase in heat production.

Tilstone and Cuthbertson (1970) have re-emphasised that there is not a generalised response of all protein to injury and that specific proteins must be studied at successive stages after injury. They have also suggested that the effect of a reduced oxygen consumption during the 'ebb' phase could be to decrease the synthesis of some sensitive proteins in the liver without affecting the increased synthesis of acute phase reactants. Liu and Neuhaus (1965) have studied rat liver polysomes after operative trauma under ether anaesthesia. The trauma stimulated glycoprotein synthesis and increased the aggregation of polysomes which became maximal at 18 hours, when the amino acid uptake of liver microsomes was also maximal. These workers suggest that injury stimulates new ribosomal and messenger (RNA) synthesis leading to increase protein synthesis. Young and Huang (1969) studied the protein synthesising activity of microsomes isolated from the injured and controlateral leg of rats with a fracture of the femur. Utilising ^{14}C-leucine these workers found a reduction in incorporation of leucine by the thigh muscle of the injured limb regardless of whether the rat had received casein at 5% or 25% of the diet before injury. The synthesis in the liver of both acute phase reactants and albumin has prompted the suggestion that export protein is synthesised by polysomes which are bound to endoplasmic reticulum, whereas protein for use within the cell is synthesised by free polysomes. In summary, the study of protein synthesis by subcellular particles shows a general depression of synthesis in muscle following fracture of the femur. Synthesis of proteins in the liver may be increased at this time, but this remains to be established.

There has long been interest but great difficulty in the problem of measuring turnover rates of protein in the intact human body. However, it seems possible that a segment of the basal energy expenditure is directly related to the turnover of body protein. Support for this concept has recently appeared from the studies of Young et al (1975), who utilised an isotopic amino acid to obtain measurements of protein turnover rates. These studies indicate a difference in values depending on age, but when one corrects the protein synthesis rate for the predicted normal energy expenditure or recommended calorie intake for that age, they find a relatively uniform relationship from infancy through adult life.

O'Keefe et al (1974) have attempted to calculate protein synthesis rates, utilising an infusion of ^{14}C-leucine in surgical patients before and after uncomplicated, abdominal surgery. These workers concluded that the increased post-operative nitrogen loss during the 'flow' or catabolic phase was correlated with a decrease in protein synthesis rates. Unfortunately, the pre-operative measurements were made while the patients were receiving nitrogen intake, whereas the post-operative studies were conducted without nitrogen intake. Unpublished studies by Duke et al (1975) and Long et al (1975) utilising ^{15}N-alanine in a single dose and a multi-compartment mathematical model, indicate minimal changes in synthesis and breakdown rates after uncomplicated operation. In contrast, synthesis of body protein appears to be increased in conditions of septic hypermetabolism and the negative nitrogen balance then occurs because the overall rate of breakdown is even more increased.

HYPERMETABOLISM AND GLUCOSE INTOLERANCE

The metabolic response to injury includes a variable degree of glucose intolerance. This has been particularly noted in burn patients (Allison et al, 1968), but presumably burns represent a severe example of a more general phenomena in injury and infection. This appears to be associated with the failure of insulin response to a glucose load during the ebb phase, and with an abnormally high insulin level during the flow phase, the latter suggesting peripheral insulin resistance (Gump et al, 1974). The ebb phase is associated with a rise in circulating glucose, fatty acids and amino acids, and with evidence of decreased ability to accept and oxidise fuel in the TCA cycle (Engel, 1952). The flow phase exhibits hyperglycaemia and glucose intolerance without any evidence from isotopic studies that the rate of oxidation of glucose is decreased. In fact, severely catabolic patients often demonstrate an increased rate of glucose oxidation (Long et al, 1971).

There is increasing evidence that hypermetabolism is associated with increased demands for gluconeogenesis. The reason for this association is in the realm of speculation, since resting hypermetabolism is commonly thought to involve tissues other than those tissues which are uniquely dependent on glucose for tissue fuel, such as the brain, red cells, etc.

Prolonged starvation is characterised by a reduction in hepatic gluconeogenesis and sparing of body protein while injury and infection cause an increase in this process at the expense of body protein. It is uncertain whether the liver is the site of the primary alteration or the primary changes occur in peripheral tissues such as muscle with the liver responding in a secondary fashion. Felig et al (1969) have shown that the decrease in hepatic glucose output is correlated with a decrease in circulating amino acids, particularly alanine. Administration of exogenous alanine during starvation results in a prompt hyperglycaemic response. Thus the provision of precursor substrate appears to be the rate limiting step in the control of hepatic glucose production in human starvation. Imamura et al (in press) have used pigs after chronic implantation of catheters, to study the behaviour of substrates across the hind limb and the liver. They found the liver clearance during injury and sepsis was normal for lactate, alanine and other gluconeogenic precursors, and concluded that the primary alteration was in the peripheral tissues, which released more substrate to produce the increased hepatic gluconeogenesis seen in injury and sepsis.

[14]C-alanine studies have provided a striking demonstration that carbohydrate formation from alanine is minimal in normal man receiving intravenous glucose at approximately 6 g per hour (Long et al, in preparation). Surgical hypermetabolism is associated with increased gluconeogenesis, despite the infusion of exogenous glucose which would normally inhibit gluconeogenesis. This increase in glucose output from the liver during hyperglycaemia has been shown in septic patients, when peripheral glucose uptake has been shown to be correlated with elevated levels of blood glucose.

POSSIBLE ROLE OF THE HYPOTHALAMUS

The author in the above discussion has attempted to consider increased protein breakdown as the cause of resting hypermetabolism, or vice versa. There is evidence that perhaps both factors may be secondary to the changes that originate from the hypothalamus. In the 'ebb' phase in the dog (Kovach, 1970), and in the rat (Stoner, 1970) changes occur in the hypothalamus following haemorrhagic shock and tourniquet injury to the hind leg. More recently, Wilmore (1974) has suggested that the hypermetabolism and other metabolic changes in the 'flow' phase after human burn injury may be the result of 'homeostatic readjustment' in hypothalamic centres. These centres may be responsible for altered neuroendocrine stimuli which influence fuel mobilisation, rates of oxidation of tissue fuel, and the thermal regulation which balances heat production and heat loss.

Summary

This presentation emphasises the association of resting energy expenditure and nitrogen excretion, where increases above normal and decreases below normal seem to parallel each other in various clinical states. The metabolic response to starvation is discussed as an example where both energy expenditure and nitrogen excretion are reduced. In contrast, severe injury and infection cause increases in both factors, which assume special significance since they occur despite some degree of starvation which is commonly associated with the hypermetabolic phase of convalescence.

Studies are reviewed which suggest that the increased nitrogen excretion in surgical catabolism is associated with accelerated breakdown of muscle protein. Conditions which are catabolic for muscle seem to be anabolic for the liver (and perhaps other visceral tissues). Evidence is discussed to support the concept that protein breakdown in muscle is to provide needs for synthesis (amino acid deamination for gluconeogenesis, amino acids for acute phase protein synthesis etc) rather than merely to provide two-carbon fragments for non-specific tissue fuel. The hypermetabolism and increased nitrogen excretion of the acute catabolic state are associated in time, but neither factor appears sufficient to be the primary cause for the other.

References

Allison, SP, Hinton, P and Chamberlain, MJ (1968) *Lancet, i,* 113
Barr, DP, Russell, LC and Du Bois, EF (1915) *Arch. int. Med., 15,* 608
Beisel, WR, Sawyer, ED, Ryll, ED and Crozier, D (1967) *Ann. int. Med., 67,* 744
Benedict, FG (1915) Publication No.203, Carnegie Institute, Washington, DC
Blocker, TG Jr, Leven, WC, Norwinski, WW, Lewis, SR and Blocker, V (1955) *Ann. Surg., 141,* 589
Brody, S (1945) In *Bioenergetics and Growth.* Reinhold, New York. Page 374

Cahill, FG Jr, Herrera, MG, Morgan, AP, Soeldner, JS, Steinke, J, Levy, PL, Reichard, BA Jr and Kipnis, DM (1966) *J. clin. Invest., 45,* 1751

Cairnie, AB, Campbell, RM, Pullard, JD and Cuthbertson, DP (1957) *Brit. J. exp. Path., 38,* 504

Caldwell, FT (1970) In *Energy Metabolism in Trauma.* (Ed) R Porter and J Knight. J & A Churchill, London. Page 7

Campbell, JA and Webster, TA (1921) *Biochem. J., 15,* 660

Campbell, RM and Cuthbertson, DP (1967) *Quart. J. exp. Physiol., 52,* 114

Cuthbertson, DP (1932) *Quart. J. Med., 1 (N.S.),* 233

Cuthbertson, DP (1942) *Lancet, i,* 433

Cuthbertson, DP and Tilstone, WJ (1967) *Quart. J. exp. Physiol., 52,* 249

Du Bois, EF (1924) In *Basal Metabolism in Health and Disease.* Lea & Febiger, Philadelphia

Duke, JH, Jørgenson, SB, Broell, JR, Long, CL and Kinney, JM (1970) *Surgery, 68,* 168

Duke, JH, Jørgenson, SB. and Kinney, JM (1975) Submitted for publication

Engel, FE (1952) *Ann. NY Acad. Sci., 55,* 381

Felig, P, Marlis, E, Owen, OE and Cahill, GF (1969) In *Advances in Enzyme Regulation, Vol. 7.* Pergamon Press, New York

Felig, P and Wahren, J (1974) *Fed. Proc., 33,* 1092

Felig, P and Wahren, J (1975) *Clin. Research* (In press)

Food and Nutrition Board, National Research Council (1974) In *Recommended Dietary Allowances, Eighth Revised Edition.* National Academy of Sciences, Washington, DC

Garber, AJ, Mendel, PH, Boden, G and Owen, OE (1974) *J. clin. Invest., 54,* 981

Graham, G and Pulton, EP (1912) *Quart. J. Med., 6,* 82

Gump, FE, Price, JB and Kinney, JM (1970) *Ann. Surg., 171,* 321

Gump, FE, Long, CL, Killian, P and Kinney, JM (1974) *J. Trauma, 14,* 5

Imamura, M, Clowes, GHA Jr. Blackburn, GL, O'Donnell, TF Jr, Trerice, M, Bhimjee, Y and Ryan, NT (In press)

Kinney, JM and Roe, CF (1962) *Ann. Surg., 156,* 610

Rovach, AGB (1970) *J. clin. Path. (Royal College of Pathology), 4,* 202

Levenson, SM, Braasch, JW, Mueller, H and Crowley, L (1957) Quoted in Levenson, SM, Pulaski, EJ and Upjohn, HL In *Physiologic Principles in Surgery.* (Ed) L Zimmerman and R Levine. WB Saunders, Philadelphia

Liu, AY and Newhaus, OW (1965) *Biochem. Biophys. Acta, 166,* 195

Lusk, G (1931) *The Elements of the Science of Nutrition, Fourth Edition.* WB Saunders, Philadelphia

Long, CL, Spencer, JL, Kinney, JM and Geiger, JW (1971) *J. appl. Physiol., 31,* 110

Long, CL, Jeevanandam, M, Kim, BM and Kinney, JM (to be submitted for publication)

Long, CL, Spencer, JL, Geiger, JW, Gump, FE and Kinney, JM (In press)

Madden, SC (1950) In *Plasma Protein.* (Ed) JBC Youman. Charles C Thomas, Springfield, Illinois. Page 62

Marliss, EG, Aoki, TT, Unger, RH, Soeldner, JS and Cahill, GF Jr (1970) *J. clin. Invest., 49,* 2256

Munro, HN and Chalmers, MI (1945) *Brit. J. exp. Path., 26,* 396

Myers, JD (1954) In *Shock and Circulatory Homeostasis.* (Ed) HD Green. HD Green, Winston-Salam, NC. Page 121

Odessey, R, Khairllah, A and Goldberg, AL (1974) *J. biol. Chem., 249,* 7623

O'Keefe, SJD and Sender, PM (1974) *Lancet, iv,* 1035
Owen, OE, Morgan, AP, Kemp, HG, Sullivan, JM, Herrera, MG and Cahill, GF Jr (1967) *J. clin. Invest., 46,* 1589
Owen, OE and Reichard, G (1971) *J. clin. Invest., 50,* 1536
Pekarek, R, Wannemacher, R, Powanda, M, Abeles, F, Mosher, D, Dinterman, R and Beisel, WR (1974) *Life Sciences, 14,* 1765
Reiss, E (1959) *Metabolism, 8,* 151
Roe, CF and Kinney, JM (1965) *Ann. Surg., 161,* 140
Saudek, CD and Felig, P (1974) In *The Combined Clinical and Basic Science Seminar.* Cornell University Medical College, October 22, 1974
Sherwin, RS, Hendler, RG and Felig, P (1975) *J. clin. Invest., 55,* 1382
Stoner, HB (1970) *J. clin. Path. (Royal College of Pathology), 4,* 47
Talbot, FB (1921) *Amer. J. dis. Children.* Page 519
Tilstone, WJ and Cuthbertson, DP (1970) In *Energy Metabolism and Trauma.* (Ed) R Porter and J Knight. J & A Churchill, London
Wannemacher, RW Jr, Dupont, HL, Pekarek, RS, Powanda, MC, Schwartz, A, Hornick, RB and Beisel, WR (1972) *J. infect. Dis., 126,* 77
Wilmore, DW (1974) *Clinics in Plastic Surgery, 1,* 4
Young, VR and Huang, PC (1968) *Brit. J. Nutri., 23,* 271
Young, VR, Steffe, WP, Pencharz, PB, Winterer, JC and Scrimshaw, NS (1975) *Nature, 253,* 192

Influence of Injury on Vitamin Metabolism

S M LEVENSON, L V CROWLEY, R RETTURA, DORINNE KAN, B A GRUBER and E SEIFTER

Departments of Surgery and Biochemistry of the Albert Einstein College of Medicine, Yeshiva University, Bronx, New York, USA

Introduction

All metabolites are interrelated and changes in one may effect functional or quantitative changes in others and the responses of certain target organs and tissues. There is increasing evidence suggesting that certain of the vitamins, notably vitamins A and D, may function as hormones.

Much of the available information regarding the relationship between injury and the vitamins is concerned with ascorbic acid and vitamin A.

ASCORBIC ACID

Most animal species can synthesise ascorbic acid, but man, other primates, and guinea pigs cannot. Ascorbic acid plays a vital role in the synthesis of collagen; the hydroxylation of proline and lysine, essential for collagen formation, requires iron, a-ketoglutarate and ascorbate. There is no dearth of wound fibro-blasts in ascorbic acid deficiency, but the arrangement of ribosomes on the endoplasmic reticulum, which is abnormally dilated, is disorganised (Ross and Benditt, 1962; Harwood, et, 1974); these changes are promptly reversible when ascorbic acid is given — the ribosomes line up in a regular order, including polysomal arrangement. Collagen synthesis occurs after ascorbic acid is given. Preliminary characterisation of the repair collagen synthesised by animals who recovered showed it to be a typical Type I collagen having the chain composition $(a_1)_2 a_2$. The extent of glycosylation of the hydroxylysine of the newly synthesised collagen was greater than that reported for either normal guinea-pig dermal collagen or dermal scar collagen (Harwood, et al, 1974). The synthesis and quality of ground substance, capillary function and integrity are also altered

253

in ascorbic acid deficiency and these influence wound healing significantly.

In normal adults, the total body pool of ascorbate is about 1.5 g as judged by studies with ^{14}C-ascorbate (Baker, et al, 1971), and can be maintained in the healthy adult by 20–30 mg of ascorbate per day.

Administered ^{14}C ascorbic acid is oxidised to $^{14}CO_2$ by the guinea pig but not by man; in man ^{14}C dehydroascorbic acid, ^{14}C deketogulonic acid, ^{14}C oxalate and ^{14}C ascorbate sulfates are found (Hodges, et al, 1969; Baker, et al, 1969).

VITAMIN A

Fat-soluble vitamin A is important for vision, reproduction, maintenance of epithelium, synthesis of mucopolysaccharides, labilisation of lysosomal membranes and certain immune, particularly cellular, responses. Recent studies of vitamin A have increased knowledge of its absorption, transport and bio-synthesis, but little is known about its mode of action other than its special role in vision (Wald, 1968) or how vitamin A is metabolised by the ill and injured or the requirements of such patients for vitamin A.

ALTERATIONS OF VITAMIN METABOLISM IN THE EBB PHASE, SPECIFICALLY IN SHOCK

During the past 14 years there has been very little investigation of possible changes in vitamin metabolism in shock and how such changes influence the progression of shock syndrome. Analytical methods are uncertain, and so are the specific actions and requirements for certain vitamins in the normal person.

Some vitamins may be active only when combined with other factors to form coenzymes, and even when 'free' vitamin is abundant there may be a deficiency of coenzyme. Hypoxia and hyponutrition of the tissues in shock may result in a 'functional' derangement and altered metabolism of certain enzymes and enzyme systems. Ionic deficiency especially of essential metals, pH, and fluid shifts may contribute to enzymic alterations during shock.

Ascorbic Acid

Soon after shock, there is an abrupt and often sustained drop in adrenal, blood and urinary ascorbic acid. Some studies have been performed with pretreatment with ascorbic acid of animals subjected to experimental shock, generally haemorrhage. When guinea pigs, which require a dietary source of vitamin C, were treated with large doses of ascorbic acid before being subjected to haem-orrhagic shock, survival rate was increased (De Pasqualini, 1946), but this did not occur in rats (Sayers, et al, 1945) or mice (Millican and Stohlman, 1956).

254

shocked by the application of a tourniquet but Strawitz, et al, (1958) found some benefit in haemorrhagic shock.

Thiamine, Nicotinic Acid, Riboflavin

Greig and associates (Greig & Govier, 1943; Lamson & Greig, 1944; Greig, 1944b) subjected dogs to fractional haemorrhage. These workers found thiamine administration resulted in a decrease of blood pyruvate (keto-acids) and an increase of both the blood pressure and survival times. They found that the pyrophosphate ester of thiamine, cocarboxylase, was being dephosphorylated in skeletal muscle, duodenum, and liver, chiefly in the former two tissues.

ALTERATIONS OF VITAMIN METABOLISM IN THE FLOW PHASE

Water-Soluble Vitamins

An abrupt decrease in plasma ascorbic acid concentration, its urinary excretion, and later a drop in white blood cell ascorbic acid concentration, and 'tissue saturation' as measured by intravenous 'load tests' have been described early after injury (Levenson, et al, 1946; Lloyd & Edge, 1973; Barton, 1972; Mason, et al, 1971) which were directly related to the severity of the injury. The changes in vitamin metabolism are parallel to the change in protein metabolism following injury. Similar changes in urinary excretion and 'tissue saturation' were reported for thiamine and nicotinamide (Levenson et al, 1946). Soon after injury there is also a decrease in urinary excretion of riboflavin, which at times is followed by a brief period of increased excretion of riboflavin. Later, during the convalescent period when the patient is in positive nitrogen balance, there is also a positive riboflavin balance (Andreae, et al, 1946).

Acute infections in man may be followed by the acute onset of clinical signs of vitamin deficiency (A, B_1, nicotinic acid, C, folic acid), and concentrations of vitamins A, B_6, or C, or folic acid in the blood may be lower than normal (Scrimshaw, et al, 1968).

EFFECT OF VITAMIN A ON WOUND HEALING

Increased Need for Vitamin A after Wounding and Other Injuries

There may be an increased requirement for vitamin A after injury under conditions where pre-existing vitamin A does not exist (Freiman et al, 1970; Seifter et al, 1975; Levenson et al, 1972). Kagan (1955) had found that rats with subcutaneous abscesses as the result of repeated injections of turpentine and sweet almond oil showed sustained decreases in serum vitamin A concentration and in liver vitamin A concentration and content. Vitamin A concentrations in the interior and periphery of the abscesses did not differ from those of uninjured subcutaneous tissue. Gastrointestinal absorption of vitamin A was not altered, but urinary excretion increased, and the kidney concentration of vitamin A was higher than normal. Recently, Chernov, et al, (1971) and Rai and Courtmanche (1975) have reported an apparent increased need for vitamin A after injury, with particular reference to the occurrence of stress ulcers. Clark and Colburn (1955) had found that large doses of cortisone result in the rapid depletion of vitamin A from the liver and kidneys of rats.

Thus while the changes in the liver vitamin A concentrations are similar in the infected and cortisone-injected rats, the kidney concentrations are different. Hunt and his associates (1969) have shown that vitamin A restored the breaking strength of incisions and the closure of open skin wounds in cortisone-treated rats towards normal, but that vitamin A had no positive effect on the healing of rats not receiving cortisone. Lee and Tong (1969) have demonstrated that the healing retardation of salicylates, hydrocortisone and prednisone can be reversed by applying retinoic acid on the wound. Our experiments suggest that vitamin A has an accelerating effect on wound healing in rats eating a nutritionally complete commercial rat chow and not given cortisone. Herrmann and Woodward (1972) also found that vitamin A given to 'non-deficient' rats resulted in increased fibroplasia as judged histologically and by hydroxyproline content of sponge granulomas. (Seifter, et al, 1975; Freiman, et al, 1970; Levenson, et al, 1972; Seifter, et al, 1976).

Effect of Marginal Vitamin A Intake on Response to Minor Wounding

Rats on a marginal intake of vitamin A, sufficient to maintain near normal growth, lost weight promptly after relatively minor wounding (dorsal skin incision and polyvinyl alcohol sponge s.c. implants) despite little difference in food intake compared with their wounded normal controls and about half of the rats on marginal vitamin A intake died. The mildly A-deficient rats formed less reparative collagen, and what collagen was formed was less cross-linked than normal as judged by the ratio of the breaking strengths of wounds treated in the fresh state and after formalin fixation.

No differences were found between the two groups of rats in terms of blood urea nitrogen (BUN) and the serum Na, K, Ca, Cl, uric acid or creatinine concentrations, all of which were within normal limits. The serum glucose, however, was 65 mg per 100 ml in the deficient rats versus 120 mg per 100 ml in the controls. It is possible that impaired glucose mobilisation may be associated with the reduced ability of the vitamin A deficient rat to survive surgical stress.

In another experiment rats were rendered moderately vitamin A-deficient as described above. After wounding, the deficient animals lost weight at a rate similar to that seen in the previous experiments. At the end of the first week postoperatively the animals were treated each day for the next 14 days with twice the daily vitamin A intake of the control rats used in this study. There was an immediate response to the vitamin A; the sluggish, moribund rats became more active, gained 8 g in weight in the first day and continued to gain weight at a very high rate for the following week. When they were killed (21 days postoperatively) their wounds were as strong as those of control rats when tested in both the fresh and formalin-fixed states.

Effect of Vitamin A Administration to Wounded, 'Non-Deficient' Rats

When supplements of vitamin A (oral and topical to margins of skin incisions and instilled in the sponges at the time of implantation) were given to healthy normal rats ingesting a commercial rat chow, but restricted in food intake by pair-feeding, and subjected to dorsal skin incisions and polyvinyl alcohol sponge implants these were significant increases in wound strength ($p < 0.001$).

Effect of Vitamin A Administration to Rats with Femoral Fractures

When rats eating a normal chow diet received a *femoral fracture in addition to the incisional wound and sponge implants,* wound healing was impaired. Vitamin A supplements (oral, topical to the incision, and impregnated in the sponges) in such rats improved the healing of the skin wound at 11 and 14 but not 10 days after injury, but did not completely obviate the adverse effects of fracture. The ratio of the breaking strengths after formalin fixation to the breaking strengths of the incisions in the fresh state was higher in the unsupple-mented rats, supporting our earlier findings that vitamin A supplementation under these conditions increases collagen cross-linking. All these differences are highly significant statistically.

For histological evaluation of the skin incisions and sponge granuloma of the rats killed at 11 days, a quantitation for each category described (collagen, ground substance and number of fibroblasts) was based on arbitrary scales of 1 to 3 and the ratios of ground substance to collagen calculated. No statistically significant differences in collagen and ground substance were found by the examination of skin wounds. Ground substance of sponge granulomas of vitamin A fractured rats compared with peanut oil group was significantly increased ($p = 0.02$) as was the ratio of ground substance to collagen ($p = 0.001$). No differences were found in the number of fibroblasts in the wounds or sponge granulomas.

In other studies to determine the *effect of injury on liver and serum vitamin A in the rats,* male rats were (1) fed a commercial chow diet, (2) fed a commercial chow diet and then adapted to a vitamin A-deficient diet, or (3) maintained from weaning on a vitamin A-deficient diet. Rats in groups 2 and 3 were given orally $60 \mu g$ vitamin A acetate per week preoperatively. All rats were subjected to wounding (dorsal skin incisions and implantation of polyvinyl alcohol sponges) with and without femoral fractures, when they weighed about 350 grams. After injury, groups of rats were maintained on various doses of vitamin A.

Supplemental vitamin A did not change the characteristic rise in adrenal weight associated with injury. Liver weights of wounded rats with or without

257

fractures were similar to or lower than those of uninjured rats regardless of the level of vitamin A supplementation. Liver vitamin A concentrations and contents were similar for a given supplemental dose of vitamin A in rats only wounded and rats wounded and subjected to femoral fracture. Within each of these groups, the level of vitamin A supplementation had little effect on serum vitamin A despite huge differences in liver vitamin A contents (5–14 fold, $p < 0.001$).

Effect of Vitamin A on the Closure of Open Skin Wounds

In rats with unilateral or bilateral femoral fracture the rate of closure of open dorsal skin wounds was not reduced nor did supplemental vitamin A have any effect.

The differences in behaviour between the healing of sutured skin incisions after fracture and the closure of open skin wounds are not surprising. The healing of open skin wounds depends on factors different in several important ways from those involved in the gain of strength of healing skin incisions. Thus, while little strength is attained by healing skin incisions in scorbutic guinea pigs (in large measure due to a failure of collagen synthesis) the closure of open skin wounds in such guinea pig proceeds at an essentially normal rate (Abercrombie, et al, 1956; Grillo & Gross, 1959).

It should be noted, though, that Ehrlich, et al, (1973) found that the rate of closure of open wounds in rats treated with cortisone is slowed and that this may be partially corrected by administration of vitamin A.

Effect of Cortisone and DOCA on Vitamin A-depleted Rats

The administration of modest amounts of cortisone or DOCA to rats mildly deficient in vitamin A (as a result of a low intake of vitamin A) results in severe weight loss, marked decrease in strength of healing wounds and decreased formation of implanted sponge granuloma collagen. All these effects are much greater than are seen in vitamin A supplemented rats given cortisone and DOCA. It will be recalled that Hunt has shown that extra-vitamin A antagonises the adverse effects of cortisone on the healing of incisions and open wounds in rats. Our experiments show that the converse is also true, that cortisone and DOCA antagonise the salutary effects of vitamin A on healing.

Effect of Vitamin A and Citral on Intra-abdominal Adhesions

In a related series of experiments the effects of vitamin A and Citral, a vitamin A antagonist, on the formation of intra-abdominal adhesions were studied in mice (Demetriou, et al, 1974). The technique of Ellis (1962) in which a knuckle of peritoneum is ligated, was used to produce the experimental intra-abdominal adhesions. The vitamin A and Citral were incorporated into the diets of the rats. We found that the vitamin A increased the number and size of the adhesions, while Citral decreased the adhesions. When the two were given together, they

258

antagonised one another as judged by the development of the adhesions.

In summary, these studies demonstrate that (1) wounding and other forms of trauma increase the requirement of animals for vitamin A, in much the same way as they increase the need for vitamin C; (2) vitamin A increases collagen synthesis and cross-linking and thereby wound strength.

Acknowledgments

Supported in part by Grants DADA—17—70—C from the Army Medical Research and Development Command, 5 KO6 GM14208 (Research Career Award, S.M.L.) from the National Institutes of Health.

References

Abercrombie, M, Flint, MH and James, DW (1956). *J. Embryo. Exper. Morph.* *4*, 167

Andreae, WA, Schenker, V and Browne, JSL (1946). *Fed. Proc. 5*, 3

Baker, EM, Hodges, RE, Hood, J, SAuberlich, HE and March, SC (1969). *Am. J. Clin. Nutr. 22*, 549

Baker, EM, Hodges, RE, Hood, J, Sauberlich, HE, March, SC and Canham, JE (1971). *Am. J. Clin. Nutr. 24*, 444

Barton, GM (1972). *Int. J. Vitam. Nutr. Res. 42*, 511

Chernov, MS, Hale, HW and Wood, M (1971). *Am. J. Surg. 122*, 674

Clark, I and Colburn, RW (1955). *Endocrinology 56*, 232

Demetriou, AA, Seifter, E and Levenson, SM (1974). *J. Surg. Res. 17*, 325

DePasqualini, CD (1946). *Amer. J. Physiol. 145*, 598

Ehrlich, HP, Tarver, H and Hunt, TK (1973). *Ann. Surg. 177*, 222

Ellis, H (1962). *Br. J. Surg. 50*, 10

Freiman, M, Seifter, E, Connerton, C, and Levenson, SM (1970). *Surg. Forum 21*, 81

Greig, ME and Govier, WM (1943). *J. Pharmacol. Exp. Ther. 79*, 169

Greig, ME (1944a). *J. Pharmacol. Exp. Ther. 81*, 240

Greig, ME (1944a). *J. Pharmacol. Exp. Ther. 81*, 164

Grillo, HC and Gross, J (1959). *Proc. Soc. Exp. Biol. Med. 101*, 268

Harwood, R, Grant, ME and Jackson, DS (1974). *Biochem. J. 142*, 641

Herrmann, JB and Woodward, SC (1972). *Amer. Surg. 38*, 26

Hodges, RE, Baker, EM, Hood, J, SAuberlich, HE and March, SC (1969). *Am. J. Clin. Nutr. 22*, 535

Hunt, TK, Ehrlich, HP, Garcia, JA and Dunphy, JE (1969). *Ann. Surg. 170*, 633

Kagan, BM (1955). *Ann. N.Y. Acad. Sci. 63*, 214

Lamson, PD and Greig, ME (1944). *TRans. Assoc. Amer. Physicians 58*, 182

Lee, KH and Tong, TG (1969). *J. Pharm. Sci. 58*, 773

Levenson, SM, Green, RW, TAylor, FHL, Robinson, P, Page, RC, Johnson, RE and Lund, CC (1946). *Ann. Surg. 124*, 840

Levenson, SM, Rettura, G, Crowley, LV, and Seifter, E (1972). *Fed. Proc. 31*,

Lloyd, EL, Edge, WG (1973). *Br. J. Anaesthesia 45*, 532

Mason, M, Matyk, PM and Doolan, SA (1971). *Am. J. Surg. 122*, 808

Millican, RC and Stohlman, EF (1956). *Am. J. Physiol. 185*, 195

Moore, T (1964). *Exp. Eye Res. 3*, 305

Rai, K and Courtemanche, AD (1975). *J. Trauma 15,* 419
Rosenthal, O, Shenkin, H and Drabkin, DL (1945). *Am. J. Physiol. 144,* 334-347
Ross, R and Benditt, EP (1962). *J. Cell Biol. 12,* 533
Sayers, G, Sayers, M, Liang, TY and Long, CN (1945). *Endocrinology 37,* 96
Scrimshaw, NS, Taylor, CE and Gordon, JE (1968). *Interactions of Nutrition and Infection* (WHO) Monograph Series no.57, World Health Organisation, Geneva. Page 88
Seifter, E, Crowley, LV, Rettura, G, Nakao, K, Gruber, C, Kan, D and Levenson, SM (1975). *Ann. Surg. 181,* 836
Seifter, E et al, (1976). Unpublished data.
Slusher, MA and Roberts, S (1957). *Endocrinology 61,* 98
Strawitz, JG, Temple, RL and Hift, H (1958). *Surg. Forum 9,* 54
Wald, G (1968). *Nature, Lond. 219,* 800

Effects of Injury on Wound Healing and Wound Infection

S M LEVENSON, L V CROWLEY and E SEIFTER

Departments of Surgery and Biochemistry of the Albert Einstein College of Medicine, Yeshiva University, Bronx, New York, USA

Introduction

Critical evaluation of the healing process is difficult. Wound healing is a complex physiologic process involving epithelisation, new capillary formation, fibroblastic proliferation, formation of intercellular substances, for example, ground substance and collagen, collagen cross-linking, collagenolysis and remodelling of the wound. Ideally, one would like to follow the healing process with serial biopsies of incisional wounds for histologic and histochemical observations and measurements of tensile strength. This is not readily accomplished in patients. Further, the problems of cell growth and wound healing are often much more complex in patients than in test tubes, tissue culture flasks or experimental animals. Specifically, the magnitude of the wound is often so great that it leads to a whole variety of metabolic and physiologica disorders which influence the healing process in important ways. Added to this, the general condition of the patient prior to wounding or injury may have profound effects. Then, too, the wounds may be inordinately complex, involving a number of different tissues and organs, complicating factors which the laboratory investigator generally assiduously avoids.

In addition to the major problems of wound healing in the seriously injured patient, the healing of simple incisions is much slower in man than in those animals generally used in laboratory investigations. For example, in the skin incisions of the rat, collagen is laid down at a rapid rate beginning on about the 5th day until about 42 days post-operatively (Levenson et al, 1965). Cross-linking of the newly formed collagen begins promptly and proceeds at greatest rates during the first 1–2 weeks. The rate of cross-linking slows rapidly during the next 4–5 weeks, but continues at a slowed rate for many months, and, in fact, continues throughout the life of

261

the rat. After the 6th post-operative week, there is a slight but progressive increase in collagen fibre calibre and compactness and a rearrangement and reorientation of the collagen fibres. Collagenolysis and new collagen synthesis proceed throughout this period of healing. Levenson et al (1962) studied the healing of small experimental sutured skin incisions (about 1 inch long) in the anterior thighs of healthy men who volunteered for the study. Even at 88 days after wounding, the amount of collagen present is far less than in unwounded skin. Although the amount of collagen in the 240-day wound is substantially more than at 88 days, it is still significantly less than in unwounded skin, and the arrangement of the collagen fibres is still far from 'normal'.

EFFECTS OF EXPERIMENTAL INJURY ON WOUND HEALING

Wound healing may be considered as a specific biological process related to the general phenomena of growth and regeneration. The various stages (including inflammation, vessel formation, fibroblastic proliferation, mucopolysaccharide, glycoprotein and collagen synthesis, collagen cross-linking, remodelling of the wound, etc) indicate that the entire process is an orderly one, showing a high degree of integration and organisation characteristic of the processes in which control mechanisms are operative. Because of this, factors which stimulate or inhibit one phase of the process have an effect on the overall process, the magnitude of the effect depending in part on how 'rate-limiting' is the facet of healing being affected. These periods are *not* sharply separated. Since wound healing and wound infection are so closely interrelated, some of our studies directed towards the prevention and control of wound infection and its local and systemic effects are also being reported here.

Effect of Thermal Burns on Healing of Laparotomy Incisions

We (Levenson et al, 1954) approached these problems a number of years ago by studying the healing of laparotomy wounds in normal and burned rats. Rats were severely scalded under light ether anaesthesia by dipping their backs for 30 seconds into hot water (85°C), a procedure which produced a third degree scald of about a third of the body surface; control animals were simply anaesthetised. Twenty-four hours later, midline laparotomy incisions were made aseptically in all animals while they were under ether anaesthesia. After operation, they ate a standard commercial rat diet and drank water ad libitum.

The healing of the laparotomy wounds of the scalded rats was strikingly different from that of the uninjured controls. During the first few post-operative days, the incisions of the scalded animals were broader, were covered by a dry sanguinous exudate, and were weaker than those of the controls. There was an immediately apparent delay in the appearance and maturation of the connective tissue (cellular and intercellular) of the laparotomy wounds in the scalded animals.

262

These microscopic differences were still evident at the end of the second post-operative week, though they were less marked by this time.

These findings were not surprising to us because in 1924, Carrel had found delayed closure of open wounds in animals with abscesses elsewhere in their bodies.

Effects of Femoral Fracture on Healing of Skin Incisions and Formation of Reparative Tissue in Implanted Polyvinyl Alcohol Sponges

We have shown in the last few years that the *healing* of dorsal skin incisions as judged histologically and by gain of breaking strength, and the formation of re-parative granulation tissue in response to subcutaneously implanted polyvinyl alcohol sponges as judged histologically and by chemical measurement of hydroxy-proline, an amino acid unique to collagen, *are impaired in rats subjected to unilateral or bilateral comminuted femoral fractures* (Crowley et al, 1972; Seifter et al, 1975; Crowley et al, 1976). The impairment in healing was somewhat greater in the rats subjected to bilateral femoral fracture than in those with unilateral fracture as judged by the formation of reparative collagen. We turned to this experimental model because (1) studies in our laboratory over a period of years have shown that dorsal skin incisions and implanted polyvinyl alcohol sponges have certain advantages over laparotomy wounds; (2) femoral fractures have some advantage over burns — the water vapour loss through the burned area and presence of bacteria with infection of varying severity introduce certain variables which complicate the study; (3) there is considerable information in the literature regarding the metabolic responses of rats subjected to femoral fracture; this has been a favourite form of experimental injury for study by Cuthbertson and his colleagues (1939).

Mechanisms Underlying the Impaired Wound Healing Associated with Severe Injury

Disturbance in Protein Metabolism

What mechanisms underlie these changes in healing? A clue was afforded by our studies of the behaviour of various tissue proteins in scalded rats which we carried out with ^{15}N-labelled glycine (Levenson et al, 1959). We fed ^{15}N-glycine, at predetermined times, to young adult male rats, scalded and uninjured, receiving by gastric tube a constant diet sufficient to maintain the uninjured rats in slight positive nitrogen balance; the tube feeding provided 0.2 kcal per gram pre-injury body weight per day. Of these kcal, 18% were from protein, 63% by carbohydrate, and 19% by fat. Unlimited drinking water was offered.

The uninjured rats remained in slight positive nitrogen balance throughout the study. Following the scald, faecal nitrogen excretion was unchanged, but urinary nitrogen excretion increased and the rat went into negative nitrogen balance. Urinary nitrogen reached a peak in 3–4 days, then gradually returned to normal in 10–14 days.

In the first set of experiments (Experiment A), a single tracer dose of ^{15}N-glycine (100 mg of glycine, 34 atom per cent excess ^{15}N) was given orally three days after scalding when the nitrogen excretion was at its peak. The rats were anaesthetised 12 hours later by ether and all blood possible withdrawn by cardiac puncture.

The total nitrogen and ^{15}N contents of the combined faeces and intestinal content were about the same in both groups, that is, about 4% of the fed tag.

TABLE I. N and ^{15}N in Urine and Faeces of Unburned and Burned Rats*
Post Injury, days 3–3½

| | URINE | | | FAECES† | | |
	mg N	Atom % Excess ^{15}N	mg ^{15}N	mg N	Atom % Excess ^{15}N	mg ^{15}N
Unburned	165	0.991	1.64	140	0.195	0.27
Burned	227	0.860	2.01	117	0.243	0.29
p	<0.001	0.9	<0.02	<0.001	<0.01	0.7
	% Ingested ^{15}N					
	URINE			FAECES†		
Unburned	24.	24.9			4.1	
Burned		30.9			4.4	
p		<0.001			0.5	

* ^{15}N-glycine, 100 mg, 30% atoms % excess ^{15}N given by gavage at start of day 3 post-burn
† Faeces plus intestinal contents

However, there was a highly significant increase (p <0.001) of 38% in urinary total nitrogen excretion after scalding (Table I). The urinary total ^{15}N excretion of the scalded rats, about 30% of the administered labelled nitrogen, was also about 25% greater than that of the controls (p <0.001).

The uninjured animals incorporated ^{15}N into their skin and carcass proteins in low concentration, and into their liver, gastrointestinal tract and plasma proteins in relatively high concentration (Table II). The same general order of incorporation was observed in the scalded animals, with ^{15}N concentration in each of their tissue proteins equal to or greater than that of the corresponding tissues of the control rats. We interpret this to mean that anabolism occurred in the tissues of scalded rats at a rate equal to or faster than in corresponding tissues of uninjured rats. Thus, the increased urinary nitrogen cannot be explained solely on the

264

TABLE II. Nitrogen Metabolism in Control and Burned Rats*

| Organ | Atom % Excess ^{15}N | | |
	Control	Burned	P Value
Skin	0.031	0.029	0.7
Carcass	0.031	0.032	0.7
Heart	0.050	0.058	<0.01
Adrenal	0.086	0.108	<0.001
Kidney	0.097	0.123	<0.01
Liver	0.116	0.142	<0.01
GI tract	0.139	0.169	<0.05
Plasma protein	0.236	0.426	<0.001

* ^{15}N glycine given by gavage 3 days after anaesthesia or anaesthesia and burning; rats sacrificed 12 hours later

basis of anti-anabolism. The carcases of the scalded rats were significantly lighter (p <0.001) than the controls, while their livers and adrenals were significantly heavier on a dry weight basis and contained more ^{15}N protein than those of the controls (Tables III and IV). The ^{15}N carcass proteins were similar in both groups.

Almost 90% of the administered ^{15}N was accounted for in the uninjured animals; the remaining 10% was doubtless in that part of the gastrointestinal tract, spleen, testes and red cells not analysed in their entirety. No total addition was made for the scalded animals since the scalded skin was not measured nor was the plasma volume estimated (Table V).

TABLE III. Organ Weights 3.5 Days Post-Injury

| Rat | Wet Weights, g | | |
	Unburned	Burned	p Value
Carcass	155	139	<0.001
Skin	40	49	<0.01
Adrenals	0.048	0.056	<0.05
Kidneys	2.09	2.21	0.4
Liver	11.57	13.52	0.1
	Dry Weights, g		
Carcass	55	50	<0.02
Skin	17	–	–
Kidneys	0.55	0.56	0.8
Liver	3.24	3.89	<0.2

TABLE IV. Effect of Severe Burns on Rat Tissue Proteins*

| | Total Protein N, mg | | | Total Protein ^{15}N, mcq | | |
	Unburned	Burned	P	Unburned	Burned	P
Carcass	4310	4100	0.3	1360	1340	0.8
Skin	1630	–	–	504	–	–
Heart	24.5	25.2	0.9	12.2	14.6	0.3
Adrenals	1.29	1.49	0.3	1.14	1.63	<0.001
Kidneys	60.5	57.4	0.3	59.4	67.7	<0.02
Liver	353	402	0.02	413	550	<0.001
Plasma†	678	–	–	1755	–	–

* ^{15}N glycine given by gavage 3 days after anaesthesia or anaesthesia and burning; rats sacrificed 12 hours later

† Plasma volume determined by the formula $PV = 0.175W^{.725}$ from Wang and Hegsted (1949)

TABLE V. ^{15}N Distribution in Rats

| | % Ingested ^{15}N* | |
	Unburned	Burned
Urine	25	30
Gut	4	4
Carcass	20	20
Skin	7	–
Heart	0.2	0.2
Adrenals	0.01	0.02
Kidneys	0.9	1.0
Liver	6	8
Plasma	27	–

* ^{15}N glycine given by gavage 3 days after anaesthesia or anaesthesia and burning; rats sacrificed 12 hours later

In a second set of experiments (B), ^{15}N glycine was given over a period of 4 days prior to scalding. The animals were sacrificed as in Experiment A at various times during the next week, and their tissues were analysed as before. In this way, an assembly of ^{15}N values was obtained which gave the rate of decline of the tag in the tissue proteins after the scald. Uninjured rats were again used as controls, they also having received ^{15}N glycine.

The decline of the ^{15}N concentration of the plasma proteins was faster in the

TABLE VI. Rat Plasma Protein*

	Atom % Excess ^{15}N		
Day	Unburned	Burned	P Value
0	0.319	–	–
1	0.258	0.205	–
3.5	0.146	0.119	<0.001
6.5	0.103	0.083	<0.01

* ^{15}N glycine given for 4 days preceding anaesthesia or anaesthesia and burning; rats killed 6.5 days later

scalded rats than in the controls (Table VI). It was found also that in the scalded animals the protein content of the liver and certain other very active organs changed little despite their markedly increased turnover rates. In fact, as mentioned above, liver protein increased in the scalded rats in the first few days after the burn. By contrast, the protein content of the carcass decreased despite a much slower turnover rate, and this decrease accounted mathematically for most of the extra urinary nitrogen loss (Table VII).

TABLE VII. Rat Carcass Protein*

	Body weight in g	Carcass weight in g	Carcass Prot.N in g	Carcass Protein ^{15}Nitorgen in g
Unburned	321	196	7.00	3.06
Burned	296	168	6.10	2.35
P value	<0.05	<0.001	<0.02	<0.001

* ^{15}N glycine given for 4 days preceding anaesthesia or anaesthesia and burning; rats killed 6.5 days later

The apparent high priority of the rapidly metabolising organs after scalding suggested to us that a liver 'wound' should heal normally in an animal with a superimposed skin injury, despite the fact that a laparotomy wound did not heal normally under the same conditions. In short, we thought that the liver should be able to heal at the expense of more slowly metabolising areas, a fact the skin wound was unable to accomplish, the skin itself being slowly metabolising.

We decided, as a practical matter, to use the regeneration of the liver following partial hepatectomy as an experimental tool rather than a wound of the liver in order to avoid the problems of bleeding and bile leakage. In our first experiment, we removed 70% of the liver of each of 24 male rats, weighing 230–250 g, while they were under light ether anaesthesia. Immediately thereafter, one half

TABLE VIII. Effect of Severe Burn on Rat Liver Regeneration (70% Hepatectomy)

	Unburned	Burned	P
Liver wt, g	4.10	4.42	0.1
Liver water, %	70.2	70.9	0.3
Liver protein N, mg	126	136	0.1

of the animals, randomly selected, were subjected to third degree scalds of 30–35% of the body. The animals were gavage fed 10 ml of 5% glucose solution and 0.9% saline six hours post-operatively and every 12 hours thereafter until sacrificed. Forty-eight hours after the hepatectomy, the animals were anaesthetised by ether and blood was withdrawn by cardiac puncture. As criteria of regeneration we measured the total weight, protein nitrogen content and concentration, water content and mitotic activity of the liver. These measurements were made 48 hours post-hepatectomy. There were no significant differences between control and scalded animals in relation to liver weight, protein concentration or content, mitotic count or water content. This result confirmed our expectation that the scald would not impair liver regeneration (Table VIII).

A 70% hepatectomy is a very powerful stimulus to liver regeneration. We felt that a 35% hepatectomy (removal of median lobe) might provide a stimulus mild enough so that the effects of a superimposed skin scald on possibly accelerating regeneration rates might come to light where none had before. The rats were fed in one experiment by gavage on glucose and saline, and in another experiment with a nutritionally complete diet beginning 24 hours after operation (this was the same diet as used in the ^{15}N experiments). The animals were again sacrificed forty-eight hours after hepatectomy. The scalded rats had livers of significantly higher weight and protein content than the uninjured rats, clearly showing that far from hindering regeneration, the scald actually accelerated proliferation (Table IX).

TABLE IX. Effect of Severe Burn on Rat Liver Regeneration (35% Hepatectomy)

	Total Liver Protein* (mg)	Liver wt (g)	Liver water (%)
Unburned	176	5.20	69.1
Burned	204	6.02	70.8
P	<0.001	<0.001	<0.05

* Rats sacrificed 48 hours after partial hepatectomy; partial hepatectomy performed one day after burning

TABLE X. Serum Proteins 48 Hours after 70% Hepatectomy (Rats)

		Unburned	Burned	P
	Albumin	2.17	1.64	<0.02
Globulins	alpha 1	0.94	0.93	0.9
	alpha 2	0.68	0.83	<0.05
	beta	1.08	1.14	0.3
	gamma	0.95	0.75	<0.05
	Total	5.82	5.28	<0.02

TABLE XI. Serum Proteins 48 Hours after 35% Hepatectomy (Rats)

		Unburned	Burned	P
	Albumin	3.02	1.38	<0.001
Globulins	alpha 1	1.08	1.08	1
	alpha 2	0.69	1.08	<0.01
	beta	0.83	1.01	<0.02
	gamma	0.32	0.20	0.2
	Total	5.95	4.76	<0.001

The levels of serum total protein and albumin were lower in the burned rats while α_2-globulin was higher. These differences were much more pronounced in the 35% hepatectomy groups than in the 70% hepatectomy groups. This is not surprising, since the changes in serum proteins which follow partial hepatectomy are proportional to the extent of the hepatectomy (Tables X, XI).

The difference in behaviour of the liver and carcass of the burned rat is strikingly different from the behaviour of these organs in the acutely starved but otherwise uninjured animal. There, liver protein drops sharply, at a rate far greater than that for the carcass protein in the starved but otherwise healthy rat. When rats are burned in addition to being starved, the loss of liver protein is slowed, as would be anticipated from our ^{15}N glycine and liver regeneration studies (Table XII).

TABLE XII. Effect of Severe Burn on Response of Rat Liver to Starvation

	Unburned	Burned	P
Liver wt, g	6.85	7.72	<0.01
Liver protein, mg	248	272	<0.01

These experiments suggest that both increased anabolic and catabolic processes go on after severe injury to the rat; all tissues do not participate equally in this response.

WOUND INFECTION

Problems of wound infection are inextricably bound to those of wound healing; when wound healing is impaired, wound infection is more common; when wound infection is present, healing is delayed.

As in the case of any infection, interrelationships between resistance, or susceptibility, of the host and the numbers and virulence of the contaminating microorganisms determine whether or not infection occurs and, if it occurs, its severity. Bacteria are by far the principal infecting microorganisms; fungi are the next most common infecting organisms, while viral wound infections are uncommon. There are some special considerations, local and systemic, related to wounds per se and the extent of wounding which condition host resistance, both local and systemic. The wounds may be accidental, operative, or physiologic, e.g. parturition. We should not forget that uterine infections occurring in women after delivery were the basis for the historic observations of Holmes and Semmelweis over a hundred years ago regarding cross-contamination and cross-infection.

Bacterial contamination, tissue necrosis, impaired blood supply, and adequacy of surgical care are clearly important in determining wound infection, but there is good evidence that animals and patients have a lowered resistance to infection following severe injury, particularly if shock has occurred (Howard & Simmons, 1974; Law et al, 1974). It has been recognised for many years that late after injury if malnutrition occurs, susceptibility to infection is increased (Burke, 1972; Taylor & DeSweemer, 1973), but, in addition, there is increasing evidence that resistance to infection is lowered early after injury, before overt malnutrition has occurred. There is general agreement that the metabolic and physiologic changes after injury, involving as they do almost every metabolite, change the resistance, local and systemic, of the injured. Resistance depends often upon the ability of the inflammatory response to create in and around the lesion a microenvironment inimicable to the infectious agent. Dubos (1955) has stated: "It is likely that disturbances in the general state of health often bring about qualitative and quantitative changes in the biochemical characteristics of the inflammatory area. These in turn may interfere with the processes which control the activities of microorganisms with the lesion. As a result, the response of the body to infection and consequently the microenvironment in which the infectious process follows its course, are under the control of factors which may be metabolic or psychic in origin. This concept accounts in part for the fact that susceptibility to infection can change independently of the immunological state of the infected individual. Since changes in susceptibility can occur rapidly and be extremely transient, the intensity of exposure to an infectious agent may be less decisive than the physio-

270

logical state of the exposed individual, determining whether infection fails to take hold, becomes established, runs an abortive course, or evolves into overt disease".

Polymorphonuclear leukocyte function, especially bactericidal capability, is impaired in a cyclical fashion after thermal injury; Alexander et al (1970, 1971) have studied principally burn patients but there is little reason to believe that their observations do not apply to patients with other injuries. In recent years Constantian et al (1975) and McLean et al (1975) have demonstrated the appearance of serum factors, not yet fully characterised or identified chemically, which interfere with polymorphonuclear cell functions. There is also growing evidence that certain immunologic functions are interfered with after severe injury; Munster et al (1973) have shown that following severe burns there is a marked depletion of certain serum immunoglobulins, particularly IgG. Butler and Rossen (1973) have shown that a short course of methyl prednisolone given to healthy male volunteers caused a sustained decrease in serum IgG due to increased catabolism of IgG during drug administration, and decreased synthesis during and for some time after drug administration. There is also some interference with complement function according to Alexander et al (1971). Munster and Artz (1974) have reported a depression of T-lymphocyte function very soon after burns, and this depression lasts for weeks. Depression of RES function after shock and injury has been known for over 20 years. For further discussion of these aspects, the reader is referred to two recent reviews (Howard & Simmons, 1974; Law et al, 1974).

There is ample evidence that in addition to protein : calorie malnutrition predisposing to certain infections (Scrimshaw et al, 1968, 1969; Axelrod, 1973; Viteri & Arroyave, 1973; Newberne, 1973; Faulk et al, 1974), deficiencies of certain vitamins (Scrimshaw et al, 1968, 1969; Axelrod, 1971, 1973;) notably vitamins A and C, and certain trace elements, e.g. iron (Baggs & Miller, 1973) and zinc, predispose the host to certain bacterial infections. A prompt lowering of serum iron and zinc in individuals with infections has been recognised for a long time. In this regard, Paterek and Beisel (1971) have presented some data suggesting that an endogenous mediator which leads to a depression of serum Zn and Fe is liberated from leukocytes which interact with microorganisms.

In the past few years, we (Gruber et al, 1974; Rettura et al, 1975) and others (Cohen & Cohen, 1973; Rogers & Newberne, 1975) have investigated the possible role of supplemental vitamin A in increasing the resistance of previously healthy, well-nourished animals to bacterial and viral infections. Our own studies in regard to bacterial infections in injured animals may be briefly summarised as follows: "....We have found that vitamin A inhibits thymic involution of mice treated with steroids or subjected to body casting and that vitamin A increases the resistance of such animals to Moloney Sarcoma Virus. Since scalded animals and patients show depression of immune responses and frequently suffer from overwhelming infection, we have conducted a series of experiments to determine

271

whether vitamin A influences the resistance of rodents to experimental infections with Candida albicans or Pseudomonas aeruginosa. Candida albicans was injected intravenously into mice: dose response curves to Candida were determined, with the mortality varying from 0 to 100% and the times of death occurring from a few days to a few weeks; both of these parameters varied in a dose dependent way. Vitamin A begun in large doses at the time of injection of Candida had *no* effect on survival. In other experiments, similar dose response curves to the topical application or intravenous injection of Pseudomonas aeruginosa to rats with third degree scalds involving 30% of their body surface were determined. The Pseudomonas aeruginosa were inoculated just after scalding in some experiments while in others the inoculations were performed 4 days after scalding. Vitamin A had no therapeutic effect under any of these circumstances ..." (Gruber et al, 1974). We pointed out at the time that these experiments do not reflect on possible positive effects of vitamin A on deaths from metabolic responses to much more severe scalds or the possible usefulness of vitamin A as adjunct therapy to the use of antibiotics, immunotherapy, or eschar excision.

We believe that further studies will demonstrate that supplemental vitamin A will be useful in the prevention and treatment of infections in severely injured animals and patients just as it has been demonstrated to be useful from the point of wound healing in injured animals.

Acknowledgments

Supported in part by Grants DADA-17-70-C from the Army Medical Research and Development Command, 5 K6 GM14208 (Research Career Award, SML) and 1RO1 GM19328 from the National Institutes of Health.

References

Alexander, JW and Wixson, D (1970) *Surg. Gynecol. and Obstet., 130,* 431
Alexander, JW, Dionigi, R and Meakins, JL (1971) *Ann. Surg., 173,* 206
Alpert, S, Gray, J, Romney, S and Levenson, SM (1969) *Lancet, i,* 841
Alpert, S, Salzman, T, Sullivan, C, Palmer, C and Levenson, SM (1973) In
   Germfree Research. Biological Effect of Gnotobiotic Environments.
   (Ed) JB Heneghan. Academic Press, New York and London. Page 87
Axelrod, AE (1971) *Amer. J. clin. Nutr., 24,* 265
Axelrod, AE (1973) In *Modern Nutrition in Health and Disease.* (Ed) RS Good-
   hart and ME Shils. Lea & Febiger, Philadelphia. Chapter 15, page 493
Baggs, RB and Miller, SA (1973) *J. Nutrition, 103,* 1554
Burke, JF (1972) In *Surgery.* (Ed) GL Nardi and GD Zuidema. Little, Brown
   and Company, Inc. Page 171
Butler, WT and Rossen, RD (1973) *J. clin. Invest., 52,* 2629
Campbell, RM and Cuthbertson, DP (1967) *Quart. J. exper. Physiol., 52,* 114
Carrel, A (1924) *Compt. Rend. Soc. Biol. (Paris), 90,* 333

Cohen, BE and Cohen, IK (1973) *Surg. Forum, 24,* 276

Coleman, W and Du Bois, EF (1915) *Arch. int. Med., 15,* 887

Constantian, MB, Menzoian, JO, Fisher, JC, Nimber, RB, Schmid, K and Mannick, JA (1975) *Surg. Forum, 26,* 1

Crowley, LV, Kriss, P, Seifter, E, Rettura, G and Levenson, SM (1972) *Fed. Proc., 31,* 730

Crowley, LV, Seifter, E, Kriss, P, Rettura, G, Nakao, K and Levenson, SM (1976a) In press

Crowley, LV, Kriss, P, Rettura, G, Nakao, K and Levenson, SM (1976b) In press

Cuthbertson, DP, McGirr, JL and Robertson, JSM (1939) *Quart. J. exp. Physiol., 29,* 13

Cuthbertson, DP, Fell, GS, Smith, CM and Tilstone, WJ (1972) *Brit. J. Surg., 59,* 925

Dubos, RJ (1955) *Lancet, ii,* 1

Faulk, WP, Demaeyer, EM and Davies, AJS (1974) *Amer. J. clin. Nutr., 27,* 638

Gruber, C, Crowley, LV, Kan, D, Seifter, E and Levenson, SM (1974) *Fed. Proc., 33,* 687

Howard, RJ and Simmons, RL (1974) *Surg., Gynec. and Obstet., 139,* 771

Law, DK, Dudrick, SJ and Abdou, NI (1974) *Surg., Gynec. and Obstet., 139,* 257

Levenson, SM, Pirani, CL, Braasch, JW and Waterman, DF (1954) *Surg., Gynec. and Obstet., 99,* 74

Levenson, SM, Crowley, LV, Oates, JF and Glinos, AD (1959) *Proc. Second Army Sc. Conf., 2,* 109

Levenson, SM, Geever, EF and Moncrief, WH (1962) Unpublished data

Levenson, SM, Geever, EF, Crowley, LV, Oates, JF, Berard, CW and Rosen, H (1965) *Ann. Surg., 161,* 293

MacLean, LD, Meakins, JL, Taguchi, K, Duignan, JP, Dhillon, KS and Gordon, J (1975) *Ann. Surg., 182,* 207

Munster, AM, Eurenius, K, Katz, RM, Canales, L, Foley, FD and Mortensen, RF (1973) *Ann. Surg., 177,* 139

Munster, AM, and Artzm CP (1974) *So. med. J., 67,* 935

Newberne, PM (1973) *Adv. Vet. Sci. Comp. Med., 17,* 265

Ogle, CK, Ogle, JD, McClellan, MA and Alexander, JW (1975) *Surg. Forum, 26,* 6

Rettura, G, Levenson, SM, Schittek, A and Seifter, E (1975) *Surg. Forum, 26,* 301

Rogers, AE and Newberne, PM (1975) *Cancer Res., 35,* 3427

Seifter, E, Crowley, LV, Rettura, G, Nakao, K, Gruber, C, Kan, D and Levenson, SM (1975) *Ann. Surg., 181,* 836

Taylor, CE and DeSweemer, C (1973) In *Food Nutrition and Health. World Review of Nutrition and Dietetics, Vol.16.* (Ed) M Rechcigl. Karger, Basel. Page 203

Viteri, FE and Arroyave, G (1973) In *Modern Nutrition in Health and Disease.* (Ed) RS Goodhart and ME Shils. Lea and Febiger, Philadelphia. Page 604.

Central Nervous System Function Following Thermal Injury

D W WILMORE, J W TAYLOR, E W HANDER, A D MASON Jr
and B A PRUITT Jr

United States Army Institute of Surgical Research, Brooke Army
Medical Center, Fort Sam Houston, Texas, USA

The reflex arc which initiates the post-traumatic metabolic response to injury consists of nervous and hormonal afferent signals to the central nervous system, with
homeostatic readjustment in the hypothalamus resulting in pituitary and sympathoadrenal discharge. This endocrine environment then directs the metabolic response
to injury and mediates alterations in flow of energy substrate. This report emphasises the importance of the hypothalamus to this reflex arc and evaluates afferent
stimuli and central nervous system mechanisms which could affect the stress response to thermal injury.

Materials and Methods

A variety of patients have been studied, most with burns greater than 35% of their
body surface area. None of the patients had blood stream infection, and most
were studied during the second or third week after injury, during the height of
their catabolic response to thermal injury. All patients were studied in an environmental chamber, at comfort temperature between 30 and 33°C unless otherwise
noted. Oxygen consumption was measured using the Douglas bag technique, and
core temperature was measured in the rectum and external auditory canal. Mean
skin temperature was calculated from multiple measurements of surface temperature in burned and unburned skin not in contact with the mattress. These
measurements were weighted mathematically by surface area to determine the
overall contribution to mean skin temperature, as previously described (Wilmore
et al, 1975a). In some patients the urinary outputs of catecholamines, glucose,
insulin, and growth hormone were measured.

THE METABOLIC RESPONSE TO COMBINED THERMAL
AND CENTRAL NERVOUS SYSTEM INJURY

Four burned patients with associated injuries of the central nervous system have
been studied (Table I). Two who sustained cerebral contusion, in association
with flame injury, demonstrated measured metabolic rates which were greater
than those predicted from the size of burn injury alone, suggesting that head injury has an additive effect to the metabolic response to thermal injury. A patient

TABLE I. Effect of CNS Injury on Post-traumatic Hypermetabolism

CNS Injury	Burn Size (% BSA)*	Age (Years)	Postburn Day Studied	Metabolic Rate $(kcal/m^2/hr)$	
				Measured	Predicted
Cerebral contusion	26	15	15	65.6	53.0
Cerebral contusion	48	23	8	88.2	68.0
Cerebral contusion T-11 spinal cord transection	60	27	3	92.0	74.4
Cerebral oedema (flat EEG)	23	19	3	30.8	56.1

* BSA = Body Surface Area

with thoracic spinal cord injury and paraplegia, 60% total body surface burn,
and cerebral contusion was markedly hypermetabolic, consistent with the degree
of his extensive trauma. This metabolic response occurred despite denervation of
a major portion of the injured skin, which was over the lower trunk and lower
extremities, and despite denervation of a large portion of the muscle mass.
Finally, a patient with a 23% burn, and brain death resulting from cerebral
oedema (determined by flat EEG) was hypometabolic with less than the normal
predicted basal levels for uninjured man and below 56.1 $kcal/m^2$/hour predicted
for individuals with thermal injury of comparable size.

INTERRUPTION OF PERIPHERAL NERVOUS STIMULATION
FROM THE INJURY

To evaluate the role of peripheral nervous stimulation from the injured area,
metabolic rate, core temperature, and urinary catecholamines were measured
in three patients during the resting state, following four hours of equilibration
in ambient comfort conditions. One per cent viscous lidocaine (Xylocaine®) was
then applied to the burn wound to achieve total anaesthesia of the second degree
areas of injury and to ensure that no afferent nervous stimulation from the other

TABLE II. Effect of Blockade of Afferent Nervous Stimuli from the Wound on
Metabolism (Mean, Range or $\pm$ SE)

Treatment	N	Burn Size (% Body Surface Area)	Age (Years)	Postburn Day Studied	Metabolic Rate (kcal/m^2/hr)	
					Before	After*
Topical anaesthesia	3	66 (53–78.5)	28 (25–30)	13 (10–17)	77.8 $\pm$ 4.2	77.5 $\pm$ 2.5
Spinal anaesthesia	1	33 (Multiple fractures)	39	33	57.3	63.8

* Mean of two–six hour measurements

areas of cutaneous injury occurred. Additional studies were then performed at 2,
4 and 6 hours following the initial application of the topical anaesthetic. Supplemental topical medication was applied periodically throughout the study period.
Although the patients were remarkably free of pain following application of the
topical anaesthetic and slept most of the time during the investigation, topical
anaesthesia exerted no effect on metabolic rate or urinary catecholamines,
measured serially throughout the study (Table II). In a single patient with a 33%
burn over his lower extremities, fracture of the right femur, right tibia, and fracture dislocation of the right ankle, a spinal anaesthetic was administered and
maintained for four hours at the T4 to T6 level. No significant effect on metabolic rate or core temperature was detected following total denervation of the
injured area (Table II).

ADMINISTRATION OF AGENTS WHICH INTERACT WITH CENTRAL TEMPERATURE REGULATION

Previous studies have demonstrated that in burned patients core and skin temperatures are raised following injury (Wilmore et al, 1974), and this hyperpyrexia
is a reflection of hypermetabolism and alterations in substrate. To determine if
the hyperpyrexia and hypermetabolism of thermal injury could be affected at the
hypothalamic level by administration of antipyretics, 20 grains of aspirin were
administered orally every four hours for two days to three patients and the resting metabolic rate was measured daily. Core temperature was measured every two
hours throughout the period of study. Aspirin exerted no detectable effect on
metabolic rate, and core temperature during the study period was also unchanged
(Table III).

L-dopa rapidly crosses the blood brain barrier, and increases concentrations of
dopamine and norepinephrine within the central nervous system. L-dopa has been
reported to reduce core temperature in 10 of 24 normal men studied in a cool

TABLE III. Administration of Agents Thought to Interact with Central Temperature Regulation (Mean, Range or ± SE)

Treatment	N	Burn Size (% Body Surface Area)	Age (Years)	Postburn Day Studied	Metabolic Rate (kcal/m²/hr)		Core Temperature (°C)	
					Before	After	Before	After
Aspirin	3	52 (41–57)	18 (14–22)	29 (13–39)	70.4±7.6	71.2±5.9*	38.1±0.3	38.2±0.4
L-dopa	7	46† (36–51.5)	28 (24–36)	16† (7–25)	54.8±5.7	57.0±5.9	37.5±0.5	37.4±0.5
Calcium infusion	3	60 (47–75)	41 (24–56)	11 [7–15]	63.9±1.9	64.9±2.0	37.7±0.4	38.1±0.5
Atropine sulphate	3	41 (35–46)	42 (24–61)	15 (9–18)	69.1±6.1	63.4±5.2	37.9±0.2	38.2±0.4

* After 48 hours of salicylate administration

† Not including two normals

277

environment (Boyd et al, 1974). L-dopa was administered by mouth in a 1.5 g dose to seven individuals in the early morning following basal metabolic studies on five burned and two normal individuals. L-dopa was absorbed in all individuals as demonstrated by an increase in serum growth hormone level (from a mean of 2.9 ng/ml to 15.7 ng/ml) two to three hours after ingestion of the drug. However, metabolic rate and core temperature were unchanged in all individuals (Table III). In fact, subsequent studies demonstrated a 10 to 15 per cent increase in metabolic rate in two patients following administration of 2—2.5 g of the amino acid.

It has been proposed that calcium exerts a braking effect on the temperature centre, which is subject to ionic modulation (Myers, 1971). Three patients, with a mean burn size of 60%, were studied before and after infusion of a dose of calcium known to evoke an endocrine response. Calcium chloride was given intravenously as a loading dose of 4 mg calcium/kg body weight, and maintained as a constant infusion over four hours; the mean serum calcium concentration increased from 7.2 mg/100 ml to 11.7 but did not affect either the metabolic rate or core temperature.

Atropine is known to inhibit cholinergic receptors in the central nervous system, and may decrease heat production by blocking central inhibitory cholinergic mechanisms (Kirkpatrick & Lomax, 1967). Atropine acts on the periphery to diminish evaporative water loss, but blockade of insensible water loss does not occur in the burn patient because of the increased vaporisational heat loss across the injured skin. Atropine sulphate administered as a single intravenous dose of 0.04 mg/kg body weight did not alter the metabolic rate or core temperature. In one patient with persistent extrapyramidal movements, the atropine diminished muscle tremors, with a decrease in metabolic expenditure from 73.3 to 62.6 kcal/m²/hour.

EFFECT OF CNS NARCOSIS ON THE SYMPATHETIC RESPONSE TO STRESS

The effects of agents known to influence the sympathetic outflow from the hypothalamus on the metabolic response to stress were also studied. Inert gases exert central narcotic effects (Schreiner, 1968), and the metabolic and respiratory response to three hours of cold exposure (14°C) was measured in 14 studies in five normal males, wearing only light cotton shorts and breathing room air, 79% helium—21% oxygen, or 79% argon—21% oxygen. Pulse rate, oxygen consumption, core temperature, urinary catecholamines, blood glucose, insulin, and HGH were serially measured. Eight additional comparison studies between room air and the helium—oxygen mixture were performed in normal individuals in a neutral thermal environment (28°C), and six other studies compared the response to intravenous infusion of epinephrine (6μg/min for one hour) during inhalation of He-O$_2$ and room air.

Heat production and core temperature were significantly lower at the end of

TABLE IV. Effect of CNS Narcosis on the Metabolic Response to Stress (Mean, Range or ± SE)

Narcotic Agent	Study Condition	N	Burn Size (% Body Surface Area)	Age (Years)	Postburn Day Studied	Metabolic Rate (kcal/m²/hour)		Core Temperature (°C)	
						Control	Narcotic	Control	Narcotic
79% Helium–21% Oxygen	Comfort (28°C)	4		28 (25–33)		37.8±1.5	35.2±3.0	36.9±0.1	36.9±0.1
79% Helium–21% Oxygen	Cold stress (14°C)	5		31 (24–37)		58.8±5.5	43.8±3.3*	36.7±0.1	36.5±0.1*
79% Helium–21% Oxygen	Comfort Epinephrine infusion	3		29 (24–37)		47.2±1.0	48.3±0.9	37.1±0.1	37.1±0.1
79% Argon–21% Oxygen	Cold stress	3		33 (28–37)		56.1±10.3	41.7±3.8	36.8±0.1	36.7±0.1*
79% Helium–21% Oxygen	Patients	4	47 (42–57)	43 (36–48)	62 (30–104)	52.8±1.5	56.4±2.5	38.4±1	38.2±1
79% Argon–21% Oxygen	Patients	2	38 (32–43)	46 (43–48)	56 (26–87)	80.4±7.7	80.8±1.2	38.2±0.0	38.6±0.2
Morphine	Patients	5	74 (59–87)	26 (21–38)	16 (7–29)	77.4±5.9	55.0±3.7*	38.2±0.1	37.3±0.1*

* $p < 0.05$

279

three hours of cold exposure during inhalation of helium—oxygen compared to the cold exposure while breathing room air (Table IV). Similar effects were noted with the inhalation of argon—oxygen mixture. No effects on metabolism were noted in the thermo-neutral studies in the normal individuals. Metabolic rate while breathing the helium and oxygen mixture was unchanged following epinephrine infusion, suggesting that helium does not act as a peripheral blocking agent but dampens central sympathetic nervous system outflow. Metabolism did not decrease with the inhalation of the inert gases in the burned patients.

In five burned patients with a mean burn size of 74% the effects of intravenous morphine on the metabolic and respiratory response were studied. An average dose of 0.38 mg morphine sulphate per kg body weight was given over one hour following basal studies, and serial oxygen consumption, pulse rate, minute ventilation, core temperature, blood pressure, and blood gases were measured. Two of

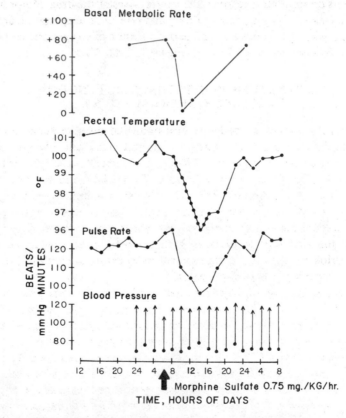

Figure 1. A prompt decrease in oxygen consumption and core temperature occurs following morphine administration. Oxygenation was normal throughout this study in this patient maintained on a ventilator

TABLE V. Alterations with Morphine Administration to Five Burn Patients (Mean ± SE)

	Before	After*
Minute volume (l/min)	21.5 ± 2.5	12.0 ± 1.0
Frequency (breaths/min)	20.4 ± 1.9	13.8 ± 1.6
Metabolic rate (kcal/m^2/hr)	77.4 ± 5.9	55.0 ± 3.7
Ventilatory equivalent (l/l)	41.2 ± 6.7	32.0 ± 4.1
Pulse rate (beats/min)	115 ± 4	104 ± 5
Core temperature (°C)	38.2 ± 0.1	37.3 ± 0.1

* $p < 0.05$

the patients on ventilators received the largest doses of the drug. Morphine significantly decreased oxygen consumption, pulse rate, core temperature, and minute ventilation, while blood pressure and partial pressure of oxygen and carbon dioxide in the blood remained unchanged (Figure 1, Table V).

ALTERATIONS IN HYPOTHALAMIC FUNCTION FOLLOWING THERMAL INJURY

Nine burn patients were studied in an environmental chamber during the second to third weeks after injury, along with five normal individuals who were approximately the same age (Wilmore et al, 1975b). The subjects wore light cotton shorts and lay on a bed in the environmental room. The initial temperature of the room was 25°C, and relative humidity maintained at 50% throughout the study. The subjects were instructed to use a bedside remote control temperature regulating unit and asked to alter room temperature to achieve comfort. All subjects remained in the room 4 to 24 hours. Ambient temperature selected at the end of the test period was recorded as the ambient temperature of comfort. Mean skin and core temperatures were also measured.

All individuals achieved subjective comfort after two to three hours by altering ambient temperature in the metabolic chamber, the rapid response of the room to adjustments allowed frequent alterations and minimised large temperature variations within the room. The mean ambient temperature selected by the normal individuals was 27.8°C and their mean skin temperature was 33.4°C, and they maintained normal core temperature. In contrast, the burn patients selected higher ambient temperatures, and their average core and mean skin temperatures were also significantly elevated above those recorded for normal man (Table VI). The ambient comfort temperature selected was related to burn size, and could be predicted from core and skin temperatures.

281

TABLE VI. Ambient Temperatures of Comfort (Mean $\pm$ SE)

	N	Ambient Comfort Temperature (^{o}C)	Mean Skin Temperature (^{o}C)	Core Temperature (^{o}C)
Normal	5	27.8 ± 0.6	33.4 ± 0.6	36.9 ± 0.1
Burn patients	9	30.4 ± 0.7	35.2 ± 0.4	38.4 ± 0.3
		$p < 0.05$	$p < 0.05$	$p < 0.01$

Human growth hormone response to insulin hyperglycaemia and arginine infusion was measured in nine additional burned patients and five normal men. Initial studies were carried out between the third and 24th day after injury and in surviving patients were repeated following wound closure and before hospital discharge. The provocative tests for human growth hormone release were performed on consecutive days in the early morning. On the first day 0.3 units/kg body weight insulin was administered to the burned patients, and 0.15 units/kg body weight to the recovered patients and normals. Serial blood samples were then obtained for estimation of blood concentration of glucose and HGH. On the subsequent morning, 30 g of a 10% solution of arginine hydrochloride was infused intravenously over 30 minutes, and blood was serially assayed for glucose, blood urea nitrogen, HGH, and insulin.

Fasting HGH was significantly elevated in the burned patients during the acute phase of injury and during recovery compared with normal basal values and the elevated HGH occurred during the period of acute injury despite the associated fasting hyperglycaemia (Figure 2). The HGH response to hypoglycaemia was more rapid, but the peak response was diminished in the burned patient when compared with recovery and with controls. The average peak HGH response of the burned patients was 12.6 ng/ml, which occurred 40 minutes following the injection of insulin, compared with a mean peak response of 27.8 ng/ml in the recovered patients, and 32.6 ng/ml in normal man ($p < 0.01$). Diminished HGH response to provocative stimuli was also observed following arginine infusion (Figure 3). HGH rose to a mean peak of 3.9 ng/ml in the acute burns compared with 9.3 and 10.1 ng/ml in the recovered patients and normal man.

Discussion

The reflex arc which initiates the post-traumatic metabolic response to injury consists of nervous or hormonal afferent signals to the central nervous system, with homeostatic readjustment in the hypothalamus resulting in pituitary and sympathoadrenal discharge. This endocrine environment then directs the meta-

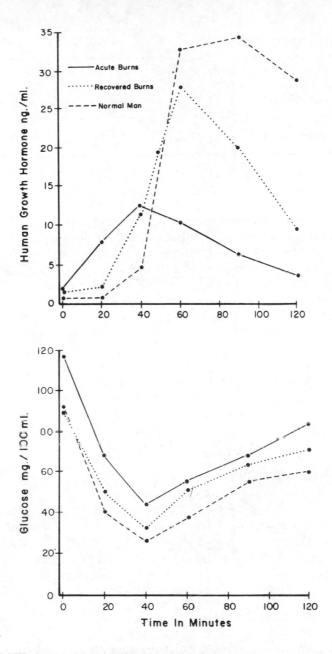

Figure 2. HGH response to insulin hypoglycaemia is more rapid in the acute burned patients, but the peak response is blunted following injury and responsiveness returns toward normal with recovery

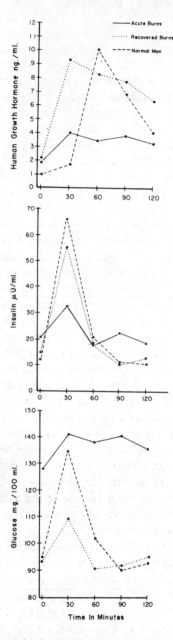

Figure 3. Infusion of 30 g arginine hydrochloride resulted in a prompt increase in levels of HGH and insulin in the recovered patients and normals, while the acute burned patients demonstrated a diminished response. Fasting insulin levels in the acute burns are appropriate for the blood glucose level, but the insulin response corrected for alterations in blood glucose and expressed as units of insulin/100 mg blood sugar is less than half as great as the response in the other groups studied

bolic response which mediates the increased heat production and alterations in substrate flow. The metabolic response to injury was absent in a patient with brain death, and studies using anaesthetics and narcotising agents demonstrated a marked reduction of the metabolic rate and catecholamine excretion associated with central nervous system narcosis. Spinal cord trauma, which interrupts the afferent nervous input from the injured area; the use of spinal anaesthesia above the injury; and application of topical anaesthetics to the injured area did not affect the metabolic response to injury. In addition, a variety of drugs, which are thought to play a central role in temperature regulation, such as salicylates, L-dopa, calcium, and atropine, exerted no detectable effect on the metabolic response to thermal injury evaluated in the short-term studies described.

Core temperature during comfort has been related to the hypothalamic set-point for physiologic thermal neutrality, which is associated with the absence of thermal regulatory effort. Normal man will achieve comfort between 28 and 29° ambient, depending upon previous acclimatisation. Thermal comfort is subjectively appreciated when central temperature sensors are not stimulated and sensory input from cold receptors in the periphery is diminished or absent. When normal man selects an ambient comfort temperature, he maintains a skin temperature above 33°C, which is considered the threshold for firing of peripheral cold receptors. However, burn patients selected a warmer ambient temperature to achieve comfort, and the room temperature selected could be roughly related to the size of injury. That a reset or readjustment in the hypothalamic temperature set may have occurred following injury is suggested by the fact that the burned patients felt comfortable at elevated ambient temperatures which were quite uncomfortable for normal man. Moreover, the patients maintained an elevated core and skin temperature while subjectively comfortable, which is similar to the central temperature readjustment which occurs with a febrile response to infection. These studies suggest that the chronic hyperpyrexia of thermal injury is a result of a readjustment in central temperature setpoint, and that the metabolic changes following injury occur because of this adjustment in setpoint, causing increased sympathetic nervous system discharge.

Human growth hormone is elevated in the early phases of injury in spite of hyperglycaemia. Growth hormone stimulation occurs with a fall in blood glucose, but is also related to a wide variety of stress-induced stimuli. Exercise, cold exposure, cardiopulmonary bypass, haemorrhage, and injury have all been associated with HGH elaboration. HGH is suppressed by hyperglycaemia, yet in burned patients, the elevated blood glucose did not suppress the HGH blood level, although blood glucose levels of 110 to 120 mg per cent will suppress HGH elaboration in normal man. Injury apparently results in an alteration in this hypothalamic function, augmenting HGH elaboration at the same time it increases sympathetic discharge, which increases substrate flow, glucose production, and nitrogen excretion.

The HGH response occurred immediately with the initial fall in blood glucose following insulin administration in injured patients, in contrast to the slower HGH response observed in recovered patients and normal man. Moreover, the overall HGH response in burned patients was markedly diminished. The relative fall in blood glucose in the acute burned patients was greater than that seen in the recovered individuals, although the absolute level of blood sugar was not as low in the acutely injured patients in spite of the increased dose of insulin administered. In spite of these levels of hypoglycaemia, there remained a marked decrease in HGH response in acute burned patients as compared with the other patients. The blunted HGH response was also observed with infusion of 30 g of arginine hydrochloride, which confirms the diminished HGH response to provocative stimuli which occurred following injury.

These studies add support to the hypothesis that the metabolic response to injury is a consequence of homeostatic readjustment within the hypothalamus, which occurs following injury. That the hypothalamus is necessary for this response is demonstrated by the studies in the patient with brain death and those of the effects following administration of potent narcotic agents. Burn patients appear to have reset their thermal regulatory setpoint upward, thus increasing the discharge of sympathetic impulses to stimulate heat production and substrate mobilisation in order to maintain new and elevated core temperature. Burned patients increase their metabolic rate in cool environments, at core and skin temperatures above the setpoints recorded for normal man. Fasting blood glucose is elevated following injury, and fasting levels of growth hormone are elevated above control values in spite of hyperglycaemia. Attempts to evaluate the afferent stimuli which caused these homeostatic readjustments within the hypothalamus have not provided a clue to the stimuli which provide this graded metabolic response to thermal injury. Further evaluation and modification of this response at the hypothalamic level, with elucidation of the afferent limb of this reflex arc, is required.

The opinions or assertions contained herein are the private views of the authors and are not to be construed as official or as reflecting the views of the Department of the Army or the Department of Defense.

References

Boyd, AE, Mager, M, Angoff, G and Lebovitz, HE (1974) *J.Appl.Physiol., 37,* 675
Kirkpatrick, WE and Lomax, P (1967) *Life Science, 6,* 2273
Myers, RD (1971) In *Primates in Comparative Physiology of Thermoregulation.* (Ed) GC Whitton. Academic Press, New York and London. Page 283
Schreiner, HR (1968) *Fed. Proc., 27,* 872
Wilmore, DW, Long, JM, Skreen, R, Mason, AD Jr and Pruitt, BA Jr (1974) *Ann. Surg., 180,* 653
Wilmore, DW, Mason, AD Jr, Johnson, DW and Pruitt, BA Jr (1975a) *J. Appl. Physiol., 38,* 593
Wilmore, DW, Orcutt, TW, Mason, AD Jr and Pruitt, BA Jr (1975b) *J. Trauma* (In press)

Catecholamines as Mediators of the Metabolic Response to Thermal Injury

D W WILMORE, J M LONG, A D MASON Jr and B A PRUITT Jr
United States Army Institute of Surgical Research, Brooke Army
Medical Center, Fort Sam Houston, Texas, USA

Introduction

Hypermetabolism characterises the metabolic response to thermal injury, and the magnitude of this post-traumatic physiological alteration is closely related to the extent of injury. Negative nitrogen balance, loss of other intracellular constituents, and a rapid decrease in body weight are consequences of the increased metabolic activity, and extensive loss of protoplasmic mass may result in severe erosion of energy and protein stores essential to optimal body function. The increased evaporative water loss from the burn wound results in surface cooling, which could stimulate metabolic activity to maintain normal heat balance and core temperature. We will review the relationship between surface cooling and hypermetabolism, present evidence implicating catecholamines as the mediator of the post-traumatic metabolic response, and discuss the role of the sympathetic nervous system in regulating heat production and substrate flow during the profound hypercatabolic response following thermal injury.

Materials and Methods

Burned patients and normal individuals were studied in an environmental chamber which is located on the Burn Ward. The burn patients were selected to represent a range in size of total surface injury, and none had significant pre-existing disease before injury. The patients did not have systemic infection, as determined by stable body temperature, absence of clinical signs of infection, and negative blood cultures and endotoxin levels before, during, and after the study period unless they were specifically included in a group of studies involving septic

287

patients. Septic patients were defined as individuals with clinical signs and symptoms of systemic infection and positive blood cultures obtained at the time of study. None of the septic patients were hypotensive or had alterations in urinary output at the time of study. The study design, methodology, and biochemical processing of specimens have been described previously (Wilmore et al, 1974).

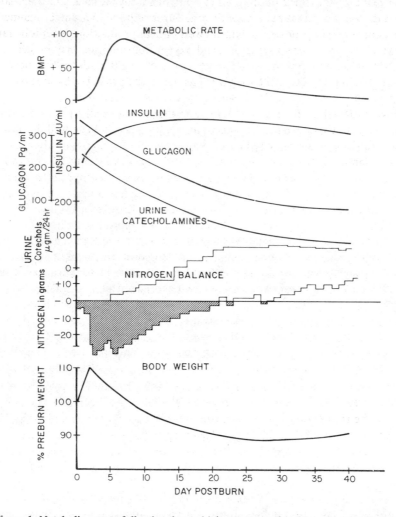

Figure 1. Metabolic events following thermal injury measured in 11 patients with an average burn size of 47 per cent total body surface. Predictive curves for insulin and glucagon are shown for a constant blood glucose of 100 mg per 100 ml. Nitrogen balance was measured in four representative patients and basal metabolic rate was derived from intermittent basal measurements and predictive equations based on burn size, day postburn and catecholamine excretion. Weight stabilisation and positive nitrogen balance are achieved as insulin returns to a normal relationship with glucagon and catecholamines

288

Increased basal metabolic rate occurs with thyrotoxicosis, infection, and major trauma, yet, the most prodigious metabolic expenditure recorded has followed thermal injury. Metabolic rate is related to burn size, and BMR increases in a linear manner with burns of up to 40 to 50% total body surface, and then flattens out, suggesting that patients with large burns respond in a similar manner by attaining maximal or near maximal levels of heat production. Metabolic rate also varies with the time after injury, and oxygen consumption may be near normal during resuscitation, then rises to a peak during the 6th to 10th postburn day, and decreases in a curvilinear manner to the predicted basal levels when satisfactory coverage of the burn wound is achieved (Figure 1).

The aetiology of the metabolic response following burn injury has been studied extensively, but the precise mechanisms have only recently been well defined. Similarities between thermally injured patients and individuals with thyrotoxicosis prompted early endocrine studies by Cope et al (1953), but the increased oxygen consumption could not be associated with abnormal thyroid function. More recent studies of T_3 and T_4 turnover, and investigations of the hypothalamic-pituitary-thyroid axis, have confirmed these earlier investigations.

Increased evaporative water loss from the burn wounds results in surface cooling, which may stimulate metabolic heat production in order to generate more heat and maintain normal body temperature. Moreover, the increased oxygen consumption and insensible water loss are both correlated with burn size. Therefore, the hypermetabolism has been related to surface cooling secondary to increased evaporative water loss from the burn wound. Covering the wound in experimental animals blocks evaporative water loss and returns metabolic rate to normal. In addition, burned rats treated at a room temperature of $30°C$ have a lower metabolic rate and lower nitrogen excretion than rats with similar burns treated at $20°C$ (Caldwell, 1962). More recently, the metabolic rate of burned patients treated in a warm environment ($32°C$) was decreased compared with those treated at $22°C$ (Barr et al, 1968). This evidence has been interpreted to support the thesis that hypermetabolism in the burned patient is a response to increased surface cooling due to increased evaporative water loss. In contrast, Zawacki et al (1970) covered the burn wound with a water-impermeable membrane, blocked evaporative water loss, but found no consistent alteration in metabolic rate in burn patients at approximately $25°C$ ambient temperature.

Our studies of burn patients in the rigidly controlled ambient conditions of an environmental chamber demonstrate a curvilinear relationship between metabolism and burn size, but a direct linear relationship between evaporative water loss and per cent total body surface burn. In the normal subjects studied with burns of less than 40% of the total body surface, metabolism at $25°C$ and 50% relative humidity was not related to surface cooling by evaporative water loss. Hence, metabolic rate was unaffected when these individuals were studied in a warmer ambient temperature. That these patients were internally warm and not externally cold was demonstrated by average core and mean skin temperatures which were consistently $1-2°C$ higher in the injured patients when compared with the control subjects, and this increase in core and skin temperature was present at all ambient temperatures studied (Table I). Burned patients demonstrated appropriate thermoregulatory control as seen by their response to a

TABLE I. Measurements from Four Normals and 20 Patients at Two Ambient Temperatures (Mean $\pm$ SE)

	Normal	Burns	p
25°C			
Metabolic rate (kcal/m^2/hr)	35.6+2.0	66.8+2.6	<0.001
Core temperature (°C)	36.7+0.2	38.4+0.2	<0.001
Skin temperature (°C)	31.4+0.2	33.1+0.2	<0.001
Core skin heat transfer coefficient (kcal/m^2/hr/°C)	6.6+0.4	13.3+1.0	<0.001
33°C			
Metabolic rate (kcal/m^2/hr)	36.3+1.6	62.6+2.3	<0.001
Core temperature (°C)	36.9 + 0.1	38.1+0.2	<0.001
Skin temperature (°C)	34.2+0.3	35.9+0.2	<0.01
Core skin heat transfer coefficient (kcal/m^2/hr/°C)	13.9+1.4	30.6+2.5	<0.001

mild cool ambient environment of 21°C. Both normal individuals and burn patients who were able to respond increased metabolic rate at these cooler temperatures, showing an ability to respond to the increased heat loss from the body.

These studies demonstrate that evaporative water loss of the burned patient is not the prime stimulator of the hypermetabolic response, but rather that increased energy production is related to an endogenous reset of metabolic activity. This basic metabolic drive is then influenced by environmental conditions. At any ambient temperature measured, the core and mean skin temperature of the burn patient is well above temperatures measured in normal man. The thermally injured patient is internally warm and not externally cold. Increased evaporative water loss provides a convenient route for transfer of this large quantity of heat generated by the body. Metabolic rate is only slightly decreased by placing patients in a warm environment, and our data, and the reports from other investigators, demonstrate that metabolic rate never returns to normal levels with treatment in a warm environment.

Hormonal stimulation of heat production occurs with elaboration of thyroid

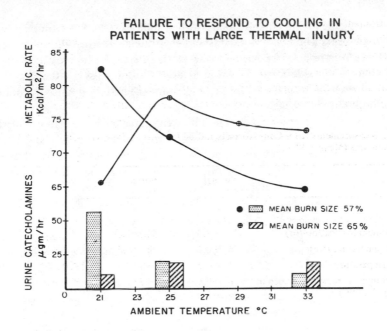

FAILURE TO RESPOND TO COOLING IN
PATIENTS WITH LARGE THERMAL INJURY

MEAN BURN SIZE 57%
MEAN BURN SIZE 65%

Figure 2. The ability to generate additional heat to cold stress is variable in patients with
large thermal injury, but appears to depend primarily on burn size. Individuals with
smaller injuries (mean burn size 57%) and available metabolic reserve respond to cooling
by increasing metabolic rate, and this response is associated with increased urinary catecholamines, while others (mean burn size 65%) lack catechol or tissue reserves, fail to
maintain heat balance and become hypothermic. These 'non-responders' are apparently
at maximal rates of energy production and cannot respond appropriately to catechol-
mediated stress, such as cooling, infection and haemorrhage

hormones or catecholamines. Thyroid function has been carefully studies, and
hyperthyroidism does not appear to be the cause of the increased oxygen consumption which follows burn trauma. Measurements of urinary excretion of
catecholamines per unit time are related to metabolic rate measured during the
same time period. This relationship appeared to be linear until metabolic rate
approached twice the basal level when the increased excretion of urinary catecholamines was associated with only a slight increase in metabolic rate, and the
predicted metabolic response never exceeded 2.5 times basal levels for normal
man. The ability to generate additional heat in response to a cool environment
was variable in patients with burns greater than 40% of the total body surface
(Figure 2). In four patients, with an average burn size of 57% BSA, there was
a marked increase in metabolic rate which maintained core temperature and
was accompanied by an increase in excretion of urinary catecholamines. However, four patients with a mean burn size of 65%, studied in a cool ambient
temperature, failed to maintain heat balance, became hypothermic with a sudden
decrease in urinary catecholamine excretion. All of these non-responding patients

291

subsequently died from complications of their injuries. Like WB Cannon's sympathectomised cats who could not withstand environmental stress (Cannon et al, 1929), the 'non-responders' lacked homeostatic reserve, for injury had reset their rates of energy production at a maximum level. Additional sympathetic nervous system reserve was unavailable for catecholamine-mediated response to cooling, infection, or haemorrhage.

To determine the precise interaction between catecholamine elaboration and heat production, nine studies were performed in six patients, before and after alpha and combined alpha and beta adrenergic blockade by the intravenous administration of phentolamine (Rogitine®), 75 mg (alpha blockade), or phentolamine, 75 mg, and propanolol (Inderal®), 75 mg, infused over 15 to 30 minutes (combined alpha and beta blockade) [Wilmore et al, 1974]. No consistent change in metabolic rate was seen with alpha blockade alone (Table II), but there was a

TABLE II. Effect of Alpha and Beta Blockade on Hypermetabolism Following Thermal Injury (Mean $\pm$ SE)

	Alpha Blockade (N=3)		Alpha and Beta Blockade (N=6)	
	Before	After	Before	After
Pulse (beats/min)	115+8	104+10	116+7	89+2*
Blood pressure (mmHg)	142/70	120/50	126+7/ 82+4	95+6/63+4*
Respiratory rate (breaths/min)	22.2+5.2·	23.4+5.9	22.2+3.7	21.3+3.7
Minute ventilation (l/min)	24.9+7.5	21.6+3.9	21.3+3.2	17.6+3.4*
Metabolic rate (kcal/m^2/hr)	70.7+7.9	68.1+4.6	69.6+5.3	57.4+5.2*
Free fatty acids (mEq/l)	1.6+0.4	5.8+2.2	4.1+0.5	2.5+0.5*

*$p < 0.02$

significant decrease in metabolic rate associated with combined alpha and beta blockade or beta blockade alone, and this response was associated with a decrease in pulse rate, blood pressure, minute ventilation, and free fatty acids. The dose of propanolol required for competitive blockade of the beta receptor system was greater than the dose required for normal man, and persistent sympathetic breakthrough occurred with smaller doses of the drug. Metabolic activity returned to its preblockade level within two to three hours.

To determine if the hypermetabolic response to injury could be reproduced by the infusion of catecholamines in normal man, 6 μg epinephrine per minute were infused in 10 studies in seven normal males. Metabolic rate increased with the infusion of epinephrine in normal man when compared with the basal periods. Hypermetabolism was accompanied by an increase in respiratory rate and minute ventilation, and these alterations in metabolic and respiratory function returned toward normal following infusion. Blood glucose, free fatty acids, and glucagon increased, growth hormone fell, and insulin and glucocorticocoids remained unchanged during the catecholamine infusion, alterations consistent with the previously reported observations. Excretion of urea nitrogen was not altered throughout the study in the fed patients, but nitrogen loss increased with infusion in the fasting patients. No significant alterations in blood urea nitrogen occurred during the study.

LOSS OF INTRACELLULAR CONSTITUENTS

Insulin appears to be central to the regulation of protein metabolism, and relative changes in plasma insulin levels are associated with muscle amino acid uptake or release. However, glucagon has potent glycogenolytic and gluconeogenic activities, hormonal properties which are precisely opposite those of insulin. The interaction between insulin and glucagon has been proposed as the determinant in both a quantitative and qualitative sense of hepatic glucose balance and gluconeogenesis (Unger, 1972).

Glucose, insulin, and urinary catecholamines were measured throughout the course of 11 patients with burns of an average size of 47% total body surface. Glucagon levels were evaluated following injury, even in the face of glucose administration and hyperglycaemia (Figure 1). Following the initial period of resuscitation, insulin levels are characteristically not in the usual proportional relationship to blood glucose, and the insulin to glucagon ratio is low following injury. As the burn heals the nutritional intake improves and in early convalescence both hormones return to normal, corresponding in time with positive nitrogen balance and weight gains. Alpha cell stimulation, and thus glucagon release, is mediated by hypoglycaemia, increased sympathetic activity, and certain amino acids. A close relationship between glucagon and catecholamines in our patients suggests that increased adrenergic activity may mediate the rise in the concentration of glucagon which occurs after injury. Catechols suppress insulin release, and low insulin levels have been reported in the immediate post-burn injury period and in severe trauma. The return of insulin and glucagon to normal levels following injury occurs with healing of the burn, when urinary catecholamines fall to normal levels. Catecholamines may therefore determine the pancreatic islet cell response, which in turn controls the disposition of key substrates. Thus increased adrenergic activity again appears to be a major mediator of the metabolic response following burn injury, not only stimulating calorigenesis but regulating substrate flow by directing the response of the alpha and beta pancreatic cells and exerting other direct hormonal effects on cellular metabolism.

ALTERATIONS IN GLUCOSE KINETICS

The rise in blood glucose level which occurs after injury and infection, and the alterations in glucose dynamics appear central to the metabolic response to stress. Long et al (1971) demonstrated an increased rate of glucose turnover in traumatised and septic patients, and Gump et al (1974) in similar patients related increased hepatic glucose production to hyperglycaemia in four of the nine patients which they studied. Glucose disappearance and glucose flow were determined in 21 patients with a mean burn size of 47% total body surface, between the 5th and 77th post-burn day, and compared with findings in 12 normal individuals of comparable age and body weight. Glucose flow (Hlad et al, 1956) was significantly elevated in the 17 burned patients studied between the 6th and 16th day post-burn when compared with normal individuals or the recovered patients (Table III). Glucose flow during the second post-burn week was related to the

TABLE III. Glucose Flow Studies (Mean $\pm$ SE)

	Normals	Burn Patients*
N	12	17
Age (years)	26 ± 2	29 ± 3
Weight (kg)	66.4 ± 3.9	67.3 ± 2.7
Glucose space (l/kg)	0.152 ± 0.010	0.177 ± 0.010
Asymptote (mg/100 ml)	70 ± 2	113 ± 5†
K (100 min^{-1})	4.01 ± 0.56	5.27 ± 0.51
Q (mg/kg/min)	3.92 ± 0.32	10.12 ± 0.95†

* 9th post-burn day average day of study

† $p < 0.001$

extent of injury, and fell with time in a curvilinear manner to normal values with healing of the burn. The increased glucose flow and elevated fasting serum glucose observed following injury did not result from prolonged glucose disappearance (Figure 3) or from alterations in the glucose space, which was equivalent to the extracellular fluid compartment. Thus, following resuscitation in burn patients, the elevated blood glucose is related to the increased entry of glucose into the extracellular fluid compartment (increased hepatic production), at a time when the proportionality constant for glucose disappearance is normal.

Simultaneous studies of glucose flow and oxygen consumption were performed in 10 normals and 17 uninfected burn patients, and showed a close relationship between heat production and glucose flow, but the patients were not utilising glucose as a primary fuel substrate, as demonstrated by low respiratory quotients (0.70–0.75) reflecting fat oxidation.

METABOLIC ALTERATIONS IN SEPTIC BURN PATIENTS

Hypermetabolism and loss of intracellular constituents have been commonly

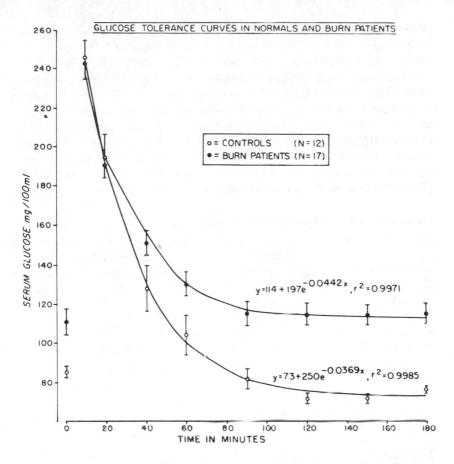

Figure 3. Comparable glucose disappearance occurred following an intravenous injection of 25 g glucose in burned patients and controls (proportionality constant is exponential in equations). The persistent hyperglycaemia of injury (asymptote the curves approach is first term of the equations) is a result of increased hepatic production of glucose, not abnormal peripheral disposal. Curves comparable to those obtained from the burn patients can be obtained by infusion of 10% dextrose to normal men, equilibrating at a steady state, and then injecting a 25 g glucose dose. Points represent mean values+ SE.

associated with infection in man, and it appears that infection exerts its catabolic alteration in body metabolism by way of the sympathetic-mediated stress response. However, patients with extensive burns die from infection and the interaction between the stress of injury and superimposed blood stream infection has not previously been described. Eighteen studies of heat production and heat loss were performed in 10 burned patients, all with positive blood cultures at the time of study. The urine output was adequate in all the patients, none of whom showed signs of hypotension or cardiovascular instability. Metabolic rate, core and skin temperature, urine and plasma catecholamines, were measured as previously described. Glucose kinetics were measured in 11 patients with positive blood stream cultures for gram negative organisms. These patients were considered to have mild or moderate infection at the time of study, and none had cardiocirculatory instability, although a decrease in core temperature was frequently noted in all individuals. The mean metabolic rate was 50.3 ± 2 kcal/m^2/ hour, compared with mean predicted or measured rates in non-septic intervals of 73 ± 1.2 kcal/m^2/hour. Urinary catecholamines were markedly elevated in these patients, averaging $910.8 \pm 406 \mu$g/hour. Glucose kinetics were markedly deranged (Table IV), a consistent finding being the significantly decreased proportionality constant for glucose disappearance into the periphery, as demonstrated by the diabetic-like glucose tolerance curves following sepsis (Figure 4).

TABLE IV. Glucose Flow in Burn Patients (Mean $\pm$ SE)

	Non-septic	Gram Negative Sepsis
N	17	11
Age (years)	29 ± 3	28 ± 3
Weight (kg)	67.3 ± 2.7	78.1 ± 2.8*
Burn size (% BS)	42 ± 5	74 ± 3†
Post-burn study day	9 ± 1	8 ± 1
Glucose space (l/kg)	0.177 ± 0.010	0.201 ± 0.012
Asymptote (mg/100 ml)	113 ± 5	113 ± 12
K (100 min^{-1})	5.27 ± 0.51	2.64 ± 0.59†
Q (mg/kg/min)	10.12 ± 0.95	4.96 ± 0.72†

* $p < 0.01$
† $p < 0.001$

In addition, glucose flow through the extracellular compartment decreased in the patients with gram negative infection. Simultaneous measurements of both oxygen consumption and glucose kinetics demonstrated that burned patients with gram negative infection have a simultaneous decrease in glucose flow through the extracellular space and a fall in oxygen consumption.

Discussion and Conclusion

Hypermetabolism, negative nitrogen balance, and weight loss characterise the metabolic response to thermal injury. Increase in sympathetic activity appears to mediate this response by elaboration of catecholamines, increasing energy

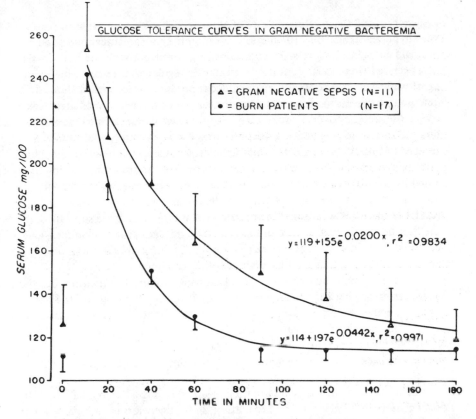

Figure 4. Glucose tolerance curves obtained from burned patients with positive blood stream culture for gram negative organisms demonstrate a decreased proportionality constant for disappearance of glucose into the periphery. The fasting blood glucose level and curve asymptote appeared to be releated to the severity of the infection and virulence of the gram negative organism, with Klebsiella and Enterobacter species causing hyperglycaemia and Pseudomonas aeruginosa associated with lower blood glucose levels (several individuals had measured fasting blood glucose levels of 70mg/100ml

production and interacting with insulin and other hormones to exert direct cellular effects on heat production and to alter substrate flow. Cold, pain, anxiety and hypovolaemia are potent afferent stimuli which augment the catecholamine response. These factors may be minised by careful clinical management. However, the basic reset in metabolic activity appears to be initiated by the burn injury, and the metabolic events do not return to normal until the cutaneous wound has healed.

Glucose flow through the extracellular space is elevated in burned patients during the peak of their hypermetabolic response. Hyperglycaemia and increased glucose flow is a result of increased glucose production, not impaired glucose disappearance, and the accelerated rate of gluconeogenesis is associated in time with hyperglucagonaemia, the increased elaboration of catecholamines, and normal fasting insulin levels. These findings are consistent with the hypothesis of Unger and Orci (1975) that insulin primarily regulates peripheral glucose disposal while glucagon controls hepatic glucose production. Increased flow of glucose to three carbon fragments,and conversion of these intermediates back to glucose, appears to occur following injury. Entry of glucose into the tricarboxylic acid cycle is limited, and fat is oxidised as the primary fuel source, a finding consistent with earlier studies which suggest a partial block in the metabolic pathways leading from three carbon to two carbon fragments during the convalescent stage of trauma (Drucker et al, 1962). Enzymes which favour conversion of three carbon intermediates to glucose are pyruvate carboxylase, and phosphoenopyruvate carboxykinase; increased synthesis of these substances in the liver occurs in the presence of high levels of glucagon, catecholamines, glucocorticoids, and low levels of insulin (Exton, 1972), precisely the hormonal environment present during the catabolic phase of injury.

Similar enzymatic adaptation occurs following prolonged starvation, but the major difference between the hormonal adaptation to starvation and the response to injury is the presence of increased sympathetic activity resulting in elaboration of catecholamines, which characterises the response in the stressed state. Catecholamines, therefore, may not only participate in directing three carbon fragment flow back to six carbon synthesis but also determine body glucose mass and the extent of glucose cycling.

Heat production at the cellular level appears to be regulated by ATP hydrolysis and ADP stimulated substrate oxidation. In heat generating biologic systems, ADP is the most critical substance for 'setting' the respiratory rate in mitochondria, a regulatory process known as acceptor control (Hochahka, 1974). The cycling of glucose requires energy and utilises ATP and generates ADP. Oxygen consumption is closely related to the rate of glucose flow through the extracellular space, and this relationship occurs at the time when glucose is not the major fuel source being oxidised. One explanation for this relationship is suggested by the hypothesis that ADP generated by the 'futile cycle' of glucose controls the oxidation of fuel, hence heat production and oxygen consumption can be related to glucose cycling through the ATP—ADP shuttle.

Increased glucose flow through the extracellular compartment is interrupted in the injured patient by gram negative infection. Our preliminary investigations suggest the metabolic block occurs at the level of glucose outflow from the liver (i.e., failure of hepatic gluconeogenesis), findings consistent with the effects of gram negative infection in animals (La Noue et al, 1968). With diminution of glucose cycling, there is a simultaneous decrease in oxygen consumption. Although administration of glucose and insulin will provide available substrate for the periphery, this therapy is not effective in relieving the specific metabolic block which interferes with hepatic production of glucose, and further therapy should be aimed toward specific correction of the altered physiology.

Finally, it should be re-emphasised that both substrate flow and heat production are controlled by the central nervous system, acting by way of the sympathetic nervous system. Increased sympathetic outflow from the hypothalamus carefully regulates mobilisation of body fuel, flow rates of substrate, and final oxidation, and this finely orchestrated metabolic response to injury is controlled and directed by the elaboration of catecholamines.

The opinions or assertions contained herein are the private views of the authors and are not to be construed as official or as reflecting the views of the Department of the Army or the Department of Defense.

References

Barr, P-O, Birke, G, Liljedahl, S-O and Plantin, L-O (1968) *Lancet, i,* 254
Cahill, GF Jr, Herrera, MG, Morgan, AP, Soelder, JS, Steinke, J, Levy, PL, Reichard, GA Jr and Kipnis, DM (1966) *J. Clin. Invest., 45,* 1751
Caldwell, FT Jr (1962) *Ann. Surg., 155,* 119
Cannon, WB, Newton, HF, Bright, EM, Menkin, V and Moore, RM (1929) *Amer. J. Physiol., 89,* 84
Cope, O, Nardi, GL, Quijano, M, Rovit, RL, Stanbury, JB and Wight, A (1953) *Ann. Surg., 137,* 165
Cuthbertson, DP (1930) *Biochem. J., 24,* 1244
Cuthbertson, DP (1932) *Quart. J. exp. Med., 25, (New Series),* 233
Drucker, WR, Craig, J, Kingsbury, B, Hofmann, N and Woodward, H (1962) *Arch. Surg., 85,* 557
Exton, JH (1972) *Metabolism, 21,* 945
Gump, FE, Long, C, Killian, P and Kinney, JM (1974) *J. Trauma, 14,* 378
Hlad, CJ Jr, Elrick, H and Witten, TA (1956) *J. clin. Invest., 35,* 1139
Hochachka, PW (1974) *Fed. Proc., 33,* 2162
LaNoue, KF, Mason, AD Jr and Bickel, RG (1968) *Computer and Biomedical Research, 2,* 51
Long, CL, Spencer, JL, Kinney, JM and Geiger, JW (1971) *A. appl. Physiol., 31,* 110
Unger, RH (1972) *Diabetes, 20,* 834
Unger, RH and Orci, L (1975) *Lancet, i,* 14
Wilmore, DW, Long, JM, Mason, AD Jr, Skreen, RW and Pruitt, BA Jr (1974) *Ann. Surg., 180,* 653
Zawacki, BE, Spitzer, KW, Mason, AD Jr and Johns, LA (1970) *Ann. Surg., 171,* 236

Aetiology and Treatment of Disorders of Fat Metabolism

J W L DAVIES and S-O LILJEDAHL

MRC Industrial Injuries and Burns Unit, Accident Hospital, Birmingham, England, and Department of Surgery, Regionsjukhuset, Linköping, Sweden

Introduction

A substantial part of the body stores of energy rich materials is contained in adipose tissue, the quantities of which may vary between 5 and 25% of body weight. The energy reserves in fat are substantial compared with those contained in either freely available protein or carbohydrate. The body content of carbohydrate (as glucose or glycogen) is very small and under normal metabolic conditions may last less than 12 hours. In conditions with a markedly elevated metabolic rate the carbohydrate reserves will only last a few hours. The potentially large reserves of energy in protein are only relatively labile since less than 1 kg of muscle or other tissue protein can be catabolised per day yielding about 30 g of nitrogen and less than 4MJ of energy. Thus in the absence of a substantial carbohydrate intake fat must provide a large part of the energy requirements. If this need is not supplied by dietary fat the body reserves of fat as triglycerides in adipose tissue will be mobilised.

This process of mobilisation of fat reserves consists of the lipolysis or hydrolysis of triglycerides to fatty acids and glycerol. The former may consist of either stearic, palmitic or oleic acids or occasionally one or more of the essential unsaturated fatty acids such as linoleic or linolenic acids. The lipolytic process is regulated by the enzyme triglyceride lipase the activity of which appears to be controlled by the amount of 3-5 cyclic AMP in adipose tissue (Carlson et al, 1970). A number of other compounds are known either to stimulate or discourage the lipolytic process. The rate of formation of fatty acids is stimulated by noradrenaline, adrenaline, thyroxine and glucagon and discouraged by insulin, prostaglandins and the various materials associated with the Krebs cycle, e.g.

300

glucose, lactate, pyruvate, acetoacetate and β hydroxybutyrate — these two latter
materials being called ketone bodies. The stimulatory effect of noradrenaline has
been studied by giving dogs a slow noradrenaline infusion (0.5 μg/kg/min) and
observing the five times increase in fatty acid production (Carlson et al, 1965).
Patients with extensive burns have high rates of noradrenaline production and
high levels of free fatty acids in serum, a relationship which statistically is highly
significant (Birke et al, 1972).

Following the lipolysis of the triglycerides the fatty acids are bound to plasma
albumin in ratios of up to 6 molecules of fatty acid per albumin molecule. The
glycerol remains available as one of the substrates required for the synthesis of
triglycerides at times when the supply of fatty acids exceeds requirements. The
concentration of fatty acids in serum is an index of the rate of fat mobilisation,
it is less than 0.5 mmol per litre under basal conditions but may exceed 1.5 mmol
per litre when energy expenditure is high. These albumin-bound fatty acids are
available to all body tissues and appear to be utilised, in direct proportion to the
concentration, as a source of energy by all tissues except those of the central
nervous system. In a normal adult male about 200 g of fatty acids are liberated
from triglycerides by lipolysis per 24 hours. A greater rate of lipolysis occurs
when the energy requirements are raised, as in patients with burns or other forms
of severe injury.

The plasma also contains other materials which have a high lipid content:

1. *Chylomicra* which are very small globules between 0.4 and 3.0 μm in diameter
consisting mainly of triglycerides but also containing relatively small amounts of
phospholipids, cholesterol and protein. The chylomicra are derived from dietary
fat and may account for the transport of about 100 g of fat per day in an adult
male eating a normal diet. As with fatty acid transport both the concentration
of chylomicra and the total quantity of fat transported in this form is raised following severe injury.

2. *Lipoproteins* which contain various amounts of lipid are synthesised in the
liver. The very low density lipoproteins (densities up to 1.006) which contain the
most lipid, transport triglycerides. The low density lipoproteins with densities
between 1.006 and 1.063 carry cholesterol around the body. Little is known
about the function of the high density lipoproteins having densities greater than
1.063.

3. *The plasma triglycerides* arise either from dietary fat via the gastrointestinal
tract (exogenous triglycerides) or from the liver as very low density lipoproteins
which contain endogenous triglycerides. Dietary fat is hydrolysed in the presence
of bile by pancreatic and intestinal lipases either completely to fatty acids or partially to monoglycerides. Glycerol and the short chain fatty acids are water soluble
and are absorbed by active transport. The fatty acids and glycerol recombine
within the intestinal cells to form triglycerides, which then aggregate to form
chylomicra.

301

4. *The phospholipids* such as choline, ethanolamine and serine are found in plasma, adipose tissue, other tissues, in cell membranes and form an important transport system in the body.

5. *Cholesterol* as the main constituent of the low density lipoproteins is the other main lipid material found in both the plasma and adipose tissue.

The following studies have shown the changes in the serum levels of triglycerides, fatty acids, phospholipids and cholesterol which result from severe injury and the treatment required to prevent, if possible, the injury having a fatal outcome.

The Relationship Between Serum Lipid Levels, Severity of Burning, Infusion of Fat, Environmental Temperature

Thirty-eight patients with burns covering a wide range of severity were divided into three groups, 7 patients had burns covering less than 15% of the body surface, 14 patients had burns covering between 15 and 30% and 17 patients had burns covering more than 30% of the body surface. The concentrations of the various lipid fractions were measured at daily intervals for the first 7 days and then at 2 or 3 day intervals for up to 6 weeks after burning. The patients were treated in wards with air temperatures around 22°C. None of the patients received any intravenous fat emulsions (Birke et al, 1965).

All patients with extensive burns (i.e. covering more than one-third of the body surface) showed raised concentrations of fatty acids in plasma during the first few days after burning. A twofold increase in concentration over that observed in normal individuals was common on the first and second days after burning when the fatty acid levels corresponded to a potential rate of energy production around 8 MJ per day. In two groups of patients with burns of 25—85% the effects were studied in subgroups of: (a) addition of 500 ml 20% Intralipid (4 MJ)/day for 8 days in addition to infused amino acids and glucose; (b) air temperature of 32°C (RH 20—25%) but without fat, the controls being around 22°C and uncontrolled humidity (Carlson & Liljedahl, 1971; Birke et al, 1972). Both the administration of fat and treatment in a warm dry environment reduced these raised fatty acid levels to nearer normal values, which corresponded to the lower potential rate of energy production around 4 MJ per day.

The two groups of patients treated either with or without infusions of fat emulsion received identical forms of treatment except with regard to energy input. The patients given mixtures of amino acids and glucose received energy inputs averaging 6 MJ per day, in contrast the mixture of amino acids and the fat emulsion provided about 10 MJ of energy per day to the other group of patients. The mechanism by which the increased energy input reduces the fatty acid levels has not yet been fully elucidated. The following observations have yet to be adequately reconciled.

302

1) The increased concentration of fatty acids suggests that the lipolysis of triglycerides occurs at a greater rate than that of the catabolism of the fatty acids to carbon dioxide and water either directly or via ketone bodies. The production of fatty acids often appears to be greater than that required for energy production (Carlson, 1970).

2) The administration of relatively large quantities of the triglyceride emulsion Intralipid reduces the plasma fatty acid levels of the patients receiving it to a greater degree than observed in patients receiving substantial amounts of carbohydrate (Carlson & Liljedahl, 1971).

3) The administration of considerable quantities of glucose reduces the level of plasma fatty acids (Roe & Kinney, 1962). This effect is probably due to the raised insulin concentration stimulated by an increasing blood sugar concentration, since insulin has a marked anti-lipolytic effect curtailing triglyceride mobilisation and the associated ketone body production (Blackburn et al, 1973). However some severely injured patients, particularly those with burns show insulin resistance (Allison et al, 1968) soon after injury. At this time a rapid intravenous input of 25 g of glucose is accompanied by a 4- or 5-fold increase in blood sugar concentration, a fall in plasma fatty acid levels and almost no change in insulin levels.

The mechanism by which treatment in a warm dry environment causes a reduction in the plasma fatty acid levels in patients with burns appears to be simply that in these conditions there is a reduced rate of energy production, as shown by a reduction in oxygen consumption (Barr et al, 1968, 1969). When the environmental temperature is within the thermoneutral zone there is a reduced need for the catabolism of the body stores of energy rich materials to maintain body temperature (Davies et al, 1969). At an environmental temperature around $32^{\circ}C$ the body heat loss by radiation, convection and conduction is minimal.

Since the administration of a fat emulsion and treatment in a warm dry environment both reduce the plasma fatty acid levels, these two beneficial forms of treatment have been combined in the treatment of burned patients during the last few years. The observed plasma fatty acids in these recent patients are lower than when fat emulsions *or* warm dry conditions were used during treatment.

As shown above patients with severe burns or other forms of injury treated without fat emulsions or in a cool environment show markedly raised plasma fatty acid levels. These raised levels lead to an accumulation of fat in the liver (Feigelson et al, 1961) if their rate of production from triglycerides exceeds their catabolism to carbon dioxide and water. In many patients the mobilisation of fatty acids appears to be excessive since many patients with injuries which have a fatal outcome have been shown to have gross fatty infiltrations in their liver tissue (Sevitt, 1957). As these high levels of fatty acids have been implicated

303

in episodes of fat embolism attempts have been made to reduce these high levels. Studies carried out in dogs with high fatty acid levels induced by either injury or the administration of noradrenaline showed that the ganglionic blocking agent guanethidine could reduce pre-existing raised fatty acid levels or prevent their rise if given immediately after injury (Carlson et al, 1965; Carlson, 1970). Human growth hormone can also be used to increase plasma fatty acid levels since it is antagonistic to the effects of glucose inputs in injured patients. Roe and Kinney (1962) gave four patients with fractures glucose infusions which raised their blood sugar levels, raised their respiratory quotients and lowered their fatty acid levels. Subsequent administration of human growth hormone lowered their respiratory quotients and stimulated further fatty acid production. Whether the reduction of high fatty acid levels or the prevention of their increase lessens the risk of fat embolism does not appear to have been conclusively demonstrated.

The changes in cholesterol concentration which halve during the first week after burning are due to corresponding falls in the concentration of low density lipoprotein which transports cholesterol around the body (Werner, 1969). It seems probable that the protein moiety of lipoprotein is either synthesised at a reduced rate or undergoes excessive catabolism rather than that there is a decrease in the synthesis of cholesterol. Whatever is the cause of the lowered plasma cholesterol concentration there appears to be a significant relationship between the concentration of cholesterol and that of albumin in each plasma sample (Birke et al, 1965).

The studies of phospholipid levels indicate that the observed fall in concentration by about 50% during the first week after burning was not related to the severity of burning. The effect of treatment in the warmer drier environment was not determined. The increased phospholipid concentration resulting from the administration of Intralipid was no doubt due to the 1.2 per cent phospholipid used in the emulsification of the soya bean oil.

The plasma triglyceride levels were raised above the normal value in patients with extensive burns during the first week after burning but then subsequently decreased to normal values. Otherwise neither less severe burning injury nor the administration of fat emulsions nor treatment in a warm dry environment significantly changed the plasma triglyceride levels.

While the lack of effect of fat emulsions on the triglyceride levels may be unexpected, since the fat emulsions mainly consist of triglycerides, the similar biological behaviour of the endogenous and exogenous triglycerides has led to an extensive range of studies in which the triglycerides of Intralipid are used to study the behaviour of triglycerides in various disease states where the endogenous triglycerides show hypo- or hyper-concentrations. Many of these studies involve the intravenous fat tolerance test (Rössner, 1974). In this test 10% Intralipid is given intravenously in volumes of 1 ml per kg body weight and the rate of disappearance of the emulsion determined by the change in plasma opacity with time over a period of 40 minutes. In normal persons the rate of reduction in opacity is biphasic. The early rate of change is linear, corresponding to a zero order reaction rate and having a rate constant K_1 expressed in μmol per minute. As the opacity decreases, a critical concentration is reached below which the rate of change corresponds to a first order reaction with a rate constant K_2 expressed as per cent of dose cleared per minute. It seems probable that K_1 reflects the total available enzyme activity for removing emulsion from the bloodstream, and K_2 a number of factors such as the rate of blood flow past the enzyme sites and the volume of distribution of the emulsion. A number of studies (e.g. Boberg et al, 1969) have shown that K_1 and K_2 are rarely, if ever, related to one another. While K_1 and the plasma triglyceride concentrations are not normally related there is often an inverse relationship between K_2 and the plasma triglyceride levels.

Both rate constants increase after a period of starvation and increase more if the starvation is associated with surgical or accidental injury. A detailed study of the rate constant K_1 by Wilmore et al (1973) has shown that starvation, stress, injury, heparin and high levels of insulin all increase K_1 and may maintain it at raised values for considerable periods of time.

Studies with labelled Intralipid have shown that this increased rate of clearance of the fat emulsion from the plasma is the result of metabolism of the triglycerides rather than clearance of foreign particles by the reticuloendothelial system. When [14] carbon labelled triglycerides are administered intravenously at least 70% of the [14] carbon appears within four hours of the injection as exhaled carbon dioxide (Walker & Johnston, 1971; Fegetter, 1974). The rate of removal of fat from the plasma has been shown by Lawson (1965) to be similar to the rate of removal of chylomicra derived from orally administered fat, and can occur at a rate of 3.8 g fat per kg body weight per 24 hours (266 g per day for a normal adult male [Wretlind, 1972]). An observed reduction in the respiratory quotient to near 0.7 strongly suggests that there is an increased rate of oxidation of fat. Following severe injury fat utilisation may exceed 5 g/kg/day.

The triglyceride content of adipose tissue appears to have a high rate of turnover, implying considerable metabolic activity. The ability to supply considerable amounts of fatty acids at short notice when carbohydrate inputs are nil or inadequate indicates that active lipolytic mechanisms must be available. Similarly adequate fat reserves can be maintained only if the synthetic mechanism causing triglyceride formation is active during periods when fatty acids and glycerophosphate are available in amounts which are greater than those immediately required for energy production. Circulating triglycerides (as chylomicra) can also be incorporated into adipose tissue, but only after breakdown by lipases in the cell membranes to fatty acids prior to entering the adipose tissue cells where they are resynthesised into triglycerides for storage. In the presence of sufficient insulin circulating glucose can enter adipose tissue cells and be then synthesised into triglycerides via pyruvate, glycerophosphate and fatty acids.

The lipolysis of triglycerides to fatty acids appears to be primarily controlled by the catecholamines. A transient increase in plasma adrenaline levels stimulates lipolysis for the production of enhanced energy reserves to satisfy those needed for the 'fright, fight, flight' reaction. The studies reported by Carlson et al (1965) who stimulated an increase in plasma fatty acid levels in dogs by infusions of noradrenaline suggests that this catecholamine is also involved in the control of energy production from fat.

As plasma adrenaline, noradrenaline and fatty acid levels are raised following severe surgical or accidental injury it has been concluded that an augmented release of catecholamines associated with sympathetic overactivity may be mainly responsible for the pattern of changes in lipids which follow injury (Liljedahl et al, 1968).

References

Allison, SP, Hinton, P and Chamberlain, MJ (1968) *Lancet, ii*, 1113
Barr, P-O, Birke, G, Liljedahl, S-O and Plantin, L-O (1968) *Lancet, i*, 164
Barr, P-O, Birke, G, Liljedahl, S-O and Plantin, L-O (1969) *Scand.J. plast. reconstr. Surg., 3*, 30
Birke, G, Carlson, L-A and Liljedahl, S-O (1965) *Acta med. scand., 178*, 337
Birke, G, Carlson, L-A, von Euler, US, Liljedahl, S-O and Plantin, L-O (1972) *Acta chir. scand., 138*, 321
Blackburn, GL, Flatt, JP, Clowes, GHA, O'Donnell, TF and Hensle, TE (1973) *Ann. Surg., 177*, 588
Boberg, J, Carlson, L-A and Hallberg, D (1969) *J. Atheroscl. Res., 9*, 159
Carlson, L-A (1970) *Ciba Foundation Symposium on Energy Metabolism in Trauma*. (Ed) R Porter and J Knight. Page 155
Carlson, L-A, Liljedahl, S-O and Wirsén, C (1965) *Acta med. scand., 178*, 81
Carlson, L-A, Butcher, RW and Micheli, H (1970) *Acta med. scand., 187*, 525
Carlson, L-A and Liljedahl, S-O (1971) *Acta chir scand., 137*, 123
Davies, JWL, Liljedahl, S-O and Birke, G (1969) *Injury, 1*, 43
Feigelson, EB, Pfaff, WW, Karmen, A and Steinberg, D (1961) *J. clin. Invest., 40*, 2171
Fegetter, J (1974) Personal communication
Lawson, LJ (1965) *Brit. J. Surg., 52*, 795
Liljedahl, S-O, Westermark, L and Wirsén, C (1968) *Combined Injuries and Shock*. Intermedes Proceedings. Page 303
Roe, CF and Kinney, JM (1962) *Surg. Forum, 13*, 369
Rössner, S (1974) *Acta med. scand. Suppl. 564*, 1
Walker, WF and Johnston, IDA (1971) *The Metabolic Basis of Surgical Care*. Chapter 13. Heinemann Ltd, London. Page 212
Werner, M (1969) *Clin. Chim. Acta, 25*, 299
Wilmore, DW, Moylan, JA, Helmkamp, GM and Pruitt, BA (1973) *Ann. Surg., 178*, 503
Wretlind, A (1972) *Nutr. and Metab., 14, Suppl.1*, 1

The Importance of Zinc and Other Essential Elements After Injury

G S FELL and R R BURNS

University Department of Pathological Biochemistry, Royal Infirmary, Glasgow, Scotland

Introduction

The degree of attention accorded to the various essential elements by clinicians is related to the ease with which deficiency or excess can be linked to a clearly recognisable clinical syndrome. Thus iron is known to be important because its deficiency leads to anaemia. Iodine deficiency is associated with cretinism, myxoedema and goitre, and excess or deficiency of potassium with cardiac arrhythmias. Other elements which have equally well established biochemical and biological importance do not appear to exert as clearly defined a clinical effect. The subtle consequences of trace element imbalances caused by dietary deficiency, in particular during intravenous nutrition, or by malabsorption or losses induced by medication and as a consequence of injury, are still imperfectly appreciated in the clinical field. The nutritional importance of essential trace elements such as zinc, chromium and manganese have been reviewed by Underwood (1971), and should lead to more intensive study of changes in essential element metabolism after injury. Analytical methods now widely available allow the measurement of almost all essential elements in blood, urine and other biological material, but the interpretation of such data in terms of clinical effect is not always possible.

The biological consequences of such minor element imbalances are interrelated and affect various biochemical pathways. Severe deficiency is associated with the failure of normal growth in children or reduced resistance to infection in adults, but clear clinical syndromes are not often recognisable. It is important to ensure an adequate supply of such elements when prolonged intravenous nutrition using the newer synthetic preparations is required. We still require more knowledge of the normal requirements of these elements and of their increased needs after injury.

Much has been written concerning the importance of zinc in intracellular bio-chemical reactions, and of the nutritional requirement of the metal for normal growth and development. Disturbance of zinc metabolism occurs in various diseases, during infection and after injury (Halsted et al, 1974). Zinc is now included in dietary recommendations (Mertz, 1974), and addition of zinc to intravenous nutritional regimes is advised by Wretlind (1972). Zinc is an integral part of some 20 metalloenzymes and therefore its deficiency could affect many different cellular processes. DNA and RNA synthesis require zinc at various stages, and protein synthesis has been shown to be reduced in the experimentally zinc depleted rat. Specific failure of individual protein synthesis by the liver has been suggested in the zinc deficient rat. Failure of the synthesis of retinal binding protein results in low levels of plasma vitamin A in spite of adequate liver stores of the vitamin. This mechanism has been postulated as the basis of vitamin A resistant night blindness in cases of alcoholic cirrhosis, which was one of the earliest conditions associated with disorder of zinc metabolism (Halsted & Smith, 1974). The average dietary intake of zinc is about 200 mmol/day, and zinc is present in many foodstuffs, and an especially rich source is animal protein. Estimates of the extent of intestinal absorption vary from 10–40%, but the regulation of absorption is not understood (Becker & Hoesktra, 1971). The initial uptake of absorbed zinc is by the liver, followed by distribution to every tissue in the body. More than 98% of zinc is intracellular and skeletal muscle contains at least 60% of the total body content by virtue of its large total mass. Some tissues such as prostate and bone have higher concentrations of zinc per unit weight.

In circulating blood most of the zinc is within the red cells in the form of the zinc metalloenzyme, carbonic anhydrase. The nucleated white cells have even higher amounts of zinc per cell, present as metalloproteins of unknown function.

Plasma zinc concentration has been extensively studied and shown to decrease in a non-specific manner in numerous diseases and after injury (Halsted & Smith, 1974). The normal range is $12-18\mu$mol Zn/litre plasma. However, numerous factors affect the values such as the age, sex, and previous diet of the subject and the manner of sample collections and technique of analysis. Comparison of observed plasma zinc concentrations with normal values therefore is of limited value without careful control of all such variables.

The zinc in plasma is distribution among three main fractions. Around 40% is firmly bound to a zinc containing α_2^- macroglobulin. This particular protein may eventually be found to have a role in zinc transport but its concentration does not alter in conditions where plasma zinc is known to be decreased. The majority of zinc in plasma, 60–80% is loosely bound to albumin and this is probably the main transport mechanism for zinc. Newly absorbed zinc binds to albumin and is transported to the liver, and thence redistributed to tissues. Deficiency of intake or failure of intestinal absorption will be reflected in lowered albumin-zinc concentrations, and estimation of this plasma fraction should provide a more informative index of zinc status than measurement of total plasma zinc concentration. A smaller, but important fraction of plasma zinc is that bound to lower molecular weight ligands, principally amino acids. This amounts to some 2–10% of the total zinc content in plasma and is in equilibrium with the albumin-bound fraction (Giroux & Henkin, 1972). The low molecular fraction is filtered by the kidney, and increases in this plasma compartment will affect urinary zinc output. Normal urinary zinc output is small, around 10 μmol zinc/day, and this is not affected by variation in the oral intake of dietary zinc, the main excretory pathway being from the gastrointestinal tract into faeces. The total filtered load of zinc per day is estimated to be some 300 mmol and less than 5% of this is found in urine. Thus it appears that renal tubular absorption is near to maximal efficiency and any increase in the filtered load presented to the renal tubules will result in increased urinary zinc losses.

Increases in the low molecular fraction of plasma zinc could arise in a number of different ways. Certain drugs could compete with zinc for binding sites for zinc on albumin, and displace the metal thus increasing the filterable plasma fraction. This may be part of the mechanism whereby steroid therapy lowers total plasma zinc and increases urinary zinc excretion. Molecules able to form stable coordination complexes with zinc which have a stronger formation constant than that of zinc-albumin will remove the metal from the protein. Such molecules may arise during alterations in metabolism after injury, in disease, or may be given as intravenous infusion as drugs, or during parenteral nutrition. During the net protein catabolism after injury amino acids are released which can form stable zinc complexes. A particularly stable compound is zinc (histidine)$_2$, and this has been shown not to bind as effectively to plasma proteins as $ZnCl_2$, and to form a readily ultrafilterable fraction in plasma. When this [65]Zn labelled complex was given orally to rats an immediate increase in urinary [65]Zn activity was noted in contrast to the delayed appearance of [65]Zn when [65]ZnCl$_2$ was administered. Increased urinary zinc losses during parenteral feeding are described (Freeman et al, 1975), and complex formation of zinc with amino-sugars is suggested as the mechanism.

During therapeutic calorie restriction in obese subjects an increased excretion of zinc in urine persists as long as therapy is continued. In spite of this negative zinc balance, plasma zinc concentrations do not decrease (Spencer et al, 1971). It is tempting to speculate that a redistribution of zinc within the plasma fractions occurs, and more zinc than normal is present as the low molecular weight complex. During the ketosis of starvation greatly increased concentrations of acids such as β-hydroxybutyric acid are present and this type of molecule is known to form suitably stable complexes with zinc at physiological pH. Such a mechanism could explain the zincuria observed in untreated diabetic patients with ketoacidosis. Furthermore, the infusion of hydroxybutyric acid, suggested as an experimental means of reducing negative nitrogen balance after injury

309

could be expected to produce pronounced zinc loss in urine.

In the injured patient an induced zinc deficiency can thus arise in a number of ways.

Inadequate Intake of Zinc

Analysis of the zinc content of some hospital diets, by Osis et al (1972) showed that the average zinc content was less than the recommended 200 mmol Zn/day. Administration of intravenous fluids, without addition of zinc, will induce a degree of tissue zinc deficiency.

Increased Loss of Zinc

Increased loss of zinc in urine occurs as part of the metabolic response to injury. The extent and duration of the urine zinc loss is dependent upon the nature and severity of the injury (Fell et al, 1973). In a case of tetanus in a 23-year old male (IM), who was in a pronounced catabolic state, with a negative nitrogen balance of some 20g N/day, a greatly increased urinary output of zinc lasted until the eventual death of this patient (Figure 1). The urinary loss which occurs in all patients undergoing elective surgery does not appear to affect significantly body zinc content, unless there are additional losses or there is an inadequate dietary zinc intake. Five patients undergoing elective surgery for replacement of diseased hip joints were given ^{65}Zn orally for some 3–4 weeks prior to surgery. This is

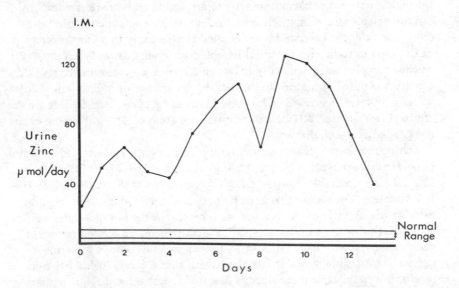

Figure 1. Urinary zinc excretion in a case of tetanus (IM). [Normal range of urine zinc is indicated by band between the horizontal lines]

sufficient time to allow equilibration of the radioisotope with all body tissues. Excretion of [65]Zn in urine and faeces, and the whole body [65]Zn activity were measured in the period before and after surgery. Although an increase in urine [65]Zn was noted during the period of negative nitrogen balance after surgery, we found no alteration in the rate of change of elimination of the whole body [65]Zn, after surgery, compared to the period prior to surgery.

Of course these patients were in good nutritional condition and were able to resume normal oral diet within 24 hr of their operation. In more seriously ill patients, with a more pronounced catabolic period, zinc losses may be greater. After severe burning injury losses of more than 10 times the normal amount of zinc in urine can persist for several weeks (Davies & Fell, 1974).

Considerable additional losses in wound exudate are likely and although oral diet was taken by these patients it may not have always provided sufficient zinc.

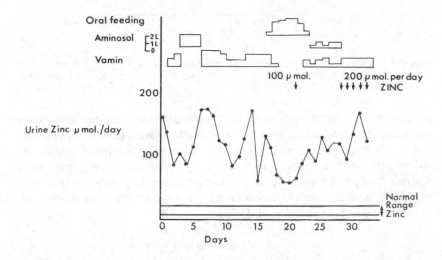

Figure 2. Urinary zinc excretion of patient DS with ulcerative colitis, while receiving periods of total parenteral nutrition. ↓ indicates intravenous infusion of zinc. Day 0 on the lower scale was the 12th day after colectomy

A 53-year old man (DS) underwent colectomy for ulcerative colitis and developed severe post-operative problems which required periods of parenteral nutrition. We found his urinary zinc to be as high as 150 μmol/day, and this loss was in addition to zinc excreted in intestinal drainage fluid, blood and sweat. The total losses were estimated as several hundred μmol Zn/day, and on this basis infusion of 200 μmol Zn/day was started (Figure 2). A basal requirement of around 20 μmol Zn/day has been recommended (Wretlind, 1972), but in such seriously ill patients this amount needs to be considerably increased. The plasma zinc level in our patient did show an increase following intravenous zinc admini-

311

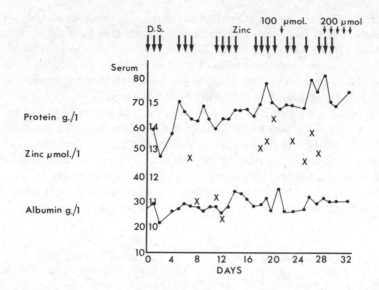

Figure 3. Changes in plasma proteins and plasma zinc in the patient (DS) following colectomy, receiving intravenous zinc. ↓ Protein infusion. ↓ Zinc infusion. x Plasma zinc concentration

stration, but was never particularly low. Although an increase in plasma proteins was seen, considerable quantities of blood products were given to the patient and it is difficult to claim an improvement in plasma protein synthesis due to the zinc therapy (Figure 3). In view of the suggestion that protein synthesis is depressed, as part of the response to injury, it is probably advisable to ensure that an induced zinc deficiency does not further reduce the efficiency of protein synthetic pathways (Fodor, et al, 1972).

MAGNESIUM

The biochemical importance of magnesium is well established, since more than 100 different intracellular enzymes require magnesium for their activation. All reactions involving phosphate transfer, including all stages of oxidative phosphorylation and the activity of ATPases are magnesium dependent. Polysomes require magnesium for stability and thus protein synthesis can be affected by magnesium deficiency. Nerve transmission and muscular contraction require magnesium and calcium ion concentrations to be in the correct ratio for normal function.

The total body content of magnesium is around 1200 mmol, and of this some 60% is in bone. Magnesium is the most abundant divalent intracellular cation and less than 1% is in the extracellular fluid. Studies with magnesium radioisotope, ^{28}Mg, show that only 15% of the total body magnesium is exchangeable within

24 hr (more than 90% of ^{42}K is exchangeable within the same period).

Recommended dietary intake is 10–15 mmol/day, and is provided by most mixed diets. About one-third of the dietary intake is excreted in urine, faecal magnesium representing mainly the unabsorbed portion of the diet. Gastrointestinal fluids, such as gastric juice or ileostomy fluid have high concentrations of magnesium. Prolonged losses of these fluids with inadequate replacement is the most common cause of magnesium deficiency. The regulation of plasma magnesium is by renal control of urinary magnesium excretion. Deficiency of intake or excessive losses are readily detected by measurement of the urinary output of the element. Changes in dietary intake from 36 mmol to less than 1 mmol mg/day resulted in no significant change in plasma magnesium but urinary output fell from 12 to less than 1 mmol mg/day (Heaton, 1969).

From detailed study of prolonged dietary magnesium depletion in normal subjects, Dunn and Walser (1966) concluded that plasma magnesium concentration was a poor guide to the degree of magnesium deficiency. Barnes (1969) records a patient with an ileostomy drainage who lost, over a four week period, 170 mmol of magnesium but whose plasma magnesium was 0.75 mmol mg/l (normal range 0.8 ± 0.15 mmol/l). The urinary excretion was less than 2 mmol mg/day.

Confirmation of reduced tissue magnesium concentration is not obtained by direct biopsy of muscle tissue, since muscle magnesium concentration does not reflect total body magnesium reserves (Alfrey et al, 1974). Indirect evidence

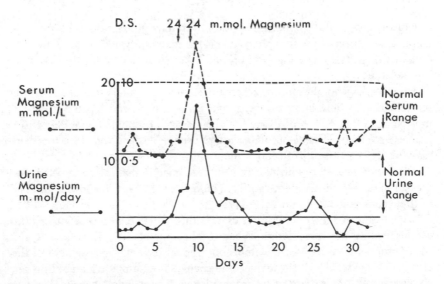

Figure 4. Changes in plasma and urinary magnesium in the patient DS following colectomy. ↓ indicates intravenous magnesium

313

of tissue deficiency may be obtained by an infusion test (Thoren, 1963). A measured amount, 0.25 mmol mg/kg, is given intravenously and more than 80% of this should be excreted in urine within 24 hours if tissue reserves are adequate.

Some measurements of plasma and urinary magnesium following surgery of the gastrointestinal tract are illustrated in Figure 4. These results were obtained for patient DS described previously, and show the initially low output of urinary magnesium suggestive of an inadequate intake to compensate for losses in intestinal fluid drainage. Infusions of magnesium were given over a two day period, and serum and urine magnesium levels increased but were not well maintained.

Shils (1973) suggests that the urinary magnesium should be kept above 5 mmol/day and that this is a suitable way to regulate the intravenous dosage. The basal intravenous requirements of 0.04 mmol/kg/day suggested by Wretlind (1972), will have to be increased in many instances, particularly when gastrointestinal surgery is required. Oral supplements of magnesium salts may be given but these correct deficiencies very slowly since the ion is poorly absorbed from the gut. Clinical effects of magnesium deficiency are not easily described. Severe deficiency resulting in low plasma magnesium concentrations can produce muscular tetany. Changes in personality, nausea, anorexia and extreme muscular weakness are also associated with magnesium lack. Long term magnesium depletion may be one additional factor in development of atherosclerotic disease (Bloch, 1973), and myocardial muscle appears selectively depleted of magnesium after sudden infarction (Behr & Burton, 1973).

PHOSPHORUS

The biochemistry of phosphorus is in part considered in relation to that of calcium, since a form of calcium phosphate is the main inorganic constituent of bone. Of the total body content of around 19 mole phosphorus, 70—80% is in the skeleton.

However, organo-phosphorus compounds are an essential component of every biochemical reaction. Energy transformations within the cell depends upon molecules such as ATP which have the high energy phosphate bond. Phosphorus is an essential part of nucleoproteins and phospholipids and therefore the element plays a part in all aspects of cellular metabolism.

Dietary deficiency of phosphorus is not recorded in man, since the element is present in readily available foodstuffs in amounts sufficient to allow an intake of the recommended 30 mmol per day.

When commercial fat emulsion is used as the main energy source during intravenous feeding extreme alterations in phosphate metabolism do not occur, since the phospholipid content of the emulsion supplies the daily requirement of the element (Vinnars, 1974). However, some changes in phosphate metabolism can be observed even in patients given fat emulsions. The sequential changes in plasma and urine phosphate for patient DS are shown in Figure 5.

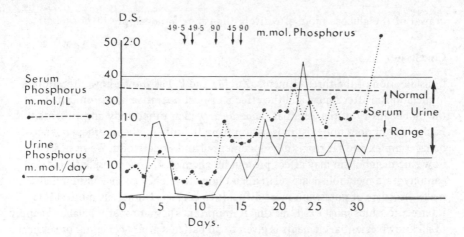

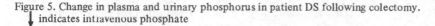

Figure 5. Change in plasma and urinary phosphorus in patient DS following colectomy. ⬇ indicates intravenous phosphate

A lower than normal urine and plasma phosphate were observed at first. It is possible that urinary phosphate will be altered during infusion of amino acids since they can block the renal tubular reabsorption of phosphate. Also it should be remembered that synthetic amino acid mixtures are deficient in phosphate compared to the preparations based upon a casein hydrolysate.

No definite clinical signs were noted in the patient DS during the period of initial hypophosphataemia and little evidence of improvement was found after infusion of phosphate, although the buffering properties of the phosphate anion did appear to help in regulation of his acid-base disturbances. The onset of renal failure in this terminal patient explains the rapidly rising plasma phosphate levels.

However, in general it would be preferable to ensure a basal input of at least 0.15 mmol P/kg/day as suggested by Wretlind (1972) rather than allow deficiency to develop. Regular estimation of plasma and urinary phosphate levels will give guidance as to whether additional amounts need be administered. After injury phosphate excretion is increased and Cuthbertson (1930) considered that this reflected the catabolic breakdown of soft tissue, since the urinary pattern of phosphate output paralleled that of nitrogen rather than calcium even in fractures. Observation of very low plasma phosphate concentration in patients fed intravenously are reported. This is especially found when 50% glucose is used as the calorie source, and the hypophosphataemia is accompanied by depression in red cell glycolytic intermediates such as 2 : 3 diphosphoglycerate (Travis et al, 1971). The clinical effects may involve depression of oxygen transport to the tissues, and Prins (1974) reports such patients have altered states of consciousness and extreme muscular flaccidity. These symptons were relieved by with-

315

drawal of the glucose more effectively than by simple supply of phosphate.

Conclusion

Consideration of the three elements, Zn, Mg and P, has shown how alterations in metabolism after injury and the effects of post-operative nutrition can affect the biochemistry of the essential elements as well as other body constituents. Each element does not exist in isolation from the others, the interdependence being complex and far from fully documented and understood. We have seen how zinc metabolism may affect protein biochemistry, how phosphate and carbohydrate metabolism are related, and how deficiency of magnesium may make disorders of potassium more difficult to correct. Numerous more subtle interrelationships must exist, making it important that a properly balanced supply of all known essential elements is given to all patients after accidental or surgical trauma. The recommendations of Wretlind (1972) supply the basis for initial therapy, and specific additions may be made based upon further experience.

References

Alfrey, AC, Miller, NL and Butkus, D (1974) *J. Lab. Clin. Med., 84,* 153

Barnes, BA (1969) *Ann. NY Acad. Sci., 162,* 786

Becker, WM and Hockstra, WC In *Intestinal Absorption of Metal Ions, Trace Elements and Radionuclides.* (1971) (Ed) SC Skoryna and D Waldron-Edward. Pergamon Press, Oxford. Page 229

Behr, G and Burton, P (1973) *Lancet, ii,* 450

Bloch, N (1973) *Brit. J. Hosp. Med., 9,* 91

Cuthbertson, DP (1930) *Biochem. J., 24,* 1244

Davies, JWL and Fell, GS (1974) *Clin. Chim. Acta, 51,* 83

Dunn, MJ and Walser, M (1966) *Metabolism, 15,* 884

Fell, GS, Fleck, A, Cuthbertson, DP, Queen, K, Morrison, C, Bessent, RG and Husain, SL (1973) *Lancet, i,* 280

Fodor, L, Eschner, J, Dick, W and Ahnefield, FW (1972) *Anaesthetist, 12,* 456

Freeman, JB, Stegnik, LD, Meyer, PD, Fry, LK and Debstein, L (1975) *J. Surg. Research, 18,* 463

Giroux, EL and Henkin, RI (1972) *Biochem. Biophys. Acta, 273,* 64

Halsted, JA and Smith, CJ (1974) *Gastroenterology, 67,* 193

Halsted, JA, Smith, CJ and Irwin, MJ (1974) *J. clin. Nutr., 10,* 345

Heaton, FW (1969) *Ann. NY Acad. Sci., 162,* 775

Mertz, W (1974) *J. Amer. Dietetic Assoc., 64,* 163

Osis, D, Kramer, L, Wiatrowski, E and Spencer, H (1972) *Amer. J. clin. Nutr., 25,* 582

Prins, JG, Schrijver, H and Staghouwer, JH (1973) *Lancet, i,* 1253

Shils, ME (1973) In *Modern Nutrition in Health and Disease, 5th Edition.* Lea & Febiger. Chap. 6, page 289

Spencer, H, Osis, D, Kramer, L and Samachson, J (1971) In *Clinical Applications of Zinc Metabolism.* Springfield Press. Chap. 8, page 101

Thoren, L (1963) *Acta chir. Scand. Suppl. 306,* 52

Travis, SF, Sugerman, HJ, Ruberg, RL, Dudrick, SJ, Delivoria-Papadopolous, M,
    Miller, L and Oski, FA (1971) *New Eng. J. Med., 285,* 763
Underwood, EJ (1971) *Trace Elements in Human and Animal Nutrition, 3rd
    Edition.* Academic Press, London and New York
Vinnars, E (1974) *Clinical Care Medicine, 2,* 143
Wretlind, KAJ (1972) *Nutr. Metabolism, 14,* Suppl.1

317

Evaluation of Complete Intravenous Nutrition—including evaluation of glucose and glucose substitutes

ARVID WRETLIND

Nutrition Unit, Medical Faculty, Karolinska Institutet, Stockholm, Sweden

Introduction

A daily supply of energy and nutrients is necessary to maintain a patient in an optimal nutritional condition to offer the best resistance to illness and trauma, such as infections, burns, surgery etc. If normal oral nutrition is impossible or can be maintained only with difficulty, essential nutrients may be provided either by tube-feeding or by the intravenous route. Intravenous feeding should be used only when oral feeding or tube-feeding is impossible. As an alternative to normal oral feeding the nutrients or their metabolites should be supplied intravenously in the same quantity and form as they are normally transferred into the general circulation from the intestine following adequate oral feeding. The amounts of energy and nutrients supplied should cover the basal requirements as well as compensate increased losses and previous deficiencies.

The intravenous supply of the nutrients required does not cause any difficulties from the practical point of view. In order to maintain or restore the normal composition of the body and to obtain normal growth in infants by intravenous nutrition, it seems to be sufficient to supply the 29 nutrients or groups of nutrients given in Table I.

When all the nutrients shown in Table I are given intravenously, this is termed by us *Complete Intravenous Feeding.* However, the energy requirement may be covered with glucose and amino acids alone without fat (*'Hyperalimentation' according to Dudrick et al, 1968, 1969*). Because hypertonic glucose solutions are used, such intravenous feeding can be performed only via a central vein catheter. Complete intravenous nutrition including fat may be given either via a peripheral vein or a central vein catheter, and now the trend is to use complete

TABLE I. Nutrients Essential for Complete Intravenous Nutrition

Fluid	Water

Sources for synthesis of body protein and for energy	Amino acids
	Carbohydrates
	Fat
Minerals	Sodium
	Potassium
	Calcium
	Magnesium
	Iron
	Zinc
	Manganese
	Copper
	Chloride
	Phosphorus
	Fluoride
	Iodide
Water soluble vitamins	Thiamine
	Riboflavine
	Niacin
	Vitamin B_6
	Folacin
	Vitamin B_{12}
	Pantothenic acid
	Biotin
	Ascorbic acid
Fat soluble vitamins	Vitamin A
	Vitamin D
	Vitamin K_1
	Tocopherol

intravenous nutrition with fat.

TREND TOWARDS COMPLETE INTRAVENOUS NUTRITION

Adequate intravenous protein nutrition can be maintained by amino acid mixtures which have the proper composition for optimal utilisation. The explanation of the observed difference in the utilisation of different types of amino acid solutions may be that certain of the non-essential amino acids are not present in some of the preparations. The degree of utilisation may also depend on variations in the concentration of the amino acids in the various solutions.

An optimal amino acid preparation for intravenous nutrition should contain both the essential and the non-essential amino acids in the L-form, and in about the same proportions as found in the aminogram of body proteins or other proteins of high biological value (Wretlind, 1972). The essential amino acids should amount to about 45—50 per cent of the total amino acids. A high content of glycine should be avoided. The future trend in the development of intravenous nutrition will be to use such properly balanced amino acid preparations.

The utilisation of amino acids given intravenously will be optimal if the energy requirement is covered by simultaneous infusion of carbohydrate solution and fat emulsions. An amino acid mixture is best utilised when the ratio between the supply of energy and amino acid nitrogen is 120 : 1 — 200 : 1. The measures that will be taken to ensure the best possible utilisation of the amino acids given are summarised in Table II.

TABLE II. Measurements for Obtaining Optimal Nutritional Effects of Intravenous Alimentation

1 Adequate amounts of amino acids for adults, minimum 0.7 g/kg/day for infants, 2.5 g/kg/day
2 Adequate energy supply
3 At least 20 cal% from carbohydrates
4 Simultaneous supply of amino acids and energy
5 Adequate supply of other nutrients
6 Mobilisation; physical activity

With intravenous fat emulsions in combination with carbohydrate, the required amount of energy can readily be supplied intravenously in a small volume of isotonic fluid. No losses are observed wither in the urine or faeces. The eggyolk phospholipid-soybean oil emulsion Intralipid seems to have the highest tolerance and to be the least toxic of all available types of fat emulsions. Thrombophlebitis is very seldom observed when the infusions of fat emulsions are given in a peripheral vein. To reduce infusion volume, most of the energy supply has been given in the form of fat. The essential fatty acids are of great importance in order to maintain all the lipid containing membranes in the body in normal conditions.

In 1832 Latta reported infusions of salts to patients with cholera. Since that time infusions of solutions containing sodium, potassium, magnesium, calcium and chloride have been used and investigated in connection with intravenous feeding. It is obvious that all 12 essential minerals or electrolytes mentioned in Table I have to be included in a complete intravenous nutrition. Of these minerals, phosphorus and zinc are of special importance for patients on intravenous nutrition.

320

TABLE III. Tentatively Recommended Daily Allowances of Energy and Nutrients to Patients on Complete Intravenous Nutrition. The allowances will cover resting metabolism, moderate physical activity of a patient and specific dynamic action, but no increased need because of trauma, burns etc. Up to about double the amount may be given to adult with burn or other condition requiring increased requirements

	ADULT Allowance per kg body weight and day		NEONATE and INFANTS Allowance per kg body weight and day	
Water	30 ml		120-150 ml	
Energy	30 kcal = 0.13 MJ		90-120 kcal = 0.38-0.50 MJ	
Amino acid nitrogen	90 mg (0.7g of amino acids)		330 mg (2.5g of amino acids)	
Glucose or fructose	2 g		12-18 g	
Fat	2 g		4 g	
Sodium	1-1.4	mmol	1-2.5	mmol
Potassium	0.7-0.9	mmol	2	mmol
Calcium	0.11	mmol	0.5-1	mmol
Magnesium	0.04	mmol	0.15	mmol
Iron	1	μmol	2	μmol
Manganese	0.6	μmol	1	μmol
Zinc	0.3	μmol	0.6	μmol
Copper	0.07	μmol	0.3	μmol
Chloride	1.3-1.9	mmol	1.8-4.3	mmol
Phosphorus	0.15	mmol	0.4-0.8	mmol
Fluoride	0.7	μmol	3	μmol
Iodide	0.015	μmol	0.04	μmol
Thiamine	0.04	mg	0.05	mg
Riboflavine	0.06	mg	0.1	mg
Nicotinamide	0.4	mg	1	mg
Pyridoxine	0.06	mg	0.1	mg
Folic acid	6	μg	20	μg
Cyanocobalamin	0.06	μg	0.2	μg
Pantothenic acid	0.4	mg	1	mg
Biotin	10	μg	30	μg
Ascorbic acid	1	mg	3	mg
Retinol	10	μg	0.1	mg
Ergocalciferol or cholecalciferol	0.04	μg	2.5	μg
Phytylmenaquinone	2	μg	50	μg
−Tocopherol	1.5	mg	3	mg

Within seven to ten days on total intravenous nutrition with solutions lacking phosphate, adult patients have been found to be significantly hypophosphatae-mic (Travis et al, 1971). The reduced amount of 2,3-diphosphoglycerate and adenosine triphosphate in the erythrocytes was accompanied by an increase in the affinity of the red cells for oxygen, causing a reduced oxygen tension in the cells of the body tissues.

Several groups of scientists have claimed that intakes of zinc accelerate the rate of wound healing. Tissue repair makes substantial demands on body reserves of zinc (Hussein, 1969; Greaves & Skillen, 1970; Pullen et al, 1971; Hallböök & Lanner, 1972; Mills, 1972; Editorial, 1973).

It is also necessary to include all the thirteen essential vitamins in an intra-venous feeding programme. Vitamin K is formed in healthy adults by certain bacteria in the intestine. In a patient being treated with antibiotics, who was on intravenous nutrition without a supply of vitaminK, signs of vitamin K deficiency were observed after 9 days (Berthoud et al, 1966). This is one example that the use of antibiotics may result in a change of the intestinal flora and a loss of intes-tinal vitamin K production, causing vitamin K deficiency, with severe or fatal

TABLE IV. Examples of Infusion Solutions and Additions for Adult on Supplementary Intravenous Nutrition. In patients with burns or other conditions with increased requirements up to about double the amounts may be used

Solution 1

a) *Solutions of crystalline amino acids (7%) and carbohydrates (19%) (Vamin)*   1000 ml
are added with an
b) *Electrolyte solution*   10 ml
containing 5mmol of Ca, 1.5 mmol of Mg, 50 μmol of Fe, 20 μmol of Zn, 40 μmol of Mn, 5 μmol of Cu, 50 μmol of F, 1 μmol of I and 13.3 mmol of Cl^-

Solution 2

Fat emulsion (20%)[Intralipid 20%]   500 ml
with an addition of an
Emulsion of Fat Soluble Vitamins   10 ml
containing 0.75 mg of retinol, 3 μg of calciferol and 0.15 mg of vitamin K_1

Solution 3

a) *Glucose 10% solution* for intravenous infusion   1000 ml
with the addition of
b) *Lyophilised Water Soluble Vitamin Mixture*   20 ml
2 ampoules, each containing 1.2 mg of thiamine, 1.8 mg of riboflavine, 10 mg of nicotinamide, 2 mg of pyridoxine, 0.2 mg of folic acid, 2 μg of vitamin B_{12}, 10 mg of pantothenic acid, 0.3 mg of biotin and 30 mg of ascorbic acid as well as
c) *Potassium phosphate solution*   15 ml
containing 30 mmol of K, 6 mmol of P and 21 mmol of acetate

bleeding. Consequently, vitamin K_1 — as well as other vitamins — should always be given daily to every patient on intravenous alimentation.

Table III summarises the tentative recommendations for the basal amount of energy and nutrients to be supplied to patients on complete parenteral nutrition (Wretlind, 1972). The recommended intravenous supply is in agreement with the recommendations for ordinary food if the biological values of normal food protein and also the inadequate absorption of some nutrients are taken into account.

TABLE V. Supplementary Intravenous Nutrition for Adults, with the solutions given in Table IV.

Energy and nutrients	Solution 1 in Table IV 1,010 ml		Solution 2 in Table IV 510 ml		Solution 3 in Table IV 1,025 ml		Total	
Water	0.94	l	0.38	l	0.97	l	2.3	l
Energy	650	kcal	1,000	kcal	410	kcal	2,060	kcal
Amino acids	70	6	–		–		70	g
Glucose or fructose	100	g	12.5	g$^{1)}$	100	g	213	g
Fat	–		106	g$^{2)}$	–		106	g
Sodium	50	mmol	–		–		50	mmol
Potassium	20	mmol	–		30	mmol	50	mmol
Calcium	7.5	mmol	–		–		7.5	mmol
Magnesium	3.0	mmol	–		–		3.0	mmol
Iron	50	μmol	–		–		50	μmol
Zinc	20	μmol	–		–		20	μmol
Manganese	40	μmol	–		–		40	μmol
Copper	5	μmol	–		–		5	μmol
Chloride	68.3	mmol	–		–		68.3	mmol
Phosphorus	–		7.5	mmol	6	mmol	13.5	mmol
Fluoride	50	μmol	–		–		50	μmol
Iodide	1	μmol	–		–		1	μmol
Thiamine	–		–		2.4	mg	2.4	mg
Riboflavine	–		–		3.6	mg	3.6	mg
Niacin	–		–		20	mg	20	mg
Vitamin B_6	–		–		4	mg	4	mg
Folic acid	–		–		0.4	mg	0.4	mg
Vitamin B_{12}	–		–		4	μg	4	μg
Pantothenic acid	–		–		20	mg	20	mg
Biotin	–		–		0.6	mg	0.6	mg
Ascorbic acid	–		–		60	mg	60	mg
Vitamin A	–		0.75	mg	–		0.75	mg
Vitamin D	–		3	μg	–		3	μg
Vitamin K_1	–		0.15	mg	–		0.15	mg
Tocopherol	–		100	mg	–		100	mg

1) Glycerol. 2) 6 g of phosphatides

However, the amounts of the water soluble vitamins for adults are twice the amounts recommended for oral use.

A practical guide for the amounts and types of infusion solutions as used in Stockholm, is given in Table IV. The amounts of energy and nutrients supplied in this way are shown in Table V and correspond to the values given in Table III. When the quantities of nutrients indicated in Table III are supplied with an energy intake adjusted to maintain weight in adults, and growth in infants, the nutritive requirements of a patient should be well covered.

In many clinical conditions there is an increased need of nutrients. After prolonged starvation, extra nutrients have to be added to replete the patient and to

TABLE VI. Recommended Daily Allowance of Water, Energy, Amino Acids, Carbohydrates, and Fat for Supplementary Parenteral Nutrition. The amounts of electrolytes should be given as indicated by electrolyte balances. The supply of water soluble vitamins may be increased to five times the amounts given in Table III

| | Per kg body weight and day to cover | | | |
	Low requirement		High requirement	
Water	25–35	ml	50–60	ml
Energy	25–30	kcal	50–60	kcal
Amino acids	1 g		2 g	
Glucose or fructose	2 g		5 g	
Fat	2 g		3–4 g	

restore the body weight. Infection, trauma, operation and burn demand a considerable increase in all nutrients — up to 200-300 per cent of the basal or normal requirement. In burns, part of the nutrients may be given orally. The necessary amounts of energy and nutrients in these conditions are indicated in Table VI. This will be further investigated and this is one of the most important tasks for scientists in the field of intravenous nutrition.

BIOCHEMICAL ASPECTS OF CARBOHYDRATE METABOLISM

The carbohydrates provide a substantial part of the energy in the human diet. The average consumption of carbohydrate in ordinary food is 45-50 per cent of the total energy intake. Most of the carbohydrate absorbed from the intestines is glucose. Fructose from our diet amounts to less than 100 g or on average about 50 g a day. Glucose has a unique position in carbohydrate metabolism. Every cell in the human body is able to metabolise glucose. The glucose produces its energy mainly by the Embden-Mayerhof glycolytic pathway. Large amounts of the energy-rich adenosine triphosphate (ATP) will be the result of the glucose oxidation.

The endocrine factors, regulating the glucose metabolism, are prevented from functioning fully in certain diseases and conditions, such as diabetes, and in shock, trauma, operations and burns. Circulatory failure may occur after severe injury but the changes in metabolism during this condition have been studied in detail only during recent years. The metabolic insufficiencies in traumatic shock have recently been reported on by Stoner and Heath (1973).

CARBOHYDRATES AND POLYOLS IN PARENTERAL NUTRITION

Carbohydrates

Glucose

Besides being one of the main energy sources, glucose is a part of or necessary for the synthesis of several substances in the body. A supply of only 100 g of carbohydrates per day reduces the nitrogen loss. The nitrogen-sparing effect of glucose is caused by insulin release from the pancreas. The insulin not only stops gluconeogenesis, but also supports glucose and amino acid transport into the cells (Cahill, 1970; Froesch & Keller, 1972); 100 g of glucose also prevents ketosis.

Dudrick and his colleagues (1968, 1969, 1972; Dudrick & Rhoads, 1971) have a vast experience of post-operative parenteral nutrition with glucose as the only non-protein, energy source. In one of their publications (Dudrick et al, 1969) they described the treatment of 300 adult surgical patients after gastrectomy, colectomy, etc. The results showed healing was rapid, nitrogen balance was positive and weight increased. They administered 525-750 g of glucose (about 10 g/kg body weight) and 100-130 g of amino acids supplemented with electrolytes and vitamins. Sanderson and Deitel (1974) have shown that the insulin response to such glucose infusions ranging from 0.4 to 0.5 g of glucose/min was adequate to keep the glucose levels in the blood within the normal range.

The amounts of glucose for paediatric patients were increased to cover the higher energy demand per kg of the infants (Wilmore et al, 1969). Up to 25 g of glucose/kg/day were given to the patients. The patients were operated for bowel atresias and burst omphaloceles. In spite of the severe operations and the large amounts of glucose, the results were good and no complications from glucose intolerance were reported.

Das et al (1970) studied an infant who was operated on for omphalocele, and who was given 27 g of glucose/kg/day. Good growth was obtained. Blood sugar levels ranged between 44 and 108 mg per cent. Less than one per cent of the total glucose infused was lost in the urine.

Shreeve et al (1956) and others (Stoner, 1970; Kinney et al, 1970) found that glucose was oxidised quite well in hyperglycaemia, even when insulin resistance occurs, and this might offer an explanation of the successful results when when glucose is used in intravenous nutrition.

325

Fructose

The hyperglycaemia after trauma, operation and in shock, is partly caused by reduced insulin secretion and insulin resistance. It has, therefore, been taken for granted that a substitute for glucose which does not increase the blood sugar level and might be metabolised independently of insulin should be of value. There is, however, no convincing evidence to prove this assumption.

Fructose does not cause hyperglycaemia or insulin release (Kosaka, 1969; Froesch & Keller, 1972). It is rapidly transformed into glycogen in the liver cells (Nilsson & Hultman, 1974; Froesch & Keller, 1972). Fructose inhibits gluconeogenesis and thus spares amino acids (Geyer, 1960; Froesch & Keller, 1972). Fructose also enters the fat cells independently of glucose and insulin (Froesch & Keller, 1972). In these cells large amounts of ketohexokinase oxidise the fructose, which thus has an antiketogenic effect (Bässler, 1970a,b; Froesch & Ginsberg, 1965; Thorén, 1963). Fructose is also more rapidly metabolised than glucose and, therefore, preferred by Bässler (1970a,b) and Thorén (1963).

In uraemia, Thorén (1963) found that fructose was better utilised than glucose. Lee et al (1972) also report uraemia as an indication for fructose — and sorbitol — infusions.

On the other hand, fructose, as such cannot be used by the brain, which is one of the principal metabolic functions of glucose.

About 70 per cent of the fructose is transformed into glucose (Ashby et al, 1965; Stoner & Heath, 1973). The part of fructose which is transformed into glucose requires insulin for its further metabolism (Keller & Froesch, 1972). The rapid metabolism of fructose produces an increase in the lactic acid level (Mendeloff & Weichselbaum, 1953; Harries, 1972). It has been shown that infusions of fructose (20% solution), in a dosage of 0.5 to 3.5 g per kg per hour to healthy individuals and also in diabetics, produce an increase of 0.9 to 8 mEq of blood lactate per litre (Bergström et al, 1969). These investigations thus show that rapid infusions of fructose produce a lactic acid acidosis. In a dehydrated child with metabolic acidosis, 20% fructose solution was infused at the rate of 3 g of fructose per kg per hour for 7 hours (Andersson et al, 1969). The child died, and it was assumed that death was caused by an acidosis during the fructose infusion. In another dehydrated child with acidosis, about the same large and rapid fructose infusions produced severe reactions with increased acidosis (Andersson et al, 1969). These and other results indicate that rapid and large infusions of concentrated fructose are contraindicated in patients with dehydration and acidosis. Fructose, in amounts of less than 0.5 g per kg per hour (12 g per kg body weight per day), seems to cause only small, or insignificant, changes in the lactate concentration in the blood.

It has also been shown that the loss of fructose in the urine is smaller than that of glucose. Some authors claim that the tolerance for fructose locally in the infused veins, is higher than that for the same concentration of glucose (Thorén,

326

1964; Job & Huber, 1961).

Maltose

Young and Weser (1971) have proposed the use of maltose in parenteral nutrition. One molecule of this disaccharide is metabolised to two molecules of glucose. It has half the osmotic activity of glucose. From this point of view, it should be possible to give a 10% maltose solution peripherally without damaging the vein more than a 5% glucose solution does. This is an obvious advantage.

Kohri et al (1972) found that maltose was metabolised as glucose in man and in guinea pig. The metabolic rates of the two carbohydrates showed a remarkable similarity. Where the rapid splitting of the maltose takes place is at present unknown. There is no maltase in the serum of man and guinea pig in contrast to other animals (Kohri et al, 1972; Yoshimura et al, 1973). Fifty per cent of infused maltose is rapidly metabolised to carbon dioxide — shown as $^{14}CO_2$ — and the other fifty per cent assimilated in the body. Other Japanese authors have reported a very low toxicity of maltose. Unfortunately, clinical investigations in man have not yet clearly shown that maltose can be used as a glucose substitute to produce the desired effects on nitrogen utilisation and on body weight.

Polyols

Sorbitol

During the last few years the sugar alcohols sorbitol and xylitol, have been used instead of carbohydrate in intravenous nutrition. Sorbitol is converted by sorbitol dehydrogenase to fructose, which is then metabolised in the way mentioned above. The enzyme sorbitol dehydrogenase in the liver is very active, even in a severely damaged organ (Hoshi, 1963). The loss of sorbitol in the urine — 4 to 25 per cent according to Principi et al (1973) — is higher than that of glucose or fructose. Investigations by Keller and Froesch (1972) have shown that only the conversion of sorbitol via fructose to glucose in the liver is independent of insulin. The further metabolism of the glucose is, however, as always only possible if insulin is available.

Xylitol

Xylitol is a pentitol and enters directly into the metabolic pentose phosphate cycle. This opens a new pathway of carbohydrate supply that may be of some metabolic interest. Schultis and Geser (1970) and Bässler (1970a,b) found xylitol more antiketogenic and more nitrogen-sparing than glucose. As xylitol is oxidised via the pentose phosphate shunt it might, theoretically, be recommendable if glucose utilisation is impaired.

327

Like fructose and sorbitol, most of the xylitol — 85 per cent according to Froesch and Keller (1972) and Müller et al (1967) — is transformed into glucose. Consequently, fat tissue and muscles need insulin to store triglycerides or glycogen from xylitol. However, liver glycogen may be accumulated without the presence of insulin (Froesch & Keller, 1972). Xylitol as well as sorbitoi and fructose seem to inhibit gluconeogenesis more efficiently than glucose (Froesch, 1972).

In several papers Schultis and Geser (1970), Schultis (1971) and Schultis and Beisbarth (1972) studied the metabolism in post-operative conditions, and found improved nitrogen balance when xylitol was administered instead of glucose. Halmagyi and Isvang (1968) have treated 1189 patients in the post-operative phase with xylitol, and found it to be equally well utilised both before and after operation. The dose was 0.79 g of xylitol/kg/30 min. The authors recommend mixtures of glucose and xylitol.

Toussaint (1968) has successfully treated infants suffering from ketonaemia, with xylitol. Elphick et al (1972) have investigated xylitol also in neonatal patients after severe gastrointestinal operations.

Many authors (Donahoe & Powers, 1970; Foerster et al, 1970; Schumer, 1971) have carefully studied the complications following xylitol infusions, such as hyperuricaemia, hyperbilirubinaemia, and renal insufficiency. The diuresis was later followed by anuria as well as liver and brain symptoms. The extensive investigations by Thomas et al (1972) also revealed other symptoms (nausea and vomiting) and lethal lesions, such as centrilobular liver necrosis and liver enzyme deficiencies. A peculiar autopsy finding was that of calcium oxalate crystals in the renal tubuli and, in one case, in the brain. The signs of intoxication were proportional to the infused dose, but even the highest dose of 0.49 g/kg/hour for, on the average, 40 hours did not affect more than 20 per cent of the patients. These symptoms appeared quite individually, and the authors make the reservation that the primary disease may be responsible for the reactions. These findings formed the basis of an Adverse Drug Reaction Report to the Australian Drug Evaluation Committee. Subsequently, xylitol was withdrawn from clinical use. An earlier accident, found to be due to a contaminated batch of xylitol, was irrelevant to this decision.

Glycerol

In dilute solutions and moderate dosage, glycerol is well tolerated in man and animals. Its metabolism and synthesis to other carbohydrate metabolites have been demonstrated. In large doses and in solutions with a concentration of 10% or more, glycerol can cause haemolysis, hypotension, central nervous disturbances and convulsions (Geyer, 1960). These effects make glycerol impossible to use as the only energy supply in parenteral nutrition. In parenteral preparations, glycerol is thus used only in fat emulsions to correct their osmotic pressure. Being a three-carbon alcohol it has twice the osmotic effects of monosaccharides. The caloric value of glycerol is almost the same as that of glucose.

Discussion

There is a difference of opinion, and very much discussion about the importance of the immediate post-operative losses of nitrogen and energy, and if they should be therapeutically compensated or not. Some have regarded the metabolic rise as a normal reaction which should not be interfered with (Moore & Ball, 1952). Many authors argue that the condition is only temporary, and that it will be normalised in a well-nourished patient after a few days (Tweedle & Johnston, 1971; Cuthbertson et al, 1972). Accordingly, for the first few days after operation only water and electrolytes should be given. Blackburn et al (1973a,b) have suggested the intravenous infusion of amino acids without any glucose or other carbohydrates in periods of negative nitrogen and energy balance. In this way, adequate fat mobilisation and starvation ketosis are produced to cover the energy requirement.

Other authors feel convinced that starving must be improper for an organism under metabolic stress, and recommend parenteral nutrition — if the patient is unable to eat — immediately after operation (Larsen & Brøckner, 1969; Owings & Mims, 1971; Sherman et al, 1971). Clark (1967) goes so far as to regard the changed metabolism as "an entirely pathological process". In all post-operative cases, where nutritional disturbance is present before or after operation, an adequate complete intravenous nutrition should be given immediately in connection with the operation according to Wretlind (1972).

Some clinical observations support the value of parenteral nutrition during the first days after surgery. Freuchen and Østergaard (1964) found that after gastrectomy their patients were in better condition and less tired if they had had parenteral infusion sufficient for a positive nitrogen balance. Brøckner et al (1962) reported no complications after major operations, and also observed shorter duration of paralytic ileus — a very important statement. Moreover, the patients were able to take their food by mouth earlier if they first had been fed parenterally.

Regarding the disturbed glucose metabolism after operation there is need for more knowledge (Stoner & Heath, 1973) before definite rules for practical work can be established. There has been extensive clinical experience of the glucose substitutes in all conditions where there is so-called glucose intolerance characterised by hyperglycaemia. These conditions are diabetes, trauma, stress and, according to Cook (1969), also liver insufficiency and pancreatitis.

Fructose, sorbitol and xylitol are metabolised together in the liver independently of insulin. The level of carbohydrate metabolites in the liver will be increased. Most of the glucose produced in the liver originates from the given glucose substitutes. In this way, less amino acids are used for gluconeogenesis. A short-lasting nitrogen-sparing effect of fructose, sorbitol and xylitol will be obtained. However, a protein anabolism in muscle and other peripheral tissues can occur only when insulin makes glucose available to these tissue cells. The

329

often repeated statement that the glucose substitutes — fructose, sorbitol and xylitol — can increase the glycogen stores in the liver independently of insulin, seems to the author to be of limited value. In insulin resistance, the body has a reduced possibility of utilising the stored glycogen, which is thus restricted from the metabolism, when the need is most urgent.

Some of the earlier described metabolic effects of glucose, fructose, sorbitol and xylitol are summarised in Table VII. Fructose, sorbitol, and xylitol, may

TABLE VII. Metabolic Properties of Carbohydrates and Polyols for Parenteral Nutrition

	Carbohydrates		Polyols	
	Glucose	Fructose	Sorbitol	Xylitol
Normal metabolite	+	+		
Metabolised by cells in all tissues	+			
Increases nitrogen utilisation	+	+	+	+
Antiketogenic	+	+	+	+
'Partial insulin independency'		+	+	+

cause acidosis which is due to a production of pyruvic and lactic acid from these substances. Keller and Froesch (1972) found a 200 per cent excess compared with glucose. The very rapid phosphorylation during the first steps of the metabolism of the fructose and sorbitol in the liver, causes a depletion of adenyl phosphates and inorganic phosphate (Thomas et al, 1972).

The advantage of glucose over fructose, sorbitol and xylitol is obvious. All tissue cells can metabolise glucose, which is a prerequisite for anabolism. The glucose is required by the brain, prevents excessive sodium and water losses, causes insulin secretion and thereby anabolic effects. However, the muscle and adipose tissue will assimilate glucose only in the presence of insulin. Exogenous insulin has thus to be given when endogenous insulin is not available. An adult patient without any metabolic disorder can easily metabolise up to 800 g of glucose per day. In severely stressed patients after operations, burns, etc, an over-stimulation of the sympathetic nervous system will block the insulin secretion. There is also a peripheral insulin resistance. When these patients have been treated with large amounts of glucose and very high quantities of insulin, the survival rate was increased significantly (Hinton et al, 1971).

Hitherto, all metabolic and clinical studies have indicated that glucose is the *carbohydrate of choice* for intravenous nutrition of patients.

Some nutritionists are of the opinion that fructose, sorbitol and xylitol should not be used as energy source in parenteral nutrition. This view is also expressed by the Swiss authorities for drugs (Fischer, 1974). They regard fructose, sorbitol and xylitol too dangerous to be used. The main objections are the resulting

330

TABLE VIII. Some Adverse Reactions of Fructose, Sorbitol and Xylitol

	Carbohydrate	Polyols	
	Fructose	Sorbitol	Xylitol
Metabolic acidosis	+	+	+
Hyperuricaemia	+	+	+
Decrease of adenine nucleotide in the liver and phosphate in the blood	+	+	+
Osmotic diuresis with electrolyte losses		+	+
Crystal deposition in kidney and brain			+

acidosis, hyperuricaemia and depletion of adenine nucleotide in the liver and inorganic phosphorus in the blood (Table VIII). As these complications occur in an unpredictable manner and cannot be controlled, these 'glucose substitutes' are now prohibited in Switzerland for intravenous nutrition. Xylitol may cause kidney damage and oxalate depositions and must not be used at all as an energy source in intravenous nutrition. Fructose or sorbitol should not be used in a paediatric clinic, in order to avoid fatal reactions in a non-identified case of fructose intolerance.

There are also some potential hazards in the use of intravenous glucose. If patients with glucose 'intolerance' receive glucose as the sole non-protein energy source in parenteral nutrition they may develop hyperglycaemia, with its potential sequelae of glucosuria and osmotic diuresis, dehydration and hyperosmolar coma. However, the blood sugar can be maintained at an acceptable level by infusing the glucose at a controlled rate, and by giving a sufficient amount of exogenous insulin to keep the blood sugar level below 200 mg% (11 mmol/l) and glucosuria less than 2 per cent of the intake. A high endogenous insulin production stimulated by hypertonic glucose may cause a reactive hypoglycaemia if the glucose infusion stops suddenly. For this reason, Moore and Ball (1952) advised (which was more than twenty years ago) a 'chaser' of 5 per cent glucose to follow hypertonic glucose infusion solutions.

Cade et al (1974) have pointed out that most hsopitals are not equipped to monitor fructose administration safely, and they are less prepared for the other glucose substitutes in clinical usage — sorbitol and xylitol. This means that most doctors instead of having a reliable support from the routine biochemistry service, find the biochemistry department equally unfamiliar with these substances and rarely equipped to make occasional blood and urine estimates of these glucose substitutes.

An increased lipolysis has been found after operations (Schultis & Geser, 1970) and after burns. The content of free fatty acids in the plasma is increased after trauma and burns (Allison et al, 1968; Wadström, 1959). Birke et al (1965) found the rise to be in direct proportion to the severity of the burn. The increased lipolysis serves a metabolic purpose. Rodewald (1962) showed that the respiratory quotient was decreased post-operatively, indicating that the high need of energy was mainly covered by fat combustion. Hallberg (1965a,b) also found that fat emulsion disappeared more rapidly than normally from the plasma after operation. This result was confirmed by Carlson and Liljedahl (1971). The great success in treatment of burns with fat emulsions is inferred from the works of Birke et al (1972) and Lamke et al (1974).

In paediatric surgery, Børresen and Knutrud (1969) and Børresen et al (1970) used a complete parenteral nutrition containing fat emulsion. They obtained a positive nitrogen balance even from the first day after operation and good healing with weight increase during convalesence. The authors conclude: "Post-operative glucose intolerance with glucosuria is no longer any problem." Since the development of non-toxic fat emulsions, a new way has been found to avoid the effect of glucose intolerance. After operation and trauma, burns, shock etc, mobilisation of free fatty acids and utilisation of fat are unimpaired. No acidosis or ketosis has been observed when glucose is supplied simultaneously.

When a solution of an amino acid mixture with carbohydrate as glucose or fructose is heat-sterilised, a destruction of the essential amino acids, such as lysine may occur ('Maillard reaction'). This will result in a decrease in the biological value of the amino acid mixture. In order to avoid this reaction, sorbitol or xylitol has been used instead of glucose or fructose. However, using a modern technique for sterilisation, and by adjusting the pH of the solutions to less than 5.5 it is now possible to prepare infusion solutions containing a mixture of amino acids and carbohydrate without any Maillard reaction occurring.

Summary

When all nutrients, absorbed from an ordinary, adequate oral food are given intravenously, this is termed *Complete Intravenous Nutrition.* Such an intravenous nutrition may be achieved by a supply of water, amino acids, carbohydrates, fat, twelve electrolytes or minerals and thirteen vitamins. With our present knowledge in this field, we can design an intravenous diet which may keep a patient on intravenous nutrition in good nutritional status for a long period up to several years.

An adequate, non-protein energy supply must form a part of complete intravenous nutrition. This supply may contain either carbohydrates or carbohydrates and suitable fat emulsion. The body cells will require a certain amount of glucose. The use of the glucose substitutes, fructose, sorbitol and xylitol does not seem to offer any significant advantages from a nutritional point of view. The disadvantages are acidosis, hyperuricaemia, hypophosphataemia and depletion of adenine nucleotide. Xylitol has also produced serious adverse reactions (osmotic diureses, oxalate deposition in kidney and brain etc) with fatal results. Hitherto, all investigations have indicated that *the carbohydrate of choice is glucose.*

References

Allison, SP, Hinton, P and Chamberlain, MJ (1968) *Lancet, ii,* 113
Allison, SP (1972) In *Parenteral Nutrition.* (Ed) AW Wilkinson). Churchill
   Livingstone, Edinburgh and London. Page 275
Allison, SP (1974) *Brit. J. hosp. Med., June,* 860
Andersson, G, Brohult, J and Sterner, G (1969) *Acta paediat. Scand., 58,* 301
Ashby, MM, Heath, DF and Stoner, HB (1965) *J. Physiol., 179,* 193
Bässler, KH (1970a) In *Parenteral Nutrition.* (Ed) HC Meng and DH Law.
   Churchill Livinstone, Edinburgh and London. Page 96
Bässler, KH (1970b) In *Balanced Nutrition and Therapy.* (Ed) K Lang, W Fekl
   and G Berg. G Thieme, Stuttgart. Page 31
Bergström, J, Hultman, E and Roch-Norlund, A (1969) *Läkartidningen, 66,* 2223
Bernard, C (1877) *Lecons sur le diabète et la glycogenèse animale.* Ballière, Paris
Berthoud, M, Bouvier, CA and Krähenbühl, B (1966) *Schweiz. med. Wschr.,
   96,* 1522
Birke, G, Carlson, LA and Liljedahl, S-O (1965) *Aca med. Scand., 178,* 337
Birke, G, Carlson, LA, von Euler, US, Liljedahl, S-O and Plantin, SO (1972)
   Acta chir. Scand., 138, 321
Blackburn, GL, Flatt, JP, Clowes, GHA, O'Donnell, TF and Hensle, TE (1973a)
   Ann. Surg., 177, 588
Blackburn, GL, Flatt, JP, Clowes, GHA and O'Donnell, TE (1973b) *Amer. J.
   Surg., 125,* 447
Børresen, HC and Knutrud, O (1969) *Acta paed. Scand., 58,* 420
Børresen, HC, Coran, AG and Knutrud, O (1970) *Nordisk Medicin, 8,* 1089
Bröckner, J, Larsen, V and Amris, CJ (1962) *Acta chir. Scand. Suppl. 325,* 67
Cade, DC, O'Donovan, JE and Galbally, BP (1974) *Clinical hazards of parenteral
   nutrition.* Lecture at the First World Congress of Intensive Care in London,
   June 1974
Cahill, GF (1970) In *Parenteral Nutrition.* (Ed) HC Meng and DH Law.
   Charles C Thomas, Springfield, Illinois. Page 85
Cahill, GF and Aoki, TT (1972) In *Intravenous Hyperalimentation.*
   (Ed) GSM Cowan Jr and WL Scheetz. Lea & Febiger, Philadelphia. Page 21
Carlson, LA and Liljedahl, S-O (1971) *Acta chir. Scand., 137,* 123
Clark, RG (1967) *Brit. J. Surg., Special Lister Centenary Number,* 445
Cook, GC (1969) *Clin. Sci., 37,* 675
Cuthbertson, DP (1942) *Lancet, i,* 433
Cuthbertson, DP, Fell, GS, Smith, CM and Tilstone, WI (1972) *Brit. J. Surg.,
   52,* 925
Das, JB, Filler, RM, Rubin, VG and Eraklis, AI (1970) *J. ped. Surg., 5,* 127
Donahoe, JF and Powers, RJ (1970) *New Eng. J. Med., 282,* 690
Drucker, WR (1972) In *Intravenous Hyperalimentation.* (Ed) GSM Cowan Jr
   and WL Scheetz. Lea & Febiger, Philadelphia. Page 55
Dudrick, SJ, Wilmore, DW, Vars, HM and Rhoads, JE (1968) *Surgery, 64,* 134
Dudrick, SJ, Wilmore, DW, Vars, HM and Rhoads, JE (1969) *Ann. Surg., 169,*
   974
Dudrick, SJ and Rhoads, JE (1971) *JAMA, 215,* 939
Dudrick, SJ, MacFadyen, BV, van Buren, CT, Ruberg, RL and Maynard, AT
   (1972) *Ann. Surg., 176,* 259
Editorial (1973) *Lancet, i,* 299
Elphick, MC, Dougall, AJ and Wilkinson, AW (1972) In *Parenteral Nutrition.*

(Ed) AW Wilkinson). Churchill Livingstone, Edinburgh and London. Page 138

Fischer, P [Ed] (1974) *Ersatzzucker für die parenterale Ernährung. Grundsatz vom 19. März*

Foerster, H, Meyer, E and Ziege, M (1970) *Klin. Wschr., 48,* 878

Freuchen, I and Østergaard, J (1964) *Acta chir. Scand. Suppl. 325,* 55

Froesch, ER (1972) In *Clinical and Metabolic Aspects of Fructose. Papers presented at a symposium in Helsinki.* (Ed) EA Nikkila and JK Hattunen. *Acta med. Scand. Suppl. 542,* 239

Froesch, ER and Keller, U (1972) In *Parenteral Nutrition.* (Ed) AW Wilkinson. Churchill Livingstone, Edinburgh and London. Page 105

Geyer, RG (1960) *Physiol. Revs., 40,* 150

Greaves, MW and Skillen, AW (1970) *Lancet, ii,* 889

Hallberg, D (1965a) *Acta physiol. Scand., 64,* 306

Hallberg, D (1965b) *Acta physiol. Scand., Suppl.65,* 254

Hallböök, T and Lanner, E (1972) *Lancet, ii,* 780

Halmagyi, M and Isvang, HH (1968) In *Kohlenhydrate in der dringlichen Infusionstherapie.* (Ed) K Lang, R Frey and M Halmagyi. Springer Verlag, Heidelberg, Berlin and New York. Page 24

Harries, JT (1972) In *Parenteral Nutrition.* (Ed) AW Wilkinson. Churchill Livingstone, Edinburgh and London. Page 266

Hinton, P, Littlejohn, S, Allison, SP and Lloyd, J (1971) *Lancet, i,* 767

Hoshi, M (1963) *Med. J. Osaka Univ., 14,* 47

Hussein, SL (1969) *Lancet, i,* 1069

Job, C and Huber, O (1961) *Arch. exp. path. Pharmakol., 241,* 53

Keller, U and Froesch, ER (1972) *Schweiz. med. Wschr., 102,* 1017

Kinney, JM, Long, CL and Duke, JH (1970) In *Energy Metabolism in Trauma. (Ciba Foundation Symposium).* (Ed) R Porter and Knight. Page 103

Kohri, H, Muto, Y and Hosoya, N (1972) *J. Jap. Soc. Food and Nutr., 25,* 641

Kosaka, K (1969) In *Pentoses and Pentitols.* (Ed) BL Horecker, K Lang and Y Takagi. Springer Verlag, Berlin, Heidelberg and New York. Page 212

Lamke, L-O, Liljedahl, S-O and Wretlind, A (1974) *Ann. Anésth. Franc., 15, Spécial, 2,* 27

Larsen, V and Brøckner, J (1969) *Scand. J. Gastroent., 4, Suppl. 3,* 41

Latta, T (1831-32) *Lancet, ii,* 274

Lee, HA, Morgan, AG, Waldram, R and Bennett, J (1972) In *Parenteral Nutrition.* (Ed) AW Wilkinson. Churchill Livingstone, Edinburgh and London. Page 121

Long, CL, Spencer, JL and Kinney, JM (1971) *J. appl. Physiol., 31,* 110

Mendeloff, AL and Weichselbaum, TE (1953) *Metabolism, 2,* 450

Mills, CF (1972) *Nutrition, 26,* 357

Moore, FD and Ball, MR (1952) In *The Metabolic Response to Surgery.* Charles C Thomas, Springfield, Illinois

Morgan, HE, Randle, PJ and Regen, DM (1959) *Biochem. J., 73,* 573

Müller, F, Strack, E, Kufahl, E and Dettmer, D (1967) *Z. f. ges. exp. Med., 142,* 338

Nilsson, L H:son and Hultman, E (1974) *Scand. J. clin. lab. Invest., 33,* 5

Owings, JM and Mims, WW (1971) *J. Sc. Med. Ass., 67,* 121

Principi, N, Reali, E and Rivolta, A (1973) *Helv. Paediat. Acta, 28,* 621

Pullen, FW, Pories, WJ and Strain, WH (1971) *Laryngoscope, 81,* 1638

Rodewald, G (1962) *Arch. klin. Chir., 301,* 532

Sanderson, I and Deitel, M (1974) *Ann. Surg., 179,* 387

Schultis, K and Geser, CA (1970) In *Parenteral Nutrition.* (Ed) HC Meng and DH Laws. Charles C Thomas, Springfield, Illinois. Page 139

Schultis, K (1971) *Z. Ernährungswiss, 10, Suppl. 11,* 7

Schultis, K and Beisbarth, H (1972) In *Parenteral Nutrition.* (Ed) AW Wilkinson. Churchill Livingstone, Edinburgh and London. Page 255

Schumer, W (1971) *Metabolism, 20,* 345

Sherman, JO, Egan, T and Macalad, FV (1971) *Surg. Clin. North. Amer., 51,* 37

Shreeve, WW, Balur, N, Miller, M, Shipley, RA, Incefy, GE and Craig, JW (1956) *Metabolism, 5,* 22

Stoner, HB (1970) *J. clin. Path., Suppl. 23 (Roy.Coll.Path.), 4,* 244

Thomas, DW, Gillgan, JE, Edwards, JB and Edwards, RB (1972) *Med. J. Austr., 1,* 1246

Thorén, L (1963) *Acta chir. Scand., 1306, Suppl.,* 1

Thorén, L (1964) *Acta chir. Scand., 325, Suppl.,* 75

Toussaint, W (1968) In *Kohlenhydrate in der dringlichen Infusionstherapie.* (Ed) K Lang, R Frey and M Halmagyi. Springer Verlag, Berlin, Heidelberg and New York. Page 38

Travis, S, Sugerman, HJ, Ruberg, RL, Dudrick, SJ, Delivoria-Papadopoulus, M, Miller, LD and Oski, FA (1971) *New Engl. J. Med., 285,* 763

Tweedle, DEF and Johnston, IDA (1971) *Brit. J. Surg., 58,* 771

Wadström, LB (1959) *Acta chir. Scand. Suppl.,* 238

Wilmore, DW, Groff, DB, Bishop, HC and Dudrick, SJ (1969) *J. ped. Surg., 4,* 181

Wretlind, A (1972) *Nutr. Metab., 14, Suppl.,* 1

Yoshimura, NN, Ehrlich, H, Westman, TL and Deindoerfer, FH (1973) *J. Nutr., 103,* 1256

Young, JM and Weser, E (1971) *J. clin. Invest., 50,* 986

Intracellular Free Amino Acids in Muscle Tissue in Normal Man and in Different Clinical Conditions

E VINNARS, P FÜRST, J BERGSTRÖM and I von FRANCKEN
St Erik's Sjukhus, Stockholm, Sweden

Introduction

Extracellular proteins and peptides cannot pass the cell membrane, and must first be hydrolysed to amino acids. The final products of digestion of dietary protein are consequently the free amino acids which are transported into the cells. The supply of free amino acids to the tissues is of primary importance in protein metabolism.

Our present knowledge of the composition of the intracellular fluid and the relationship between extra- and intracellular amino acid concentrations is mainly based on animal studies of the amino acid composition of tissue under varying experimental conditions. Muscle has been most frequently analysed and, from the quantitative point of view, gives the best estimation of the average intracellular amino acid composition in the whole organism by far since skeletal muscle is the most abundant cellular tissue and relatively uniform as to cellular composition.

Herbert et al (1966) investigated the total free amino acid pool in different tissues of rats and showed that the concentration of most of the amino acids was considerably higher in the tissues than in plasma and also that the size of the pools of individual free amino acids differed widely. About 80% of free amino acids in the total body were in skeletal muscle. Considerable differences have been observed between different species (Hamilton, 1945; Friedberg & Greenberg, 1947; Herbert et al, 1966; Munro, 1970). Many of these investigations are of basic biochemical importance, but because of species variation the results are not reliable in human muscle.

Weakness and easy tiring are the most common symptoms of surgical convalescence. The last thing to return in convalescence after major injury or sepsis is the ability to work a full day without fatigue. This disability is more severe and prolonged than can be accounted for by bed rest and decreased nutrition. A prominent feature of acute surgical catabolism is a negative nitrogen balance associated with protein breakdown and increased urea synthesis and excretion, but the underlying mechanism and physiologic significance remain obscure. The clinical weakness and fatigue may be the result of muscle protein breakdown which is reflected in a negative nitrogen balance. The accelerated muscle protein breakdown in injured or septic patients may therefore suggest an increase in cytoplasmic amino acids in muscle. An increased release of free amino acids from muscle cells may also result in the observed increased gluconeogenesis and urea synthesis in the liver.

By direct determination of intracellular free amino acid concentrations in muscle tissue obtained from human subjects it may be possible to extent our knowledge of amino acid metabolism under different conditions and such findings could serve as a basis for guiding the development of more adequate nutrition. Sampling and analysis of muscle tissue in man is still difficult and so far this is probably why so few intracellular amino acid determinations in human muscle have been done. The only available results were reported by Zachman et al (1966) who estimated the total concentration of amino acids in muscle obtained in biopsies during minor operations following cortisone administration. Such procedures are not suitable where repeated sampling of muscle for longitudinal studies in one single individual is required. To overcome this difficulty a technique for percutaneous needle biopsy of skeletal muscle was worked out by Bergström (1962), which permits repeated sampling of muscle tissue.

A brief review of the methodology, the problems of interpretation, and results obtained in normal individuals and in different clinical conditions will be given.

METHODOLOGY

Tissue Sampling

The needle consists of a sharp-tipped hollow outer needle with a small opening near the tip. A cylinder with a sharp edge fits tightly into the needle. The needle is introduced under local anaesthesia into the quadriceps femoris through a minor incision of the skin, the inner cylinder is pulled back and then pushed in again, punching out a small piece of muscle bulging into the opening of the needle. With a needle having a diameter of 4.5 mm one can obtain 30–150 mg of muscle tissue for analysis.

The wet biopsy material is dissected very carefully to remove all visible fat and connective tissue. This material is divided into different sections (8–15 mg). Two sections are used for determination of water, fat, and electrolytes and two other sections for measurement of free amino acids and DNA.

Analytical Technique

Determination of water, fat, and chloride. The muscle samples are weighed repeatedly on an electro balance (Cahn RG) for 5 min after biopsy and the wet weight is estimated by extrapolation to zero time. Water is determined by weighing before and after drying at 90°C. Natural fat is extracted with petroleum ether. The dried fat free pieces are extracted in 0.25 ml 1 N HNO_3. 100 μl of extract are treated during 16 h with 20μl sodium borate solution in alkali (0.6% sodiumborate in 10 N NaOH) for removing the SH-groups which interfere with Cl-ions and disturb the determination. The extract is then neutralised with 30 μl 7.5 N HNO_3. 100 μl of the oxidised and pH adjusted extract are titrated with 5 mmol $AgNO_3$ solution of 150 mV, using a microtitrator (Radiometer ABU 12) modified for ultramicro purposes. The coefficient of variation of the method as determined from analysis of duplicate specimens is 4.3%.

The plasma chloride is determined according to Zall et al (1956), the total plasma proteins using a biuret method.

Determination of free amino acids in muscle tissue and in plasma. The weighed muscle tissue specimen is homogenised in a Potter-Elvehjem glass homogenisor. The protein is directly precipitated with 0.5 ml ice-cold 16% sulphosalicylic acid. Peripheral vein blood is obtained from the forearm in parallel with the muscle biopsy. After immediate centrifugation 1 ml plasma is precipitated with 30 mg sulphosalicylic acid.

The free amino acids are determined either on a modified Beckman 120 C amino acid analyser, or on a Labotron CHR-2 analyser using one-column lithium-buffer system (Kedenburg, 1971; Bergström et al, 1974).

The extra- and intracellular distribution of water is based on the chloride space and Nernst equation. Using the chloride distribution constant the intracellular concentrations of the different parameters can be expressed. The distribution constant is a function of membrane potential at 87.2 mV (Bolte et al, 1963). The calculations are presented in the section headed *Calculations.*

Bolte et al (1972) have studied the membrane potential in skeletal muscle in uraemic patients in different states of uraemia. Only in the terminal state did he observe a decreased membrane potential. Bergström et al (1971) in a number of papers reported skeletal membrane potential measured in vivo in the rat embryo. The low membrane potential became normal with increasing age. It should be pointed out that the measurement was done in connection with an operation on rats and consequently during post-operative catabolism.

On the other hand, observations have been made in certain clinical and experimental conditions indicating that increasing amounts of chloride may enter the cells (for references, see Bergström, 1962). A constant and sustained fall in membrane potential has also been demonstrated during acute haemorrhagic shock (Campion et al, 1969; Shires et al, 1970). However, individual deviations of ± 10 mV do not influence the estimated intracellular water content more than

2% (Bergström et al, 1974).

References for muscle data presentation. Measurements of amino acids, electrolytes, and water are usually expressed as amount per *weight of wet tissue*. However, this reference may be unreliable since the tissue content of fat and water can vary considerably. Therefore, *dry fat free solids (DFFS)* may be more useful than wet weight to express the results. DFFS was introduced very early (Darrow et al, 1939). In normal subjects the amount of fat and connective tissue consists of a relatively constant fraction of the total fat free solids. However, during pathological conditions such as inactivity (Eichelberger et al, 1956), starvation (Hurth & Elkinton, 1959), and protein deficiency (Mendes & Waterlow, 1958), the ratio between muscle cells, solids, and connective tissue may be changed. Similar changes might also be expected in severe catabolism. These reasons emphasise the need to develop a more standard reference like *alkaline soluble protein (ASP)* or *DNA* which is independent of the content of connective tissue. Since DNA is thought to be constant per cell in a given tissue, the calculation of intracellular material per amount of DNA reflects the amount per cell. There are theoretical advantages in using *intracellular water* as a basis of reference, especially when considering the relationship between extra- and intracellular electrolyte concentrations and osmotic water transport between cells and their environment. However, the difficulties of determining exactly the extra- and intracellular water distribution in biopsies have already been pointed out.

Calculations. The determination of extra- and intracellular water was based on the chloride method. Chloride is freely diffusible across the skeletal muscle fibre membrane and is distributed according to the Nernst equation (Wilde, 1945; Conway, 1957):

$$E = \frac{R \cdot T}{F} \ln \frac{[Cl]_e}{[Cl]_i}$$

where E = membrane potential, R = general gas constant, F = Faraday's constant, T = absolute temperature, and $[Cl]_e$ and $[Cl]_i$ = the chloride concentration in extra- and intracellular water, respectively.

Assuming a normal membrane potential of 87.2 mV (Bolte et al, 1963), the ratio between the chloride distribution is

$$87.2 = 61.5 \log \frac{[Cl]_e}{[Cl]_i}$$

which gives

$$\frac{[Cl]_e}{[Cl]_i} = \frac{26}{1}$$

339

The extracellular chloride concentration $[Cl]_e$ was calculated from the plasma concentration $[Cl]_p$ by correction for a Donnan factor (0.96) and the plasma water content, which was indirectly estimated from the total protein content using the regression formula of Eisenman et al (1936). $[H_2O]_p = 984 - 7.18 \times$ plasma protein concentration g/100 ml plasma

$$[Cl]_e = \frac{[Cl]_p \cdot 1,000}{0.96 \cdot [H_2O]_p}$$

With the assumptions quoted above, the extracellular water content (H_2O_e, ml/kg muscle) was calculated from the muscle water content (H_2O_m, ml/kg muscle), and the concentration of chloride (mmol/l) in extra- and intracellular water (Graham et al, 1967).

$$H_2O_e = \frac{1,000 \cdot Cl_m - H_2O_m \, [Cl]_i}{[Cl]_e - [Cl]_i}$$

The intracellular water content $H_2O_i - H_2O_m - H_2O_e$.

The intracellular concentration of each amino acid $[AA]_i$ was calculated by subtracting the free extracellular part from the total amount (AA_m) assuming the plasma concentration $[AA]_p$ to be equal to the concentration in the interstitial fluid.

$$[AA]_i = \frac{1,000 \cdot AA_m - H_2O_e \cdot [AA]_p}{H_2O_i}$$

It is assumed that all natural free amino acids except tryptophan are not significantly bound to plasma proteins (Gulyassy et al, 1971).

NORMAL VALUES

In 23 healthy volunteers the total water content in muscle tissues was 763 ± 5.9 ml/kg muscle (mean ± SD), the extracellular water content was 99 ± 29.9 ml/kg muscle, and the intracellular water content was 663 ± 28.7 ml/kg muscle. These figures are in agreement with earlier results from our laboratory (Bergström & Bittar, 1969).

The extra- (EC) and intracellular (IC) concentration and the IC/EC gradient for each amino acid were calculated. The free amino acid concentration in plasma and in intracellular muscle water, expressed in mmol/l, for each amino acid are presented in Figure 1. The amino acid concentrations in plasma were essentially in agreement with results presented by other investigators (Peters et al, 1968; Young & Parsons, 1970).

The majority of the amino acids had a much higher concentration in intracellular water than in plasma. The concentration gradient was especially high for

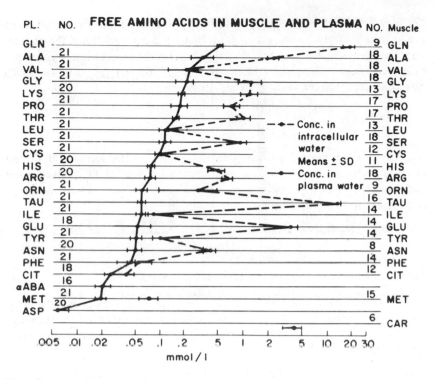

Figure 1. Comparison between aminograms in plasma water and intracellular muscle water. Means ± SD are given (n = 32)

taurine, glutamic acid, and glutamine. The essential amino acids valine, leucine, isoleucine, and phenylalanine and the non-essential amino acids citrulline and tyrosine had a gradient below 2. The remainder showed a gradient between 5 and 10.

The results of the present study confirm earlier findings in experimental animals, which show that the intracellular concentrations of free amino acids are much higher than the concentrations in plasma (Herbert et al, 1966; Munro, 1970; Adibi, 1971). However, there seem to be consistent differences in the amino acid pattern between different species. Thus the concentration of glycine is considerably higher than glutamine in the caiman and about equally as high as glutamine in the rat (Herbert et al, 1966), whereas in man the intracellular concentration of glycine is low and the concentration of glutamine is higher than all the other amino acids combined, except taurine (Figure 2). The dipeptide carnosine occurs in relatively high concentration. Another dipeptide, anserine, found in dog and rat muscle, is present only in trace quantities in human muscle tissue. In man, as well as in other species investigated, a few non-essential amino acids, glutamine, glutamic acid, and alanine represent the bulk of the intracellular free amino acids.

341

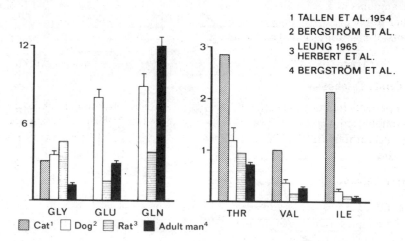

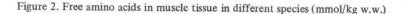

Figure 2. Free amino acids in muscle tissue in different species (mmol/kg w.w.)

The Size of the Intracellular Free Amino Acid Pool

As skeletal muscle contains the largest pool of intracellular free amino acids it is of interest to estimate the size of this pool. Based on direct determinations in man 1 kg skeletal muscle contains 230 g dry solids, 120 g extracellular water, and 650 g intracellular water .

The total determined free amino acid concentration was found to be about 34.5 mmol/l intracellular water, corresponding to 4.8 g amino acids. Taurine is present in the concentration of about 15 mmol/l intracellular water coresponding to 1.9 g. Free peptides, such as carnosine, are not taken into consideration.

For a normal man with a body weight of 70 kg and a muscle mass of 40% of the body weight, the total volume of intracellular muscle water is 18.2 litres and the total intracellular amino acid content in muscle is 86.5 g. Of this total pool of free amino acids the eight essential amino acids represent only 8.4%, whereas free glutamine constitutes 61%, glutamic acid 13.5%, and alanine 4.4%. In fact the total pool of intracellular free amino acids in muscle tissue consists mainly of these three amino acids, which constitute about 79% of the total pool.

We have concluded that the muscle cells contain higher concentrations of amino acids than are found in the plasma. No consistent property, such as pK value, polarisation, or charge, seems to be common to the different groups. The existence of a marked concentration gradient for some of the amino acids requires that free diffusion through the muscle fibre membrane be restricted. The fact that the intracellular amino acid pattern is reproducible from one individual to another suggests that the concentration of each individual amino acid in the

342

cell is precisely regulated by biophysical and biochemical mechanisms. The relative amounts of free amino acids found in the muscle tissue bear no relationship either to the average composition of muscle proteins or to the known requirements of man for essential amino acids.

CHANGES IN RELATION TO SEVERITY OF CATABOLISM

Moderate Catabolism

Five patients in moderate catabolic state were studied 2–3 days after routine uncomplicated operations. The patients were maintained by intravenous feeding with carbohydrate (1500 kcal daily), electrolytes and vitamins, nitrogen was not given.

Severe Catabolism

The influence of severe trauma and sepsis was studied in seven patients who had severe complications, such as sepsis or severe peritonitis after major surgery. The patients were fed intravenously with carbohydrates, fat and amino acids corresponding to about 2,200 kcal and 8.5 g nitrogen per day; muscle biopsies were taken one to six weeks after the complications following surgery and trauma had set in. As direct measurements of the membrane potential were not made in this group of subjects a computer program was developed to estimate the effect of a decreased potential on the water distribution and the distribution of the different substances studied.

The relations between the different investigated variables (water, electrolytes and free amino acids) and the membrane potential are expressed according to exponential functions where the membrane potential is used as a stepless function from −50 to −100 mV.

$$[A_i] = \frac{1000\,A_m - \dfrac{[A_p] \cdot Cl_m \cdot 0.96\,(984 - 7.18\,P)}{[Cl_p]} + \dfrac{[A_p] \cdot H_2O_m - 1000\,A_m}{e^{E/26.7}}}{H_2O_m - \dfrac{Cl_m \cdot 0.96\,(984 - 7.18\,P)}{[Cl_p]}}$$

where A_i is the concentration of the amino acid in intracellular muscle water
A_m is the content of the amino acid in muscle
A_p is the concentration of the amino acid in plasma
Cl_m is the content of chloride in muscle
Cl_p is the concentration of chloride in plasma
P is the concentration of protein in plasma
H_2O_m is the content of water in muscle
E is the membrane potential
e is the base of the natural logarithms

343

Moderate Catabolism

The extracellular water content was markedly increased and the intracellular water content was slightly decreased in comparison to findings in healthy subjects.

The total amount of the free essential amino acids recovered in plasma and muscle did not differ from the corresponding mean obtained in normal subjects or the values obtained pre-operatively. The total amount of non-essential amino acids, however, was decreased in muscle which resulted in a decreased intracellular pool size. No significant change in the total plasma free amino acid pool was observed.

The amino acid profiles differed in many respects from those observed in normal subjects (Figure 2). The most significant changes in plasma compared with normal controls were an increase in phenylalanine and tyrosine and a decrease in isoleucine and histidine concentrations. The concentrations of serine and proline showed a more moderate decrease while the level of leucine increased slightly.

Many of the changes which could be demonstrated intracellularly were not reflected in the plasma. In muscle tissue there was a highly significant decrease in the concentrations of glutamine, arginine and lysine and a significant fall in proline and glutamic acid concentrations. The increases in the concentrations of taurine, valine and phenylalanine were all highly significant. A significant rise occurred in the concentrations of serine, glycine, alanine and leucine whereas the rise in tyrosine and citrulline concentrations was almost significant.

Compared with the normal transmembrane gradient there were marked increases for glycine, valine, serine, alanine, isoleucine and leucine. The ratio phenylalanine to tyrosine was increased significantly in muscle compared with values found in normal subjects. The ratio glycine to valine was unchanged both in plasma and muscle compared with normals (Figure 3).

Severe Catabolism

The total water content was further increased compared with the patients after moderate trauma, and the increase was related both to the elevated extracellular water content and to the severity of the catabolic state. The intracellular water was significantly decreased in four of the patients and was slightly increased in two patients when calculated at a membrane potential of −50 mV.

In contrast to moderate trauma the size of the essential free amino acid pool was reduced both in plasma and muscle. The total quantity of non-essential amino acids was further decreased in plasma but was in the same order of magnitude in muscle as in moderate trauma. Consequently the total amino acid pools were reduced both in plasma and muscle.

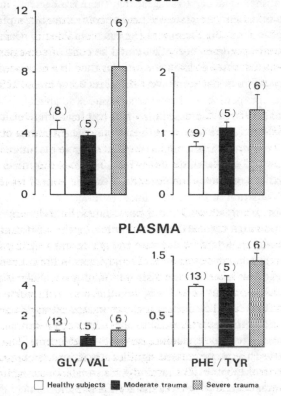

RATIOS GLY/VAL AND PHE/TYR
IN HEALTHY SUBJECTS AND IN
CATABOLIC PATIENTS
Mean ± SE

MUSCLE

PLASMA

GLY/VAL   PHE/TYR

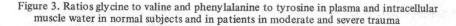
☐ Healthy subjects ■ Moderate trauma ▦ Severe trauma

Figure 3. Ratios glycine to valine and phenylalanine to tyrosine in plasma and intracellular
muscle water in normal subjects and in patients in moderate and severe trauma

In plasma all of the essential amino acids were highly significantly decreased
except for phenylalanine which was increased. Among the non-essential amino
acids the decrease in asparagine, serine, glycine, histidine, arginine, citrulline and
ornithine was highly significant. The decrease of proline was almost as significant
as the increase of cystine. In muscle, phenylalanine was significantly increased
and lysine decreased. Early significant increases in aspartate, asparagine, glycine
and alanine and decreases in glutamine, histidine and arginine concentrations
were found. An almost significant increase in taurine, aspartate, asparagine, glycine
and alanine concentrations was observed. The phenylalanine/tyrosine ratio was

345

markedly increased in both plasma and muscle. The increased ratio of glycine to valine was not significant in either plasma or muscle (Figure 3).

DISCUSSION

There is no published evidence to suggest that there is a decrease in transmembrane potential in patients in moderate post-operative catabolism following routine surgery without complications. The calculated distribution constant, assuming a normal membrane potential, could be considered to give reliable results for the reported water distribution and for the intracellular amino acid concentrations. On the other hand, in severe diseases (Bolte et al, 1972; Cunningham et al, 1971) and in experimental haemorrhagic shock in animals (Campion et al, 1969; Shires et al, 1970) a decreased membrane potential has been demonstrated.

The same method can be used to estimate the concentrations of the free amino acids in the intracellular compartment at variable membrane potentials between -50 to -100 mV, without direct measurement of actual membrane potential. Deviations of membrane potential from the normal value will strongly influence the calculation of the extracellular water content and all those substances which are mainly present in the extracellular fluid. An assumed fall in the membrane potential with -10 mV may influence the estimated extracellular water content more than 10%. A decrease to $-$mV means a 50% reduction of the extracellular water content. On the other hand, changes in transmembrane potential will have negligible effect on the distribution of intracellular water and of compounds which are mainly present in the intracellular compartment. Individual deviations of ± 10 mV will not influence the estimated intracellular water content by more than 2%. Furthermore, a drop of the membrane potential down to -50 mV will never effect the concentration of the free intracellular amino acids more than $1-7\%$. This can be ignored in comparison with the errors inherent in the determination of the individual amino acids, which ranges from 2.8 to 9.1%.

In earlier communications the free intracellular amino acid concentrations were reported in normal man. Also the pool size and the difference between the intra- and extracellular concentrations were discussed (Bergström et al, 1974). In trauma significant changes were observed from these normal patterns. The observed deviations in intra- and extracellular concentrations from the normal means were similar in moderate and severe trauma in muscle. However, the differences were more pronounced in severe trauma compared with moderate catabolism.

Munro (1970) suggested that the abnormal plasma amino acid pattern may be a sign of protein catabolism. It can therefore also be expected that protein catabolism will be reflected in the free muscle amino acid pattern. However, abnormalities in intracellular free amino acid concentrations found in different types of catabolism, such as untreated uraemia (Bergström et al, 1975), starvation (Bergström et al, to be published) and diabetes (Bergström et al, to be published) were not consistently found in post-traumatic catabolism. From our studies we

346

conclude that there seems to exist a specific free intracellular amino acid pattern, which is characteristic for the disease rather than a general catabolic process.

In untreated uraemia the low plasma concentrations of valine, isoleucine and leucine indicate protein malnutrition; the intracellular pool of valine was decreased. In uraemic muscle, however, leucine and isoleucine were found to be normal or slightly increased. These findings strongly indicate amino acid imbalance in the intracellular space. In contrast to uraemia a decrease in valine concentration was not observed in surgical catabolism. In addition to valine depletion, decreases in tyrosine and threonine concentrations were characteristic findings in uraemia, but were not found in surgical catabolism. Phenylalanine, which was elevated in post-traumatic catabolism, was found in low concentrations in muscle of untreated diabetics and after starvation but was found to be high in plasma in all three conditions. The most important changes in post-traumatic catabolism were consistent falls in lysine and glutamine. The pronounced decrease of lysine was also found in starvation and may be considered as a sign of general muscle catabolism. The unique decrease in glutamine observed in trauma, on the other hand, seems to be characteristic of post-traumatic catabolism.

By maintaining our patients on at least 300 g of carbohydrates daily, the basic non-protein energy requirements were supplied, and it is not likely that the results were influenced by caloric deficiencies. By supplying an adequate amount of electrolytes we tried to avoid electrolyte deficiency. Intracellular potassium depletion is known to raise the concentrations of the basic amino acids lysine, arginine and histidine in skeletal muscle of rats and dogs (Brandt et al, 1960; Iacobellis et al, 1956; Leibholz et al, 1966) and arginine, lysine and ornithine in man. The changes in the amino acid pool in severe trauma were more pronounced despite giving 8.5 g of nitrogen as amino acids compared to the subjects with moderate trauma who were not given nitrogen post-operatively. This quantity of nitrogen, however, may not have been sufficient to put these patients with severe trauma into a positive nitrogen balance. On the other hand, the typical depression of the E/N amino acid ratio seen in protein deficiency (Munro, 1970) was not observed in severe or moderate trauma. In fact we observed an increase in the E/N ratio.

These differences in the intracellular amino acid pattern indicate that the specific abnormalities found in post-traumatic catabolism cannot simply be explained as an effect of inadequate nutrition. The described changes may be due to an endocrine imbalance initiated by the trauma or surgery. It is known that corticosteroids increase the levels of most free amino acids in muscle in mice and rats (Betheil et al, 1965; Kaplan & Shimizu, 1963; Ryan & Carver, 1963). These effects seem to be due to inhibition of muscle protein synthesis (Wool & Weinshelbaum, 1960). Even if the corticosteroid effect is of importance this cannot be the only explanation since both increases and decreases in the intracellular concentration of individual free amino acids were observed.

Insulin causes a rapid reduction in the plasma levels of amino acids whereas in muscle it leads to an increase of 6 amino acids while 13 others remain unchanged (Wool, 1964). Carbohydrate infusions have a similar effect (Munro, 1970). In order to avoid these hormonal or nutritional effects in our investigation the muscle samples were taken after eight hours' fasting.

The increased phenylalanine/tyrosine ratio found in kwashiorkor and uraemia has been considered to be an early sign of catabolism (Padilla et al, 1971; Snyderman et al, 1973; Bergström et al, to be published). We found that in post-traumatic catabolism the same phenomenon occurred but this was due more to an increase in phenylalanine than to a decrease in tyrosine. In fact the tyrosine concentration was, in most cases, also increased in trauma but to a lower extent than phenylalanine.

CONCLUSIONS

It has been demonstrated that a marked increase in the glycine to valine ratio occurs during starvation (Lindblad, 1971). This increase was due to a significant elevation of the glycine concentration and a simultaneous decrease in the valine concentration. In the post-traumatic state a highly significant increase in the glycine concentration was found both in muscle and plasma, indicating that a similar metabolic change was observed. However, the valine concentration was found to be normal or slightly increased, resulting in an unchanged ratio of glycine to valine.

The different concentrations of the individual free amino acids between specific catabolic states may be of importance in the overall nutritional state of the patients. It has also been demonstrated that the recommended proportions and minimum requirement of the essential amino acids based on data from healthy subjects (Rose, 1949) cannot be directly applied in uraemia (Bergström et al, to be published). Hegsted (1973) stated in a review on amino acid and protein requirements "We cannot afford to be too confident of the applicability to man of results with rats." This implies that proteins, such as egg elbumin or lactalbumin, which are very efficient in promoting growth in young rats may not be as good for maintenance of adult humans in catabolic states. This in turn means that we may not use either 'good' proteins or the requirements of healthy adults for designing amino acid solutions for maintenance of catabolic patients. We hope that increased knowledge about the conditions during surgical catabolism in the largest, metabolically active amino acid pool in the body, the intracellular muscle pool, will serve as a basis for designing amino acid solutions specially adapted to requirements in specific catabolic states.

Acknowledgments

This investigation was supported by grants from the Swedish Medical Research Council (Project No.B74-19X-1002-09; B75-03X-4210-02), Tore Nilsson's Fund for Research, and Semper's Fund for Nutritional Research.

References

Adibi, SA (1971) *Amer. J. Physiol., 221,* 829

Bergström, J (1962) *Scand. J. clin. lab. Invest., Suppl. 68*

Bergström, J and Bittar, EE (1969) In *The Biological Basis of Medicine, Vol.6.* (Ed) EE Bittar and N Bittar. Academic Press, New York. Page 495

Bergström, J, Furst, P, Josephson, B and Noree, LO (1970) *Life Sci. (II)9,* 787

Bergström, J, Boethius, J and Hultman, E (1971) *Acta physiol. Scand., 81,* 164

Bergström, J, Furst, P and Noree, LO (1972) In *Proceedings of the European Dialysis and Transplant Association, Vol.8.* (Ed) JS Cameron, D Fries and CS Ogg. Pitman Medical, London. Page 393

Bergström, J, Furst, P, Noree, LO and Vinnars, E (1974) *J. appl. Physiol., 36,* 693

Betheil, JJ, Feigelson, M and Feigelson, P (1965) *Biochem., Biophys., Acta, 104,* 92

Black, DAK and Milne, MD (1952) *Clin. Sci., 11,* 397

Bolte, HD, Riecker, G and Rohl, D (1963) *Klin. Wochenschr., 41,* 356

Bolte, HD, Becker, E and Volker, W (1972) In *Uremia.* (Ed) R Kluthe, G Berlyne and B Barton. Thieme Verlag, Stuttgart. Page 14

Brandt, IK, Matalka, VA and Combs, JT (1960) *Amer. J. Physiol., 199,* 39

Campion, DS, Lynch, LJ, Rector, FC Jr, Carter, N and Shires, GT (1969) *Surgery, 66,* 1051

Ching, S, Rogoff, TM and Gabuzda, GJ (1973) *J. lab. clin. Med., 82,* 208

Conway, EJ (1957) *Physiol. Rev., 37,* 84

Cunningham, JN Jr, Carter, NW, Rector, FC Jr and Seldin, DW (1971) *J. clin. Invest., 50,* 49

Curran, PF (1972) *Arch. intern. Med., 129,* 258

Darrow, DC, Harrison, HE and Taffel, M (1939) *J. biol. Chem., 130,* 487

Eichelberger, L, Akeson, WH and Roma, M (1956) *Amer. J. Physiol., 287,*

Eisenman, AJ, MacKenzie, LB and Peters, JP (1936) *J. biol. Chem., 116,* 33

Friedberg, F and Greenberg, DM (1947) *J. biol. Chem., 168,* 405

Fürst, P (1974) *Scand. J. clin. lab. Invest., 30,* 307

Giordano, D, de Pascale, C, de Santo, NG, Esposito, R, Cirillo, D and Stangherlin, P (1970) In *Proceedings of the 4th International Congress of Nephrology, Vol.2.* (Ed) N Alwall, F Berglune and B Josephson. Karger, Basel. Page 196

Graham, JA, Lamb, JF and Linton, AL (1967) *Lancet, ii,* 1172

Gulyassy, PF, Peters, JH and Schoenfeld, P (1971) *Abstr. Amer. soc. Nephrol.* Washington DC, November 1971. Page 29

Hamilton, PB (1945) *J. biol. Chem., 158,* 397

Hegsted, DM (1973) In *Proteins in Human Nutrition.* (Ed) JWG Porter and BA Rolls. Academic Press, London. Page 356

Herbert, JD, Coulson, RA and Hernandez, T (1966) *Comp. biochem. Physiol., 17,* 583

Hurth, EJ and Elkinton, JR (1959) *Amer. J. Physiol., 196,* 299

Iacobellis, M, Muntwyler, E and Dogen, CL (1956) *Amer. J. Physiol., 185,* 275

Kaplan, SA and Shimizu, CSN (1963) *Endocrinology, 72,* 267

Kedenburg, CP (1971) *Anal. Biochem., 40,* 35

Leibolz, JM, McCall, JT, Hays, VW and Speer, VC (1966) *J. animal Sci., 25,* 37

Lindblad, BS (1971) In *Metabolic Processes in the Foetus and Newborn Infant.* (Ed) HP Jonxis, HKA Visser and JA Troelstra. HE Stenfort Kroese NV, Leiden. Page 111

Munro, HN (1970) In *Mammalian Protein Metabolism., Vol.4.* (Ed) HN Munro.

Academic Press, New York. Page 299

Mendes, CB and Waterlow, JC (1958) *Brit. J. Nutr., 12,* 74

Noree, LO, Bergström, J, Fürst, P and Hallgren, B (1971) In *Proceedings of the European Dialysis and Transplant Association, Vol.7.* (Ed)JS Cameron, D Fries and CS Ogg. Pitman Medical, London. Page 182

Padilla, H, Sanchez, A, Powell, RN, Umezawa, C, Swendseid, ME, Prado, PM and Sigala, R (1971) *Amer. J. clin. Nutr., 24,* 353

Peters, JH, Gulyassy, PF, Lin, SC, Ryan, PM, Berridge, BJ Jr, Chao, WR and Cummings, JG (1968) *Trans. Amer. Soc. artif. intern. Organs, 14,* 405

Rose, WC (1949) *Fed. Proc., 8,* 546

Ryan, WL and Carver, MJ (1963) *Proc. Soc. exp. biol. Med., 114,* 816

Sanslone, WR, Muntwyler, E, Kesner, L and Griffin, GE (1970) *Metabolism, 19,* 179

Shires, GT, Carrico, CJ, Baxter, CR, Giesecke, AH and Jenkins, MJ (1970) In *Principles in Treatment of Severely Injured Patients, Vol.4.* (Ed) CE Welch. Advances in Surgery, Year Book. Page 255

Snyderman, SE, Holt, LE Jr, Norton, PM, Roitman, E and Finch, J (1963) *Amer. J. clin. Nutr., 12,* 333

Wilde, WS (1945) *Amer. J. Physiol., 143,* 666

Wool, IG (1964) *Nature, 202,* 196

Wool, IG and Weinshelbaum, EI (1960) *Amer. J. Physiol., 198,* 1111

Young, GA and Parsons, FM (1970) *Clin. chim. Acta, 27,* 491

Young, GA and Parsons, FM (1973) *Clin. sci. mol. Med., 45,* 89

Zachman, M, Cleveland, WW, Sandberg, DA and Nyhan, WL (1966) *Amer. J. dis. Child., 112,* 283

Zall, DM, Fisher, D and Garner, MO (1956) *Anal. Chem., 28,* 1665